Thermal Agents in Rehabilitation

Contemporary Perspectives in Rehabilitation

Steven L. Wolf, PhD, FAPTA
Editor-in-Chief

PUBLISHED VOLUMES

Thermal Agents in Rehabilitation

Third Edition

Susan L. Michlovitz, MS, PT, CHT
Adjunct Associate Professor
Department of Physical Therapy
Allegheny University of the Health Sciences
Philadelphia, Pennsylvania
and
Physical Therapist and Hand Therapist
Temple University
Department of Orthopaedic Surgery
Philadelphia, Pennsylvania

F. A. DAVIS COMPANY • Philadelphia

F. A. Davis Company
1915 Arch Street
Philadelphia, PA 19103

Printed in the United States of America

Last digit indicates print number: 10 9 8 7 6 5 4 3

Publisher, Allied Health: Jean-François Vilain
Developmental Editor: Crystal McNichol
Production Editor: Glenn L. Fechner
Cover Designer: Louis J. Forgione

As new scientific information becomes available through basic and clinical research, recommended treatments and drug therapies undergo changes. The author and publisher have done everything possible to make this book accurate, up to date, and in accord with accepted standards at the time of publication. The author, editors, and publisher are not responsible for errors or omissions or for consequences from application of the book, and make no warranty, expressed or implied, in regard to the contents of the book. Any practice described in this book should be applied by the reader in accordance with professional standards of care used in regard to the unique circumstances that may apply in each situation. The reader is advised always to check product information (package inserts) for changes and new information regarding dose and contraindications before administering any drug. Caution is especially urged when using new or infrequently ordered drugs.

Library of Congress Cataloging-in-Publication Data

Thermal agents in rehabilitation / [edited by] Susan L. Michlovitz.—
3rd ed.
    p. cm.—(Contemporary perspectives in rehabilitation)
    Includes bibliographical references and index.
    ISBN 0-8036-0044-5 (alk. paper)
    1. Thermotherapy. 2. Cold—Therapeutic use. 3. Physical therapy.
I. Michlovitz, Susan L. II. Series.
    [DNLM: 1. Cryotherapy. 2. Heat—therapeutic use. 3. Physical
Therapy—methods. WB 469 T411 1996]
RM865.T47 1996
615.8'32—dc20
DNLM/DLC
for Library of Congress   95-39679
                                        CIP

To my mom (in memory) and my dad for laying a good foundation. . . .
Thanks. . . .

Foreword

It seems virtually impossible for me to fathom that a decade has passed since the inception of the *Contemporary Perspectives in Rehabilitation* series. An image that has also become clouded by time is Sue Michlovitz's desire, albeit shrouded in a cloak of uncertainty, to undertake our first volume. After all, although Sue's knowledge about thermal agents was extraordinary, her writing experience was limited. However, through some coaxing by my colleagues at F.A. Davis and an occasional thought from me, Sue was able to create a product that was well received.

Still, if someone had told me that 10 years later we would be producing the third edition of what now has become an international standard in the therapeutic use of thermal agents, I would have had a hard time believing him. The reality is, however, that over this decade I have been fortunate to witness Sue's personal development and her persistent conviction that *Thermal Agents* can never rest on its past laurels but must continue to serve as a premier resource for students, their teachers, and the clinical community. Toward this end Sue and her ensemble of contributors have never lost sight of the primary mission in this series, to educate and inform in a decisive, decision-making, and documented mode.

When I first reviewed this latest edition, I thought that perhaps Sue had deleted information that was still relevant and important. For example, had a discussion on therapeutic ultrasound units disappeared? Were the methods for applying shortwave diathermy or dosage considerations deleted? These and other concerns were quickly allayed when I realized that they were not deleted but, rather, expressed within more contemporary and relevant constructs. The fact is, Sue continues to approach this book as though each edition is a new venture, obligating her to convince her contributors to express contemporary information in a manner that is relevant to changes in practice and accountability. The extent of those changes I leave to her to express in the Preface.

Suffice to say that this third edition is even stronger than its highly successful predecessors. It has never lost sight of its target audience and is sensitized to the belief that students and clinicians have much to learn (and review) when using temperature gradients to effect physiological change. The challenge arises in presenting this material in new and innovative ways that include new topics, updated references, and clarity of expression. Once again, the challenge has been met. What follows is a premier work that will soon acquire the unique attributes ascribed only to "classic" texts.

Steven L. Wolf, PhD, FAPTA
Series Editor

Preface

Health care delivery has been rapidly changing and increasingly scrutinized since the last publication of this text in 1990. However, thermal agents continue to be widely used in clinical practice to reduce pain, promote tissue healing, and reduce stiffness of joints. These techniques can be an integral part of the total treatment plan for many patients with musculoskeletal dysfunction. Since the book's inception, I have stressed that these agents are an adjunct to the total treatment plan and not the treatment *in toto*. The use of thermal agents alone or in combination with each other in lieu of exercise and patient education is, in my opinion, simply not appropriate.

Unfortunately, there have been practitioners who have chosen to overuse these modalities, creating clever billing schemes in order to collect for the menu of services "rendered." It is this practice, I presume, that has left a bad impression on those responsible for paying these bills, that is, third-party payers, and for the scrutiny under which thermal agents are falling.

Therefore, in order to further strengthen this text to assist the student and clinician in clinical decision making and rationale for judicious use of thermal agents, many case scenarios have been added in this edition. In addition, studies that support the scientific rationale have been updated through diligent literature reviews by all the authors.

Another new feature of this edition is the addition of Chapter 13 "The Use of Heat and Cold in Hand Rehabilitation." This chapter is added to the last section of the book on clinical decision making. These final four chapters of the book are designed so that the student and clinician are able to tie together and further integrate the underlying principles discussed in the first nine chapters of this book. Instructors that incorporate problem-based learning should be able to use information from these chapters in appropriate units throughout their programs. A final addition to this book is the listing of study objectives at the end of each chapter. This should assist the student in organizing and reviewing pertinent information that has been presented in each chapter.

Susan L. Michlovitz

Preface to the First Edition

Thermal agents are used in physical therapy and rehabilitation to reduce pain, to enhance healing, and to improve motion. The physical therapist should have a solid foundation in the normal physiological control of the cardiovascular and neuromuscular systems prior to using an agent that can alter the function of these structures. In addition, a background in the physiology of healing mechanisms and of pain serves as a basis for the rationale of using thermal agents.

Often, the decision to include a thermal agent in a therapy plan or to have the thermal agent *be* the sole treatment rendered (as in the case of the frequently used "hot packs and ultrasound combination" for back pain) is based on empirical evidence. The purpose of this book is to provide the reader with the underlying rationale for selection of an agent to be included in a therapy program, based on (1) the known physiologic and physical effects of that agent; (2) the safety and use of the heat/cold agent, given the conditions and limitations of the patient's dysfunction; and (3) the therapeutic goals for that particular patient. The authors have been asked to review critically the literature available that documents efficacy and effectiveness of each thermal agent. A problem-solving approach to the use of thermal agents is stressed throughout the text.

The primary audience for this text is the physical therapist. The student will gain a solid foundation in thermal agents, the clinician will strengthen his or her perspective of thermal agents, and the researcher is given information that will provide ideas for clinical studies on thermal agents. Athletic trainers and other professionals who use thermal agents in their practice should find this text of value.

The text is in three parts. Part I, Foundations for the Use of Thermal Agents, includes information from basic and medical sciences that can serve as a framework for the choice to include thermal agents in a rehabilitation program. A discussion of the proposed mechanisms by which heat and cold can alter inflammation, healing, and pain is included in these chapters.

Part II of the text, Instrumentation: Methods and Application, incorporates concepts of equipment selection, operation and maintenance, and clinical application. The leading chapter in this part is on instrumentation principles and serves to introduce concepts of electrical circuitry and safety as applied to equipment used for thermal therapy. Physical therapists have become responsible for product purchase and making recommendations about products through the expansion of consultation services, private practices, sports medicine clinics, extended care facilities, and home health care. Therefore, we must be prepared to engage in dialogue with manufacturers, product distributors, and other colleagues about the safety and quality of these products. To this end, some practical suggestions are provided in Chapter 3, intended to assist with purchase decisions.

Chapters 4 through 8 discuss the operation and application of heat and cold agents. Numerous principles of clinical decision making are included within each chapter. There are certain principles that are inherent to all agent applications: (1) The patient must be evaluated and treatment goals established; (2) contraindications to treatment must be known; and (3) the safe and effective use of equipment must be understood.

Chapter 9, on low-power laser, deviates somewhat from the overall theme of thermal agents. Low-power laser is not expected to produce an increase in tissue temperature, so its effects could not be attributed to thermal mechanisms. Therefore, this cannot be categorized as a thermal agent. However, I believe this topic is worthy of inclusion in this text because (1) the indications for its use overlap those of thermal agents; (2) laser is a form of non-ionizing radiation as are diathermy and ultrasound, which are used for pain reduction and tissue healing; and (3) laser would most likely be included in a physical therapy student curriculum in the coursework that includes thermal agents. At the time of this writing (summer 1985), low-power laser is still considered by the U.S. Food and Drug Administration as an investigational device. Only carefully designed clinical studies will help determine the laser's clinical efficacy—perhaps contributing to the body of knowledge needed to change the laser's status from an investigational to an accepted therapeutic product.

Part III, Clinical Decision Making, is designed to assist the student and clinician in integrating basic concepts that have been presented throughout the entire book, emphasizing problem solving and evaluation.

Much information has been published in the medical literature on the effects or clinical results of heat and cold application. Oftentimes, the therapist is called upon to justify the use of a certain modality. A careful review of the research literature may be necessary to provide an explanation for treatment.

There are many areas that require further investigation. For example, contrast baths (alternating heat and cold) are often used in sports medicine clinics. But a careful review of the literature reveals that only scanty information supports the use of contrast baths for any patient population. It is important for the clinician to be able to interpret accurately and to apply the methods and results that are presented in the literature. The inclusion of a chapter (Chapter 10) on techniques for reviewing the literature and establishing a paradigm for clinical studies of thermal agents provides the clinician with such a background on which to build.

Chapters 11 and 12 are devoted to specific patient populations in which thermal agents are commonly used. The chapter on sports medicine is representative of a population with a known cause of injury and predictable course of recovery. The majority of these patients are otherwise healthy. On the other hand, the chapter on rheumatic disease presents a model for a patient population that can be expected to have chronic recurrent—sometimes progressive—dysfunction associated with systemic manifestations.

An appendix is included—temperature conversion scales (this text uses the centigrade scale).

Susan L. Michlovitz, MS, PT

Acknowledgments

Kudos are extended to:

The authors who have contributed their clinical and academic wisdom to this edition.

Sue Giangrasso who has plugged along with manuscript typing and preparation since we began with an IBM typewriter (with scant memory) in 1984 for edition one. (We no longer use the typewriter!)

Maureen McBeth for the new photographs in Chapters 5, 7 and 13.

Kathy Hemsley for the new photographs in Chapter 11.

The editorial and production staff at F.A. Davis Company, particularly to Crystal McNichol who had to keep after me again and again . . . .

Sue Michlovitz

Contributors

Stacie L. Collender, PT
Instructor and Academic Coordination of Clinical Education
Department of Physical Therapy
University of Delaware
Newark, Delaware

Dennis M. DePace, PhD
Associate Professor of Anatomy and Neurosurgery
Allegheny University of the Health Sciences
Philadelphia, Pennsylvania

Jane M. Fedorczyk, MS, PT, CHT, ATC
Assistant Professor
Department of Physical Therapy
Allegheny University of the Health Sciences
Philadelphia, Pennsylvania
and
Consultant, Hand and Orthopedic Rehabilitation Services
Levittown, Pennsylvania
and
Philadelphia Hand Center
King of Prussia, Pennsylvania

Kathryn Hemsley, MEd, ATC, PT
Senior Staff Therapist
Temple University Sports Medicine Center
Fort Washington, Pennsylvania
Bryn Mawr Rehabilitation Hospital
Malvern, Pennsylvania
Adjunct Instructor
Beaver College
Program in Physical Therapy
Philadelphia, Pennsylvania

Luther C. Kloth, MS, PT
Professor
Program in Physical Therapy
Marquette University
Milwaukee, Wisconsin

Theresa McDiarmid, MSc, RPT, MCSP
Rehabilitation Consultant
Dynamic Rehabilitation
North York, Ontario
Canada

Susan L. Michlovitz, MS, PT, CHT
Adjunct Associate Professor
Department of Physical Therapy
Allegheny University of the Health Sciences
Philadelphia, Pennsylvania
and
Physical Therapist and Hand Therapist
Temple University
Department of Orthopaedic Surgery
Philadelphia, Pennsylvania

Roberta A. Newton, PhD, PT
Professor
Department of Physical Therapy
College of Allied Health Professions
Temple University
Philadelphia, Pennsylvania

Brian V. Reed, PhD, PT
Associate Professor
Department of Physical Therapy
University of Vermont
Burlington, Vermont

G. A. (Sandy) Rennie, MSc, BPT
Associate Professor
Department of Physical Therapy
University of Alberta
Edmonton, Alberta
Canada

H. T. M. Ritter, III, BA, CBET
Senior Project Engineer
ECRI
Plymouth Meeting, Pennsylvania

Judy R. Sotosky, MEd, PT
Private Consultant
Virginia Beach, Virginia

xvi

Wayne Smith, MEd, PT, ATC, SCS
Assistant Professor and Academic Clinical Coordinator
Program in Physical Therapy
Kirksville Osteopathic Medical College, Southwest Center
Phoenix, Arizona

Lynn Snyder-Mackler, PT, ScD, SCS
Associate Professor
Department of Physical Therapy
University of Delaware
Newark, Delaware

Kristin Von Nieda, MEd, PT
Assistant Professor and
Assistant Director
Department of Physical Therapy
Allegheny University of the Health Sciences
Philadelphia, Pennsylvania

Mark T. Walsh, PT, MS, CHT
Co-owner Hand & Orthopedic Rehabilitation Services P.C.
Levittown, Pennsylvania
and
Adjunct Assistant Professor
Philadelphia College of Pharmacy and Science
Philadelphia, Pennsylvania

Mary P. Watkins, MS, PT
Research Associate Professor
Program in Occupational Therapy and Surgery
Washington University
School of Medicine
St. Louis, Missouri

Marvin C. Ziskin, MD, MS BmE
Professor of Radiology and Medical Physics
Temple University Medical School
Philadelphia, Pennsylvania

Contents

SECTION II: Instrumentation: Methods and Application

Chapter 11. The Application of Cold and Heat in the Treatment of Athletic Injuries 304

Kathryn Hemsley, MEd, ATC, PT, and
Wayne Smith, MEd, PT, ATC, SCS

Chapter 12. Use of Heat and Cold in the Management of Rheumatic Diseases 331

Judy R. Sotosky, MEd, PT, and Susan L. Michlovitz, MS, PT, CHT

Chapter 13. Heat and Cold in Hand Rehabilitation 355

Jane M. Fedorczyk, MS, PT, CHT, ATC

Foundations for the Use of Thermal Agents

CHAPTER 1

Wound Healing and the Use of Thermal Agents

Brian V. Reed, PhD, PT

Injury to vascularized tissue initiates a series of responses collectively known as inflammation and repair. These processes serve to control the effects of the injurious agent and return the tissue to a normal state. Inflammation occurs first and includes vascular, hemostatic, cellular, and immune responses. These serve to dispose of microorganisms, foreign material, and dead tissue in preparation for the subsequent repair process. Tissue repair is characterized early by proliferation of new blood vessels and by the formation of new connective tissue. This re-establishes tensile strength and

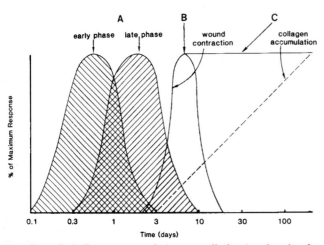

FIGURE 1–1. Phases of wound repair. Healing of a wound has been arbitrarily divided into three phases: (*A*) inflammation (early and late), (*B*) granulation tissue formation, and (*C*) matrix formation and remodeling. These phases overlap considerably with one another and are plotted along the abscissa as a logarithmic function of time. Inflammation is divided into early and late phases, denoting neutrophil-rich and mononuclear cell-rich infiltrates, respectively. The magnitude of wound contraction parallels granulation tissue formation, as indicated. Collagen accumulation actually begins shortly after the onset of granulation tissue formation, continuing throughout the phase of matrix formation and remodeling. (From Clark,[3] p 4, with permission.)

makes the repair tissue viable. Later in the repair process, remodeling of the connective tissue takes place, and this serves to further increase tissue strength. The exact duration of each of the phases of inflammation and repair is not distinct because the phases overlap and because there is variability from one case to another. However, it is useful to have a concept of the timing of the phases. A diagram of the approximate timing of these events is presented in Figure 1–1.

Unfortunately, not all repair ends in restoration of normal tissue. Certain human tissues, including epidermis, liver, bone, skeletal muscle, adipose tissue, alimentary tract epithelium, and tracheobronchial epithelium, can regenerate to varying degrees, but other tissues cannot. To the degree that damaged tissue cannot regenerate, the nonspecific process of scar formation takes place. Scar tissue provides tensile strength but is otherwise devoid of physiologic function. Because scar tissue tends to become tight, extensive scarring can be disfiguring and may affect organ function.

It is important to have an understanding of the processes of inflammation and repair and how they can be modified. Physical therapists and other rehabilitation specialists often must deal with acute inflammatory conditions (e.g., sprains), chronic inflammatory conditions (e.g., rheumatoid arthritis), open wounds (e.g., decubitus ulcers), surgical incisions, or problems secondary to the healing process (e.g., peripheral edema or limited joint mobility). When appropriate, heat and cold may be used in the course of treatment to modify the inflammatory response. For example, cold is often the first line of defense to minimize the pain and swelling of acute musculoskeletal injuries. Heat, on the other hand, is sometimes used to resolve subacute sequelae of inflammation and repair, such as hematomas.

The intent of this chapter is to provide the reader with a basic understanding of the processes of tissue inflammation and repair, describe clinical problems associated with excessive or chronic inflammation and repair, and review the potential therapeutic role of thermal agents in the processes of inflammation and repair.

TABLE 1-1 Some Common Causes of
Injury That Produce Inflammation

Trauma (e.g., sprains, burns)	Autoimmune diseases:
Bone fractures	Rheumatoid arthritis
Foreign bodies	Polymyositis
Bacteria and fungi	Scleroderma
Decreased blood supply	

INFLAMMATION (DAYS 1 TO 10)

Nearly 2000 years ago, Celsius first described four signs associated with inflammation: swelling, heat, redness, and pain. Another characteristic, loss of function, was later added, and these five signs came to be called the "cardinal signs of inflammation." A boil occurring in the skin as a reaction to invasion by bacteria is a good example of the cardinal signs of inflammation.

Inflammation begins when injury or disease causes a disruption in the normal physiology of a tissue. Table 1-1 lists some common causes of injury that will trigger inflammation. Although the inflammatory reaction follows the same pathway regardless of the cause of the injury, some causes will tend to emphasize certain events more than other events. For example, anoxia (such as occurs in peripheral vascular disease) tends to result in dry necrotic tissues, whereas bacterial invasion typically causes pus formation.

The inflammatory process involves a vascular response, a hemostatic response, a cellular response, and an immune response. These are controlled by a complex interaction of neural and humoral mediators not yet fully understood.

Vascular Response

The initial stages of inflammation are characterized by vascular changes. Transient vasoconstriction of arterioles occurs, lasting a few minutes. During this time, the vessel walls of the capillaries, and especially the postcapillary venules, become lined with white blood cells (leukocytes), a process known as *margination*. Vasoconstriction is followed by vasodilation, which causes an increase in blood flow and an increase in vessel hydrostatic pressure. Coincident with vasodilation, increased permeability of the microvessels (capillaries and venules) occurs. This happens because the endothelial cells "round up," creating gaps between the cells. This allows the escape of cells, macromolecules, and fluid from the vascular system (Fig. 1-2). Edema occurs because the escaping cells and macromolecules create an osmotic gradient, which causes fluid to move into the interstitial spaces. The lymphatic vessels, which normally clear the interstitium of osmotically active particles, are overwhelmed.

To better understand edema formation, fluid balance can be considered in terms of a balance of forces. Four forces are described in Starling's hypothesis[1]: capillary hydrostatic pressure (P_c), interstitial oncotic pressure (π_i), interstitial hydrostatic pressure (P_i), and colloid oncotic pressure (π_c). The first two forces tend to drive fluid out of the exchange vessels (filtration), while the latter two forces tend to drive fluid into the exchange vessels (reabsorption). An equilibrium of fluid exchange is reached according

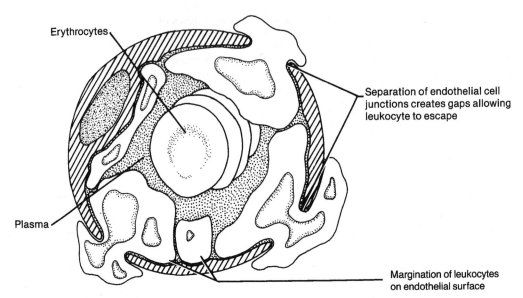

FIGURE 1–2. Vascular response to wound healing. (Adapted from Bryant,[2] p 7.)

to the algebraic sum of these forces. The concept of this balance of forces is schematized in Figure 1–3*A*.

Lymphatic vessels also play a role in determining compartment fluid volume. The lymphatics are capable of returning modest amounts of fluid and leaked plasma proteins to the vascular system. The peripheral edema caused by inflammation is a result of increased capillary hydrostatic pressure, increased interstitial oncotic pressure, and overwhelmed lymphatics.

The vascular response to injury probably is caused by local mediators released at the site of injury. Most notable among these are histamine, bradykinin, prostaglandins, and complement fractions. Each of these substances causes vasodilation. Histamine, in particular, has been implicated in the alteration of microvessel permeability. Histamine is released from mast cells and blood platelets at the injury site.

The type of edema fluid varies with the stage of inflammation. Initially, the permeability of the microvessels is only slightly altered and, therefore, no proteins or cells escape. The edema fluid formed is called a *transudate* and consists mainly of water and dissolved electrolytes. It is clear in appearance and contains very few cells. As microvessel permeability increases, cells and plasma proteins escape. The edema fluid, which was at first clear, becomes more viscous (owing to the protein) and cloudy (owing to the leukocytes); the fluid is called an *exudate*. When an exudate contains large numbers of leukocytes, it is called pus. A diagrammatic representation of these events is presented in Figure 1–3*B*.

The edema that occurs with wounds is usually a localized event, but edema can also occur systemically. For example, in congestive heart failure, there is a buildup of pressure in the veins that is due to the heart's inability to maintain cardiac output. Blood accumulates in the veins, and the resulting pressure is backed up into the postcapillary venules and the capillaries. This increase in hydrostatic pressure causes a net fluid flux in the interstitium. Another example of systemic edema occurs with

FIGURE 1–3. Schematic representation of edema production. (*A*) Normal state—fluid balance is maintained by the balance of the (Starling) forces of filtration and reabsorption across the vessel wall. Relative influence of forces is indicated by the size of arrows. P_c = Capillary hydrostatic pressure: blood pressure in the capillaries; P_i = interstitial hydrostatic pressure: normally low due to low volume of fluid in the interstitium; π_c = capillary oncotic pressure: normally high due to high concentration of osmotically active entities (cells, proteins, electrolytes) in the blood; π_i = interstitial oncotic pressure: normally low due to low concentration of osmotically active entities (cells, proteins, electrolytes) in the interstitium. (*B*) Inflammed state—in response to injury, mediators are produced, arterioles dilate, blood volume and pressure in the capillaries increase, outward filtration increases, and edema forms (transudate); white blood cells marginate. As inflammation becomes more intense, neutrophils, and other blood cells migrate into the surrounding tissue to form thick edema fluid (exudate). P_c = Capillary hydrostatic pressure: increased due to vasodilation; P_i = interstitial hydrostatic pressure: increased as interstitium reaches its fluid capacity; π_c = capillary oncotic pressure: reduced as concentration of osmotically active entities decreases; π_i = interstitial oncotic pressure: increased as concentration of osmotically active entities in the interstitium increases.

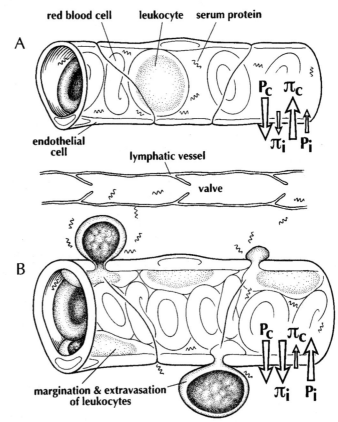

renal pathology in which serum proteins are lost in the urine. The result is that capillary oncotic pressure decreases and, once again, fluid is lost to the interstitium. In cases of systemic edema, treatment must also be systemic and usually involves pharmacologic intervention. With either localized or systemic edema, the presence of edema for long periods, especially if it occurs in an area of poor circulation, as in peripheral vascular disease, will interfere with proper oxygenation. So-called stasis ulcers, common in peripheral vascular disease, heal poorly in the presence of persistent edema.

The clinical manifestations of inflammation can be explained by the sequence of vascular events. Vasodilation causes the characteristic redness and warmth associated with inflammation. Overexpansion of the interstitial spaces accounts for the observed swelling and accompanying discomfort. Production of bradykinin and prostaglandins augments the pain stimulus.

Hemostatic Response

The hemostatic response functions to control blood loss when blood vessels are ruptured. The small blood vessels retract, helping to seal themselves off. Platelets aggregate and deposit fibrin, which traps red blood cells, creating a blood clot. The fibrin also occludes local lymphatic channels, preventing drainage of fluid from the injured area, thereby localizing the inflammation. When bleeding is internal, confined to a tissue or organ, a mass of clotted blood known as a *hematoma* can develop. Hematomas may cause tenderness, and, in muscle tissue, they may limit range of motion or function.

Cellular Response

Leukocytes play a critical role in the inflammatory process, clearing the injured site of microorganisms and setting the stage for tissue repair. There are several types of leukocytes, including neutrophils, lymphocytes, monocytes, basophils, and eosino-phils. It is useful to note that neutrophils, eosinophils, and basophils are sometimes classified as polymorphonuclear leukocytes, because they have a nucleus consisting of several lobes.

The various leukocytes are specialized, thus different types of leukocytes are predominant in the early and late phases of the process. Initially, all types of leukocytes migrate to the site of inflammation in numbers proportionate to their concentration in circulating blood.[2] Because neutrophils are the greatest in number, they characterize early inflammation (Fig. 1–1). As with all the leukocytes, neutrophils are attracted to the inflamed site by chemotactic agents released at the time of injury. The major function of the neutrophils is to rid the site of contaminating bacteria and debris. They accomplish this by phagocytosis. As some neutrophils disintegrate, their digestive enzymes are released into the tissue. These chemicals perpetuate the inflammatory reaction by acting as irritants and as chemotactic agents, attracting other leukocytes into the area of inflammation.

Late inflammation, which begins within a few hours of injury, is characterized by the predominance of mononuclear leukocytes (monocytes) and lymphocytes. This is at least partially because these cells live longer than neutrophils and the other polymorphs. In the interstitium, monocytes have the ability to convert into large cells called macrophages, which, like neutrophils, are phagocytic. In fact, they are remarkable for their ability to engulf large amounts of bacteria and cellular debris. In contrast to neutrophils, however, the appearance of monocytes seems to be critical to the initiation of tissue repair.[3] Lymphocytes also are present in the later phase of inflammation. Lymphocytes play a major role in mediating the body's immune reaction, supplying antibodies for specific antigens. It is not surprising, therefore, that they are prominent in chronic inflammatory conditions. An example of this is rheumatoid arthritis, a disease characterized by chronic inflammation in various joints. The characteristic cell types in tissue biopsy of this disease are lymphocytes and monocytes.

For the most part, basophils and eosinophils are involved only in certain types of inflammation and will not be discussed further.

Immune Response

The immune response is both a cell-mediated and a humorally mediated response. The roles of lymphocytes and the phagocytic leukocytes in the immune response have already been described. Another aspect of the immune response, however, is the complement system. Complement is a series of enzymatic proteins that are activated by bacterial toxins or immune complexes. Various activated components are involved in many steps in the inflammatory process, including phagocytosis, increasing vascular permeability, and providing chemotactic attraction for leukocytes.

In diseases of autoimmunity, the inflammatory response is not beneficial. Because the body perceives certain tissues as foreign, there is an antigen-antibody reaction that results in a chronic inflammatory response against the tissues. Rheumatoid arthritis is one example of an autoimmune disease. In rheumatoid arthritis, chronic synovial inflammation causes destruction of articular cartilage. Table 1–1 contains examples of some other autoimmune diseases that affect the musculoskeletal system. In addition, Chapter 12 of this text details the use of thermal agents with rheumatic diseases.

Some conditions, such as autoimmune diseases or the presence of a foreign body, can cause chronic inflammation. Chronic inflammation creates unique problems and, therefore, is discussed separately later in this chapter. Chronic inflammation is one indication for intervention in the inflammation and repair process.

TISSUE REPAIR

Proliferative Phase (Days 3 to 20)

The first phase of tissue repair is a proliferative one involving both epithelial and connective tissues. Epithelium is a covering; it is the layer(s) of cells that form the epidermis of the skin and the surface layer of mucous and serous membranes. Connective tissue, on the other hand, is the cement that connects and supports other tissues. Under normal conditions, connective tissue is relatively acellular, composed of fibrous strands and ground substance that make up an intercellular matrix. Connective-tissue strength and elasticity varies in tissues such as bone, tendon, ligament, and skin, according to its makeup and degree of organization.

Certain epithelial tissues have a high regenerative capacity and undergo a process known as *re-epithelialization*. In the case of an open wound where the skin has been broken, for example, epithelial cells around the periphery of the wound proliferate and migrate across the wound site until the compromised area is covered. The epithelial cells appear to be surrounded by other epithelial cells, so they migrate in the direction where there are none (into the wound) until they contact other epithelial cells. The cells then stop migrating and undergo mitosis, reforming layers of epithelial cells.

In connective tissue, fibroplasia takes place. Cells known as *fibroblasts* develop from undifferentiated mesenchymal cells, migrate into the inflamed area along fibrin strands, and begin to synthesize scar tissue. Scar tissue is a type of connective tissue, and as such, it is composed primarily of the protein *collagen* and mucopolysaccharides. The fibroblast secretes both of these and through this process, a connective-tissue matrix is re-established. By means of successive wrappings, collagen acquires strength. The basic structural element of collagen is a triple helix chain of amino acids known as tropocollagen. Bundles of tropocollagen strands form collagen filaments. Groups of collagen filaments become wrapped into fibrils; the fibrils are in turn wrapped into primitive collagen fibers; and the primitive collagen fibers are wrapped into collagen fibers (Fig. 1–4). The final collagen fiber has a ropelike appearance when examined microscopically (Fig. 1–5). At first the amino acid chains are held together by weak

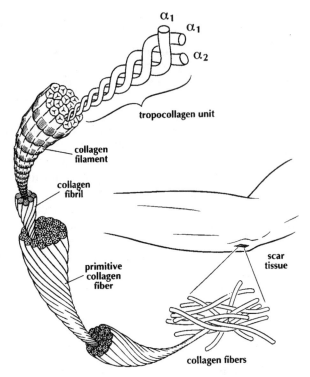

α_1
α_1
α_2

tropocollagen unit

collagen
filament

collagen
fibril

scar
tissue

primitive
collagen
fiber

collagen fibers

FIGURE 1–4. Illustration of collagen composition: tropocollagen to collagen fibers.

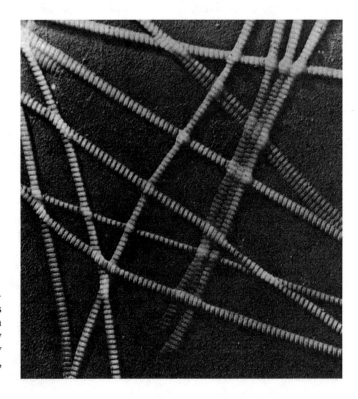

FIGURE 1–5. Electron micrograph of collagen fibers from human dermis. (From Fitzpatrick, TB: Dermatology in General Medicine. McGraw Hill, New York, 1987, p 260, with permission.)

electrostatic bonds. These are later replaced by strong intramolecular and intermolecular covalent bonds, which give the scar tensile strength. With time, collagen strands become organized into bundles that acquire a particular "weave."

At the same time, endothelial buds develop from intact capillaries. The endothelial buds eventually connect with other buds, forming patent vessels that supply the area. Endothelial buds and developing scar give the healing wound a characteristic red, granular appearance; hence the term *granulation tissue* is applied to this type of wound tissue. The appearance of granulation tissue is a sign of good progress in a healing wound. Endothelial budding and other noted events of the proliferative phase are illustrated for skin in Figure 1–6.

Wound contraction is a phenomenon that begins to occur in the connective tissue at this point. Actin-rich fibroblasts known as *myofibroblasts*, which have the ability to contract, accumulate at the margins of the wound. The myofibroblasts move toward the center of the wound, pulling the edges of the wound together, anchoring to each other and to collagen strands, and helping to reduce the size of the area to be covered. Figure 1–7 illustrates wound contraction. As previously mentioned, extensive scar contraction can be disfiguring and may limit function.

Remodeling Phase (Day 9 Onward)

The second phase of tissue repair is a remodeling of the connective-tissue matrix. This period of scar maturation, which may last for years, is marked by the disappear-

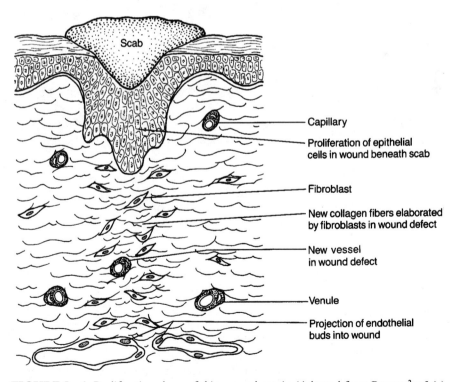

FIGURE 1–6. Proliferative phase of skin wound repair. (Adapted from Bryant,[2] p 14.)

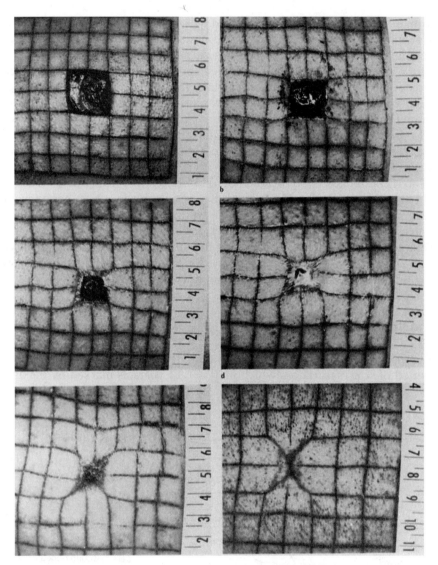

FIGURE 1-7. Illustration of wound contraction. Photographs of full-thickness excisional wound made on an 8 × 8 cm tattoed grid on domestic pig skin over a 45-day period. This sequence depicts healing by both granulation and wound contraction. (From Fitzpatrick, TB: Dermatology in General Medicine. New York, McGraw Hill, 1987, p 330, with permission.)

ance of fibroblasts. The collagen fibers initially laid down by fibroblasts are randomly oriented so that the connective-tissue matrix is fragile (Fig. 1–8*A*). During remodeling, the collagen fibers become more organized with interwoven bundles of parallel fibers (Fig. 1–8*B*). The weak hydrogen bonds are replaced by stronger covalent bonds; these changes provide greater tensile strength. The final characteristics (i.e., loose and mobile compared with dense and immobile) of a scar are dependent on the amount of collagen, the type of collagen, and the weave of the collagen bundles. It is important to note, however, that despite remodeling, scar tissue is never as strong as the tissue it re-

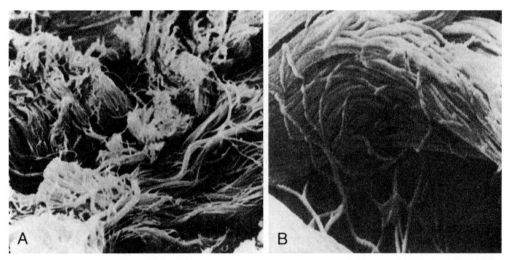

FIGURE 1-8. Collagen strand orientation with wound maturation. Photomicrographs illustrating collagen organization in a wound over time. (*A*) Disorderly arrangement of collagen in a new wound. (*B*) Well organized collagen from normal dermis. (From Hunt, TK, and Dunphy, JE [eds]: The Fundamentals of Wound Management. New York, Appleton-Century Crofts, 1979, p 36 and p 38, with permission.)

places. At maximal strength, mature scar tissue is only 70% as strong as intact tissue.[4] In addition, it is less vascular, creating a diffusion barrier to oxygen and nutrients, and making the tissue less able to dissipate applied heat. As scar matures, blood vessels disappear until the repair is relatively avascular; the scar goes from a rosy appearance to a white, shiny appearance.

The mechanism of remodeling is through collagen turnover. Collagen is taken up and laid down again along strands of fibronectin.[5,6] Collagen is destroyed by the enzyme collagenase, which is derived from polymorphonuclear leukocytes, granulation tissue, and migrating epithelium.[7,8] Collagenase is capable of cleaving the covalent bonds within and between collagen molecules, allowing metabolism of the scar collagen.[7] The factors that dictate exactly how a scar will be remodeled are not completely clear, but somehow the remodeling process tries to mimic the connective tissue structure of the tissue being repaired;[9] in addition, the type of tension applied to the scar will affect how it remodels.[10] This phenomenon probably involves a piezoelectric effect, that is, an electrical charge induced along collagen fibers, which helps to orient them parallel to lines of stress.[11,12] Repeated range-of-motion and/or prolonged low-load stretching techniques such as dynamic splints, serial casting, positional heat-and-stretch techniques, and neuromuscular electrical stimulation are examples of clinical techniques that can change scar configuration.[13]

As a means of summarizing the processes of inflammation and repair, Table 1-2 outlines the major events, and Figure 1-9 presents a graph of the normal inflammation and repair processes over time and the cells predominant at various stages.

ABNORMAL SCARRING

Excessive scarring may develop when there is an imbalance between collagen production and uptake. Overproduction of collagen can result in a hypertrophic scar or

TABLE 1-2 Summary of Events in Inflammation and Repair

	Inflammation
Vascular response	Vasodilation, margination of leukocytes, increased microvessel permeability, edema formation
Hemostatic response	Vessel retraction, clot formation
Cellular responses	Leukocyte infiltration—predominantly polymorphs (e.g., neutrophils) early and monocytes and lymphocytes later on
Immune responses	Via leukocytes and complement system
	Repair
Proliferative phase	Re-epithelialization, fibroplasia in connective tissues, development of granulation tissues via capillary budding, wound contraction
Remodeling phase	Collagen fibers taken up and reformed in a nonrandom orientation that increases tissue tensile strength

keloid scar. The biologic differences between these two types of scars are still being defined, but the clinical distinction is that a hypertrophic scar is contained within the boundaries of the original wound, while a keloid scar extends beyond the borders of the original wound.[14] In both cases, collagen synthesis exceeds collagen lysis. Hypertrophic scarring frequently occurs with severe burn injuries because of the large area involved and the full thickness depth of injury. An accelerated rate of metabolism is induced by the demands of inflammation and repair. Collagen synthesis is oxygen dependent while lysis is not, and because of this, postburn scarring can be controlled with pressure garments. The garment induces a state of ischemia that helps to reduce collagen synthesis while lysis continues, allowing a balance between synthesis and lysis to be re-established. Keloid scarring is related to a genetic inhibition of collagen lysis, and treatment of keloid scars with surgery, pressure, radiation, corticosteroids, and other drugs has had limited success.[15] An example of keloid scarring is shown in Figure 1-10.

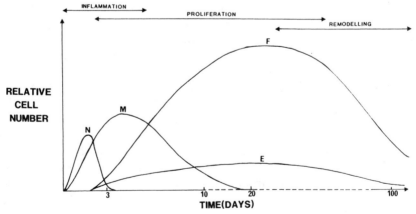

FIGURE 1-9. Relative cell concentrations over time in wound healing. E = endothelial cells; F = fibroblasts; M = macrophages; N = neutrophils. (From Dyson, M: Role of ultrasound in wound healing. In McCulloch, JM, Kloth, LC, Feedar, JA [eds]: Wound Healing: Alternatives in Management, ed 2. Philadelphia, FA Davis, 1995, p 340, with permission.)

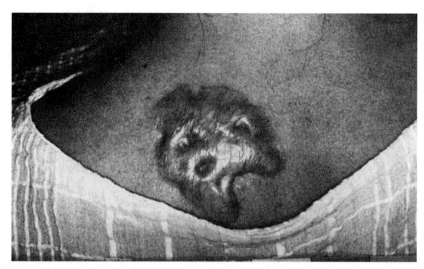

FIGURE 1–10. This keloid scar of the left posterior scapular area is a result of thermal injury to the back. This thermal injury occurred as the result of carbon dioxide laser treatment of a decorative tattoo. (Courtesy of David B. Apfelberg, MD, Palo Alto, CA.)

Scar Mutability

In rehabilitation, the therapist is often concerned with trying to induce change in scar tissue. For example, in cases of adhesive capsulitis or joint contracture, the therapeutic goal is to lengthen dense connective tissue in joint capsules, ligaments, and tendons. Dermal scarring is also treated as with burn scar or at surgical incision sites. As previously mentioned, common treatment techniques include prolonged low-load stretching, positional heat and stretch, joint mobilizations and deep friction massage. To develop an optimal treatment plan, it is important to understand the maturation process that scar undergoes.

Tillman and Cummings[11] have outlined the following stages of scar maturation. These phases focus on scar characteristics, but of course the stages of inflammation coexist, especially early on.

Days 2 to 4   *Initial scar formation:*   The scar is weak and may rupture with even low levels of physical force.

Days 5 to 21   *Fibroplasia and contraction:*   There is a high concentration of cells in the developing scar (fibroblasts, macrophages, neutrophils, lymphocytes, and other cells). Much collagen is laid down, and remodeling ensues; blood vessels invade, and as a result the scar takes on a characteristic rosy appearance. With remodeling, collagen bundles become larger and more organized. Wound contraction takes place. Measures to increase motion may be most effective due to the process of scar remodeling, which is most active during this phase.

Days 21 to 60   *Consolidation:*   Cells disappear; the scar becomes more fibrous and develops more strength with covalent bonding. Scar also becomes progressively less responsive to treatment.

Days 60 to 360   *Final maturation:*   Cells and blood vessels become very sparse; remodeling tapers off to a low level, and scar assumes its final appearance. Scar is relatively nonresponsive to treatment at this point.

Thus, to have the most influence on scar outcome, treatment should occur during peak remodeling—between 1 and 8 weeks postinjury, except in the case of burn scar. Current theory holds that stretching and physical stress influence scar by directing the remodeling process.[11,16] High loads can rupture dense connective tissue. Rather than destroy connective tissue structures, repeated, prolonged low loads can bring about gradual elongation by causing new collagen to be laid down in elongated form and in the direction of the applied stress, as old collagen strands are taken up.[10,11,16] The rationale for heat is that heat can alter the viscoelastic properties of connective tissues, at least in vitro. Heating between 37°C and 40°C can elongate rat tail tendon in vitro,[17-20] although heating above 40°C causes melting of tropocollagen and consequent denaturation of collagen, and irreversible effect.[19] Currently, clinical research to support the efficacy of heat-and-stretch techniques is lacking. The long-term use of compressive garments is a proven method for modifying burn scars.[21]

HUMAN IMMUNODEFICIENCY VIRUS AND INFLAMMATION AND REPAIR

The human immunodeficiency virus (HIV) can affect wound healing. HIV is a major worldwide health problem, with millions of people infected. The virus compromises the immune system, eventually making the host susceptible to a variety of opportunistic infections, a clinical condition known as acquired immune deficiency syndrome (AIDS), and delayed wound healing.

With HIV, macrophages and T (thymus-dependent) helper lymphocytes or T cells are preferentially affected. T cells play a critical role in coordinating an antibody response in conjunction with other lymphocytes known as B lymphocytes. The virus attaches to a receptor known as CD4, which is prevalent on the T cells and macrophages. With the destruction of T cells and macrophages, the immune response is impaired by inadequate antibody formation and by decreased phagocytosis. Because T cells and macrophages also help regulate fibroblast and endothelial cell activity, their depletion impairs collagen deposition and granulation tissue formation, and consequently, wound tensile strength and vascularity are less than optimal.[22-24] Persons with HIV or AIDS may have impaired wound healing ability and may require immediate wound care because of increased susceptibility to infection.[25] For further information on wound care for patients with HIV or AIDS, the reader is referred to the excellent article by Tucker[25] and Chapter 6 of this text.

INFLAMMATION AND REPAIR IN SPECIAL TISSUES

It has been convenient to this point to consider the model of dermal wound healing, but the general processes of inflammation and repair are similar in all tissues. In some other tissues, unique cells are involved and the type of collagen and its organization vary considerably. In bone, for example, osteoblasts and osteoclasts carry out remodeling to create new Haversian systems. In injured peripheral nerves, Schwann cells act to phagocytize nonviable nerve axons and form a neurilemmal tube to receive new axon buds. In skeletal muscle, satellite cells are involved in the regeneration of damaged tissue. A detailed discussion of inflammation and repair in these special tissues is beyond the scope of this chapter. For such information, the reader should consult textbooks that deal specifically with bone, nerve, muscle, tendon, or ligament.

CHRONIC INFLAMMATION

Normally, the acute inflammation reaction is virtually complete in 2 weeks. If the reaction continues for more than 4 weeks, it is called *subacute inflammation*. If it continues for months or years, it is called *chronic inflammation*. Chronic inflammation may occur as an autoimmune response or as an extension of acute inflammation, as may occur if a joint is repeatedly traumatized. An overuse syndrome such as shoulder impingement syndrome is an example of chronic inflammation caused by repeated minor trauma. It is thought that inadequate time for repair and nutritional replenishment perpetuates inflammation and can lead to eventual failure of connective tissue such as a tendon rupture. Unlike acute inflammation, in which the major cell type is the neutrophil, the predominant cells involved in chronic inflammation are lymphocytes, monocytes, and macrophages.

Another major difference between acute inflammation and chronic inflammation is the extent of fibroblastic proliferation. As the chronic process continues, more fibro-blasts are formed, more collagen is produced, and scar formation becomes extensive. In chronic inflammation, therefore, the usual result is replacement of normal tissue with scar, even in organs that have the ability to regenerate. In the musculoskeletal system, this can mean the development of adhesions. Adhesions are simply scar tissues, especially internal scar tissues, that limit mobility. These may occur in or around joint capsules, tendons, or muscles. For optimal function of healed articulating and gliding tissues, a delicate balance between adequate tensile strength and adequate mobility is required, and chronic inflammation does not lend itself to such a balance. Lack of movement within the available range of motion promotes the development of adhesions, therefore active and passive range-of-motion exercises are important for maintaining motion in patients with chronic inflammatory diseases of the musculoskeletal system.

CLINICAL EVALUATION OF WOUNDS

There are qualitative and quantitative distinctions that are useful in the clinical evaluation of wounds. What is evaluated will vary considerably according to whether the wound is open or closed, acute or chronic, present in soft tissues or bone or joint. The following is a synopsis of key indicators. The detailed evaluation of wounds is an entire discipline for each of the various tissues, and the reader should seek other sources for further information in addition to some information provided in Chapter 6 of this text.

Closed Wounds

• *Edema: Pitting edema* is edema in soft tissues in which applied pressure leaves a sustained depression of the overlying skin. This results from the temporary displacement of fluid and indicates that permanent changes in soft tissues have not oc-curred. *Brawny edema* is a swelling in which the soft tissues have become thickened and firm as a result of connective tissue infiltration and fibrosis. The tissues usually have a dusky, mottled appearance. Brawniness, which is the result of a chronic ede-matous condition, is often associated with venous stasis ulcers as previously noted. *Joint effusion* is swelling within a joint. Typically there is pain and limited motion. Joint effusion can be diagnosed by means of a ballottement test in which applied pressure causes movement of fluid inside the joint capsule.[26]

- Presence, age, and appearance of scar tissue; mobility of the scar and surrounding tissues.
- Other appropriate clinical tests and laboratory findings from x-rays, active and pas-sive range of motion, selective tissue tension tests, joint accessory motion tests, and special tests.

Chronic Open Wounds

- Location
- Surface area
- Depth or volume
- Symptoms of infection (presence of pus, odor, pain)
- Presence of drainage and its appearance
- Presence and quality of granulation tissue (color, texture, amount)
- Evidence of re-epithelialization or wound contraction
- Presence of necrotic tissue

FACTORS THAT MODIFY THE INFLAMMATION AND REPAIR PROCESSES

A number of factors may modify all or some of the steps in the inflammation and repair processes. Factors such as advanced age, malnutrition, anemia, peripheral vas-cular disease, and the presence of infection hinder inflammation and repair. A few of these factors will be considered in greater detail.

Nutrition

Injury causes physiologic stress, which induces a hypermetabolic state. Wound healing depends on an available supply of amino acids, proteins, vitamins and miner-als, and water, as well as sufficient calories from foodstuffs to fuel the inflammation and repair processes. Thus, individuals who are malnourished will not heal well. Ma-jor burns are once again a special consideration. Recovery from major burns entails a prolonged hypermetabolic state. Detailed descriptions of nutritional requirements and diets for patients with chronic wounds have been described by Frank.[27] Certain vita-mins are of interest because of their known roles in wound healing. Vitamin C is criti-cal for hydroxylation reactions during collagen synthesis.[28] Vitamin A enhances macrophage availability and thus aids in inflammation and wound closure.[29] Zinc is important in facilitating epithelialization.[30]

Diabetes Mellitus

Metabolic disorders may also interfere with wound healing. This is especially true for people with diabetes mellitus. People with diabetes are prone to peripheral vascular disease in both macrovessels and microvessels. In addition, peripheral neuropathies are common in diabetes, increasing the probability of traumatic injury to the limbs. Finally, a dampened immune response exists, which compromises the ability to combat infection. For all these reasons, people with diabetes are prone to soft-tissue ulcers that are slow to heal. There is now evidence that with non–insulin-dependent diabetes, excellent control of blood glucose and insulin levels is critical to preventing these secondary effects.[31]

Drugs

Certain drugs can inhibit inflammation. Corticosteroids, such as prednisone and cortisol, are powerful anti-inflammatory drugs that stabilize cell membranes, thereby inhibiting production of prostaglandins and related thromboxanes and leukotrienes. These drugs are sometimes used for very severe acute inflammatory conditions or for chronic inflammatory conditions. In the latter case, however, they are not always the first choice because of their strong side effects. Nonsteroidal anti-inflammatory drugs (NSAIDs), such as aspirin and ibuprofen, also inhibit inflammation by interrupting the production of prostaglandins, but in this case, the mechanism is interruption of the pathway by which prostaglandins are synthesized from arachidonic acid. NSAIDs have fewer side effects than corticosterioids and are often used to reduce inflammation.

Immobilization

Prolonged immobilization promotes the development of adhesions and limited motion, even after normal healing.[32] There is little doubt that immobilization aids early inflammation and repair. The need to apply a limb cast to immobilize a bone fracture or to suture a gaping soft-tissue wound seems self-evident, and there is good experimental evidence that immobilization produces faster healing.[33,34] Immobility, however, is necessarily accompanied by adhesions and stiffness. Studies of animal models have demonstrated that immobilization for up to 9 weeks has caused adhesions in all areas of synovial joints and that the connective tissue has been biochemically altered, having abnormal collagen cross-linking and decreased elasticity.[32] Remobilization is critical to recovery of function after inflammation and repair. For this reason, continuous passive motion (CPM) by machine is often employed as soon as possible after the injured area is stable. This is usually supplemented with active and passive range-of-motion exercises. Studies on dogs with tendon lacerations have demonstrated superior functional outcome with immobilization and early CPM, compared with immobilization only.[32,35]

Physical Agents

Some physical agents can also affect wound healing. These include electrical stimulation, total-contact casting, hyperbaric oxygen, ultraviolet C, low-intensity laser, and thermal agents, including therapeutic ultrasound. The role of thermal agents in inflammation and repair will be considered here.

EFFECTS OF THERMAL AGENTS ON INFLAMMATION AND REPAIR

In general, cold applications (cryotherapies) are used to treat closed acute inflammatory conditions, such as sprains, and heat therapy for subacute or chronic inflammatory conditions, such as chronic tendinitis. The rationale for these tenets has been that cold minimizes acute edema and hemorrhage and provides a good analgesic effect, whereas heat increases blood flow and thereby assists in the reabsorption of late inflammatory exudates and debris.

There are some experimental data to justify this approach to treatment. The effects of heat and cold in experimentally induced inflammation were studied by Schmidt and coworkers[36] and were summarized in a review article. Edema was induced by injecting various noxious substances into rat paws and measuring the degree of swelling. Models of both acute arthritis and chronic arthritis involving antigen-antibody reaction were studied. Heat was either administered as whole-body hyperthemia or was applied to the paws and tail only. Cold was applied as whole-body hypothermia. The effects of heat or cold varied according to the stage of inflammation. Heat inhibited inflammation in the model of chronic inflammation. Cold inhibited the more acute types of inflammation.

The premise that cold is beneficial for acute inflammation is supported by other basic research. Investigators have demonstrated that cooling decreased the effects of histamine on capillary permeability, presenting a rationale for the use of cold with edema.[37,38] Studies of postburn edema in rodents demonstrated that immediate cooling did, indeed, minimize edema formation.[39,40] Dorwart and colleagues[41] reported that in dogs, synovial fluid leukocytes exposed to cold had reduced phagocytic activity, another indication of dampened inflammation.

The basic research findings on cold are complemented by clinical-research findings. Application of cold in acute inflammatory conditions has been associated with reduced edema,[42–45] lowered leukocyte counts,[42,46] reduced analgesic intake,[42,47] increased pain threshold,[48,49] reduced indices of muscle spasm and soreness,[50] and shorter recovery times.[51] It seems logical that while cold can interrupt edema formation, existing edema must be reduced by compression, although this point has not been proved. Compression theoretically increases P_i, thereby aiding reabsorption of fluid. Thus, with acute orthopedic trauma, we have the addage of RICE: *rest, ice, compression, and elevation.*

Although deep heat, such as diathermy, has traditionally been used to aid in the reabsorption of subacute hematomas, evidence for the efficacy of this treatment is equivocal. Fenn[52] induced hematomas in rabbit ears and treated them with daily shortwave diathermy for 30 minutes. The area of the treated hematomas was significantly reduced by the 6th day of treatment. Lehmann, Dundore, and Esselman,[53] on the other hand, studied the clearance of radioactively labeled red blood cells injected into pigs treated with microwave diathermy. No difference in the clearance of the red blood cells was observed between the treated and the nontreated sides of the animals.

A different rationale for the use of heat modalities in chronic inflammatory conditions comes from in vitro observations that heat combined with stretch can alter the viscoelastic properties of connective tissue, making it more extensible.[17-20,54] Thus, "heat and stretch" is a logical strategy for helping to overcome adhesions. Proof for the clinical efficacy of this strategy is presently lacking. Wessling and coworkers[55] did study heat (with ultrasound) and stretch on triceps surae length using conventional goniometric measurements of ankle dorsiflexion in normal humans. They found small, but statistically significant, increases in motion with stretch alone and with heat and stretch, and the increase was greatest with heat and stretch. Patients were not tested, however, and in any case, it would seem that the connective tissue most affected in these experiments was skeletal muscle rather than dense connective tissue.

Heat may be beneficial in chronic inflammatory conditions, but it exacerbates acute inflammation.[36,56] In soft-tissue infections such as boils, superficial heat in the form of warm compresses or soaks is a traditional treatment. These treatments localize the inflammation and accelerate abscess formation so the abscess can be drained. For acute musculoskeletal inflammations, however, there is a general consensus that heat applications should be avoided for fear they will exacerbate hemorrhage and edema.[56] The presumed mechanism for this is that heat will produce increased blood flow and thereby increase microvascular hydrostatic pressure. Indeed, in clinical studies, investigators found that heat aggravated edema formation and prolonged recovery time in acute orthopedic injuries.[57,58]

The generalization about the effects of heat on chronic inflammation may not apply with deep heats in rheumatoid arthritis. Harris and McCroskery[59] studied the effect of temperature on degradation of cartilage by rheumatoid synovium. They demonstrated a fourfold increase in enzymatic lysis of human cartilage in vitro with a temperature increase of 5°C. This marked increase in damage might be caused by an elevated metabolic rate of the macrophages and the destructive enzymes in this autoimmune disease.[59,60] An increase in joint temperature might increase cartilage destruction in patients with rheumatoid arthritis, and because the deep-heat modalities (continuous wave ultrasound, diathermies) would be most likely to elevate joint temperature, it may be best to avoid the deep-heat treatments in patients with rheumatoid arthritis.[56,60] By contrast, superficial heats, such as hot packs, have not been associated with rheumatoid cartilage destruction. Horvath and Hollander[61] made intra-articular temperature measurements in normal individuals and patients with arthritis and found that joint temperature actually fell in response to hot packs. It has been postulated that this was caused by a reflex shunting of blood flow away from the joint to the more superficial tissues.[60,61]

In contrast to its deep-heating capabilities, low-intensity ultrasound has been associated with claims of improved wound healing in various tissues including skin,[62-64] tendon,[65] bone,[66] and bursae.[67] Pulsed, "low-wattage ultrasound applications are now in common clinical use for a variety of inflammatory and open wound conditions. Recently, when applied in combination with ultraviolet C, low-intensity ultrasound has even been associated with improved wound healing.[68]

Presumably, these effects are caused by nonthermal phenomena in the tissues. The exact mechanisms by which ultrasound influences tissue healing are not well understood but may involve free radical formation,[69] altered blood flow,[70] mast cell degranulation,[71] or other effects on humeral mediators. It has been suggested that ultrasound may also stimulate protein production synthesis in fibroblasts.[72] As Maxwell points out, it is possible that ultrasound's effects on tissue healing vary according to tissue type, dosimetry, and unique circumstances.[73] Thus, it is important to better define the specific effects of low-intensity ultrasound so that rational treatment strategies can be developed.[73]

CASE STUDY 1

Ms. X is a 57-year-old female directory assistance operator who has adhesive capsulitis of the right glenohumeral joint. She first noticed an insidious onset of discomfort and limited motion about 6 weeks ago. She has difficulty sleeping at night and is awakened when she rolls onto her shoulder. She has difficulty with activities of daily living (ADLs) such as donning a coat or other articles of clothing.

During the initial evaluation it is found that active range of motion (AROM) is limited as noted below in flexion, abduction, and internal and external rotation. There is a capsular end-feel during passive range of motion (PROM). Accessory joint motions are limited. X-rays are reported to be "normal," and there are no indications of rotator cuff tendinitis.

Given an absence of contraindications, Ms. X's physical therapist, after discussion with the patient, decides to implement a program of heat and stretch, joint mobilizations, and AROM and contract-relax exercises. Heat is applied via 1 MHz ultrasound at 1.5 W/cm^2 continuous wave for 10 minutes to the anterior and inferior glenohumeral joint. The patient is seen in the clinic twice weekly.

The treatment rationale is to alter the joint capsule's viscoelastic properties, at least temporarily, in order to potentiate stretching techniques, and to facilitate remodeling of the dense connective tissues of the joint capsule to allow increased AROM (i.e., elongation of collagen fibers and altered weave of collagen bundles). Data are collected as noted in the flowchart (Table 1–3). The patient is seen biweekly and undertakes the prescribed home exercise program; by the end of 5 weeks, all short-term goals have been achieved.

CASE STUDY 2

Mr. Y is a 36-year-old man with acute rotator cuff tendinitis of the right shoulder, of 3 days' duration. Mr. Y is a firefighter by occupation, and he often "pumps iron" at the fire station, when not out on calls. He also enjoys playing league softball. The clinical presentation is one of limited AROM in flexion, extension, abduction, and internal and external rotation. PROM is normal. Resisted isometric contractions are strong but painful in the motions mentioned. Joint accessory motions are pain-free and are judged to be normal in magnitude. The rotator cuff is tender to manual palpation.

After discussing the pathophysiology of the problem and treatment options with Mr. Y, the physical therapist initiates a treatment program that includes 1 MHz ultrasound at an intensity of 0.5 W/cm^2, pulsed in a 20% duty cycle (p 20%) for 5 minutes; AROM exercises; strengthening exercises; deep friction massage; and ice pack applications for 10 to 15 minutes. At first, the strengthening exercises are isometric only; however, as the patient recovers, the exercises are made resistive using a stretch band. Mr. Y applies ice packs three to four times a day on his own and carries out the prescribed exercises twice daily, five repetitions each. At his physical therapist's urging, he temporarily discontinues weight lifting and softball.

Text continued on p. 27

TABLE 1–3 Flowchart, Case Study 1

Analysis	7/28/95	8/4/95	8/11/95	8/18/95	8/25/95	9/1/95
SUBJECTIVE	Right shoulder hurts: achy, sharp pains at end-ranges of motion and with sudden or jarring movements	Shoulder was sore after last treatment; feeling better now. Shoulder feels more loose.	"I'm feeling much better; gaining every day."	Still improving, although at a slower rate. Can do all ADL pretty well.	"I feel good. I'm much better than when I started."	"I feel 100%. No problems at work or with ADLs."
OBJECTIVE PROM						
Flexion	112°	130°	145°	165°	175°	180°
Abduction	90°	115°	130°	150°	163°	170°
External Rotation	15°	33°	48°	61°	73°	80°
Internal Rotation	20°	37°	56°	64°	68°	70°
Function	Difficulty donning jacket, other clothing	Still having difficulty, although less so	Mild discomfort with dressing, ADLs	Can perform all ADL without discomfort	Functioning well	Full function
Pain Level (0–10 scale)	9 = worst, 2 = best	6–7 = worst, 1 = best	5 = worst, 1 = best	4 = worst, 5 = best	2 = worst, 0 = best	0 pain

Continued

TABLE 1-3 Flowchart, Case Study 1 (*Continued*)

Analysis	7/28/95	8/4/95	8/11/95	8/18/95	8/25/95	9/1/95
Treatment	1) 1 MHz CW-US at 1.5 w/cm² × 10' anterior and inferior right shoulder	1) X	1) X	1) X	1) X	Developed a revised home exercise program: AROM and self mobilizations. To be performed 1 × daily for maintenance of regained ROM and function
	2) Grade 1 at 2 joint mobs, R G-H jt	2) X	2) X	2) X	2) X	
	3) A/PROM	3) X	3) X	3) X	3) X	
	4) PNF: Contract-relax: flexion, abduction, external rotation	4) X	4) X	4) X	4) X	
	5) Home exercise program including A/PROM, self mobilizations	5) X Gave technique pointers		5) X Added isotonic resistance ex: 3#wt, 3 sets 10 reps. To do 1 × day		
ASSESSMENT	Adhesive capsulitis; will benefit from heat and stretch, manual techniques, PNF, AROM exercises.	Good improvement; treatment seems effective	Continued improvement; joint capsule apparently loosening/remodeling	Doing well; rate of improvement has declined	A/PROM continues to improve; hope to regain full motion, symmetrical to LUE	All short-term goals achieved; good recovery. Patient is ready for discharge.
PLAN	See 2 × week; CW-US; PROM; joint mobilizations; contract/relax; home exercise program	Continue present treatment plan	Continue present treatment plan	Continue	Continue	Discharge with home program of maintenance exercises

CW-US = continuous mode ultrasound; PNF = proprioceptive neuromuscular facilitation.

TABLE 1–4 Flowchart, Case Study 2

Analysis	8/9/95		8/16/95	8/23/95	8/30/95	9/13/95
SUBJECTIVE	Right shoulder hurts: pain is sharp, present with all motions, especially reaching overhead; little pain at rest.		Shoulder was sore for a couple hours after last treatment (only); better now. Ice helps a lot. D/C'd resistance exercise and softball.	"I'm feeling better; gaining every day; anxious to resume resistance work and sports."	Still improving, pleased with progress. Can do all ADL fairly easily. Tried throwing—mild discomfort.	"I feel fine—good as new. Have tried throwing again on a few occasions without problems. Have also begun light resistance exercises."
OBJECTIVE A/PROM	PROM	AROM	AROM	AROM	AROM	AROM
Flexion	170° (soft end-feel)	120°	135°	143°	168°	175°
Abduction	160° (soft end-feel)	110°	125°	135°	152°	163°
External Rotation	80° (soft end-feel)	40°	50°	57°	63°	85°
Internal Rotation	70° (soft end-feel)	35°	45°	56°	64°	72°
Function	Sharp pain with motions involving right shoulder; particular difficulty with overhead tasks (e.g., shampooing, combing hair [per patient]).		Still having difficulty, although not as much.	Mild discomfort with dressing, ADLs per patient Able to perform "towel exercise" behind back	Can perform all ADL with very mild discomfort.	Functioning well—no problems
Resisted isometric Contractions						
Abduction	Strong, painful		Strong, painful	Strong, mildly painful	Strong, pain very mild	Strong, pain-free
External rotation	Strong, painful		Strong, painful	Strong, mildly painful	Strong, pain very mild	Strong, pain-free
Pain level (0–10 scale)	8 = worst, 1 = best		7 = worst, 1 = best	4 = worst, 1 = best	4 = worst, 5 = best	5 = worst, 0 = best

Continued

25

TABLE 1–4 Flowchart, Case Study 2 (*Continued*)

Analysis	8/9/95	8/16/95	8/23/95	8/30/95	9/13/95
Treatment	1) 1 MHz US @ 0.5 w/cm² × 5, p 20%, R rot. cuff 2) Cross-fiber friction masage to R rotator cuff tendons 3) AAROM with PNF: Contract-relax: flexion, abduction, external rotation 4) Ice pack × 10 min 5) Home exercise program including AROM, isometric exercises for rotator cuff	1) X 2) X 3) X 4) X 5) X Gave technique pointers	1) X 2) X 3) X 4) X 5) D/C'd isometrics; Began Theraband (yellow), exercises for flexion, extension, abduction, adduction, external rotation, and internal rotation motions, 10 reps/day each.	1) X 2) X 3) X 4) X 5) X Added isotonic resistance exercise: 3 # wt, 3 sets × 10 reps. To do 1 × day, progress to 2 ×/day	1) X 2) X 3) X 4) Discussed status and risk factors re: recurrence of RCT problem, and practical measures to avoid eg. pre game stretches, etc. Agreed to D/C
ASSESSMENT	Rotator cuff tendinitis; Will benefit from interventions to decrease acute inflammation, stretch & strengthen RC. Pt. needs to decrease stress on RC. Expect good response over 4–5 weeks	Subjective & objective improvement	Continued improvement; inflammation subsiding. Appropriate to begin strengthening throughout AROM.	Doing well	Apparently good resolution of problem. Pt is at some risk of recurrence due to his desire to resume competition and resistive work.
PLAN	See 3X week; P-US; AAROM; contract/relax; friction massage, home ex. program	Continue present treatment plan	Continue present treatment plan. Discourage premature resumption of sports, etc.	Continue	Discontinue. Follow-up with patient in 2 weeks to reinforce measures to avoid recurrence.

For this overuse syndrome, the rationale for treatment is to decrease inflammation via the anti-inflammatory modalities of cold and low-intensity ultrasound, as well as by allowing the involved structures to be at rest. Isometric exercise can help to maintain the strength of the contractile elements without loading the articulating structures through the range of motion. As inflammation subsides, gradual strengthening through the available range of motion is advisable. Data are collected as noted in the flowchart, Table 1–4. Within 4 weeks, Mr. Y has regained full AROM. Mr. Y's shoulder is now pain-free, and he can carry out all ADLs, including throwing a ball.

SUMMARY

The processes of inflammation and repair are normal, desirable responses to injury, serving to restore tissue integrity. The inflammatory process is a complex event involving vascular, hemostatic, cellular, and immune responses that are controlled by numerous neural and humoral mediators, which clean the wound area, preparing it for the subsequent repair process. Tissue repair involves proliferation of new connective tissue and blood vessels and, over time, remodeling of the scar.

Intervention in the processes of inflammation and repair with thermal agents or other modalities is appropriate only when the intervention will facilitate or accelerate the process, or when undesirable effects of the processes must be controlled. When the inflammation or repair processes become excessive or chronic, therapy is directed at attenuating the process.

Several physical agents can affect inflammation and repair, including the thermal agents. In general, cryotherapy is used in acute inflammatory conditions, and heat is used in chronic inflammatory conditions. The various heat and cold applications are reviewed in subsequent chapters of this text. *It should be apparent that thermal agents are not best used in isolation from other forms of therapy. Rather, they should be one part of the treatment plan.* The therapist must assess the state of inflammation and repair, decide on the appropriate thermal agent, and then incorporate it into the overall treatment plan, continually monitoring the clinical outcome.

Study Objectives

Having completed this chapter, the reader should now be able to:

1. List the phases of inflammation and tissue repair.
2. Explain how edema forms as a result of injury.
3. Explain the qualitative differences in types of edema.
4. Characterize the leukocyte cell types and their functions in acute inflammation; in chronic inflammation.
5. Describe patient problems that result from chronic inflammation.
6. Describe qualitative and quantitative indicators of wound status.
7. List characteristics of scar that have importance in patient management.
8. Describe the maturation of scar and periods when scar is most mutable.
9. List four patient factors that can modify the inflammation and repair processes.
10. List physical agents that can promote wound healing.

REFERENCES

1. Starling, EH: On the absorption of fluids from the connective tissue spaces. J Physiol (London) 19:312, 1896.
2. Bryant, WM: Wound Healing. Clinical Symposia (Ciba) 29(3):9, 1977.
3. Clark, RAF: Overview and general considerations of wound repair. In Clark, RAF and Henson, PM (eds): The Molecular and Cellular Biology of Wound Repair. Plenum Press, New York, 1988, p 4.
4. Levenson, SM, et al: The healing of rat skin wounds. Ann Surg 161:293, 1965.
5. Bryant, WM: Wound Healing. Clinical Symposia (Ciba) 29(3):15, 1977.
6. Clark, RAF: Overview and general considerations of wound repair. In Clark, RAF and Henson, PM (eds): The Molecular and Cellular Biology of Wound Repair. Plenum Press, New York, 1988, p 17.
7. Riley, WB and Peacock EE: Identification, distribution and significance of a collagenolytic enzyme in human tissues. Proc Soc Exp Biol Med 124:207, 1967.
8. Agren, MD, et al: Collagenase in wound healing: Effect of wound age and type. J Invest Dermatol 99(6):709, 1992.
9. Madden, JW: Wound healing: The biological basis of hand surgery. Clin Plast Surg 3:3, 1976.
10. Arem, AJ and Madden, JW: Effects of stress on healing wounds: I. Intermittent noncyclical tension. J Surg Res 20:93, 1976.
11. Tillman, LJ and Cummings, GS: Biologic mechanisms of connective tissue mutability. In Currier, DP and Nelson, RM (eds): Dynamics of Human Biologic Tissue. FA Davis, Philadelphia, 1992, p 1.
12. Flint, MH: The basis of the histological demonstration of tension in collagen. In Longacre, JJ (ed): The Ultrastructure of Collagen. Charles C Thomas, Springfield, IL, 1976, p 60.
13. Hardy, MA: The biology of scar formation. Phys Ther 69:12 1014, 1989.
14. Peacock, EE, Madden, JW, and Triea, WC: Biologic basis for treatment of keloids and hypertrophic scars. South Med J 63:755, 1970.
15. McPherson, JM and Piez, KA: Collagen in dermal wound repair. In Clark, RAF and Henson, PM (eds): The Molecular and Cellular Biology of Wound Repair. Plenum Press, New York, 1988, p 488.
16. Cummings, GS and Tillman, LT: Remodeling of dense connective tissue in normal adult tissues. In Currier, DP and Nelson, RM: Dynamics of Human Biologic Tissue. FA Davis, Philadelphia, 1992, p 45.
17. Gersten, JW: Effect of ultrasound on tendon extensibility. Am J Phys Med 34:362, 1955.
18. Lehmann, JF: Effect of therapeutic temperatures on tendon extensibility. Arch Phys Med Rehabil 51:481, 1970.
19. Rigby, BJ: The effect of mechanical extension upon the thermal stability of collagen. Biochem Biophys Acta 79:634, 1964.
20. Warren, CG, Lehmann, JF, and Koblanski, JN: Heat and stretch procedures: An evaluation using rat tail tendon. Arch Phys Med Rehabil 57:122, 1976.
21. Staley, MJ and Richard, RL: Burn Care Rehabilitation: Principles and Practice. FA Davis, Philadelphia, 1994, p 391.
22. Banda, MH, Hunt, TK, and Silver, IA: Fibrosis. Clin Symp 37:12, 1985.
23. Leibovich, SJ and Ross, R: The role of the macrophage in wound repair. A study with hydrocortisone and anti-macrophage serum. Am J Pathol 78:71, 1975.
24. Peterson, MJ, Barbul, A, and Breslin, RJ: Significance of T-lymphocytes in wound healing. Surgery 102:300, 1987.
25. Tucker, RS: Wound care in patients with HIV. Clin Management 12:73, 1992.
26. Wallace, LA, Mangine, RE, and Malone, TR: The Knee. In Gould, JA (ed): Orthopaedic and Sports Physical Therapy. CV Mosby, St Louis, 1990, p 334.
27. Frank, GC: Nutritional requirements for patients with chronic wounds. In McCulloch, JM, Kloth, LC, and Feedar, JA (eds): Wound Healing: Alternatives in Management, ed 2. FA Davis, Philadelphia, 1995, p 87.
28. Kanzler, MH, Gorsulowsky, DC, and Swanson, NA: Basic mechanisms in the healing cutaneous wound. J Dermatol Surg Oncol 12(11):1156, 1986.
29. Hunt, TK: Vitamin A and wound healing. J Am Acad Dermatol 15(4):817, 1986.
30. Bobel, LM: Nutritional implications in the patient with pressure sores. Nurs Clin North Am 22(2):379, 1987.
31. Diabetes Control and Complications Trial Research Group: The Effects of Intensive Treatment of Diabetes on the Development and Progression of Long-Term Complications in Insulin-Dependent Diabetes Mellitus. N Engl J Med 329(14):977, 1993.
32. Woo, SL-Y, et al: The importance of controlled passive mobilization on flexor tendon healing: A biochemical study. Acta Orthop Scand 52:615, 1981.
33. Frank, C, Amiel, D, and Akeson, WH: Healing of the medial collateral ligament of the knee: A morphological and biochemical assessment in rabbits. Acta Orthop Scand 54:1917, 1983.
34. Nystrom, B, and Holmlund, D: Experimental evaluation of immobilization in operative and nonoperative treatment of Achilles tendon rupture: A radiographic study in the rabbit. Acta Chir Scand 149:669, 1983.
35. Gelberman, RH, et al: Effects of early intermittent passive immobilization on healing canine flexor tendons. J Hand Surg 7:170, 1982.

36. Schmidt, KL, et al: Heat, cold and inflammation. Rheumatology 38:391, 1979.
37. Rippe, B and Grega, GJ: Effects of 150 prenaline and cooling on histamine-induced changes of capillary permeability in the rat hindquarter bed. Acta Physiol Scand 103:252, 1978.
38. Wolf, MB, et al: Effects of cold on vascular permeability and edema formation in the isolated cat limb. J Appl Physiol 73(1):166, 1992.
39. Biomgren, I, et al: The effect of different cooling temperatures and immersion fluids on post-burn oedema and survival of the partially scalded hairy mouse ear. Burns 11(3):161, 1985.
40. Jakobsson, OP and Arturson, G: The effect of prompt local cooling on oedema formation in scalded rat paws. Burns 12(1):8, 1985.
41. Dorwart, BB, et al: Effects of heat, cold and mechanical agitation on crystal-induced arthritis in the dog. Arth Rheum 16:540, 1973.
42. Schaubel, HH: Local use of ice after orthopedic procedures. Am J Surg 72:711, 1946.
43. Basur, R, Shepard, E, and Mouzos, G: A cooling method in the treatment of ankle sprains. Practitioner 216:708, 1976.
44. Cote, DJ, et al: Comparison of three treatment procedures for minimizing ankle sprain swelling. Phys Ther 68(7):1072, 1988.
45. Weston, M, et al: Changes in local blood volume during cold pack gel application to traumatized ankles. J Orthop Sports Phys Ther 19(4):197, 1994.
46. Farry, PJ, et al: Ice treatment of injured ligaments: An experimental model. New Zealand Med J 12:12, 1980.
47. Conolly, WB, Paltos, N, and Tooth, RM: Cold therapy: An improved method. Med J Aust 2:525, 1972.
48. Benson, TB and Copp, EP: The effects of therapeutic forms of heat and ice on the pain threshold of the normal shoulder. Rheumatol Rehabil 13:101, 1974.
49. Gammon, GD and Starr, I: Studies on the relief of pain by counterirritation. J Clin Invest 20:13, 1941.
50. Prentice, WE: An electromyographic analysis of the effectiveness of heat or cold and stretching for inducing relaxation in injured muscle. J Orthop Sports Phys Ther 3:133, 1982.
51. Hocutt, JE, et al: Cryotherapy in ankle sprains. Am J Sports Med 10:316, 1982.
52. Fenn, JE: Effect of pulsed electromagnetic energy (Diapulse) on experimental hematomas. Canad Med Assoc J 100:251, 1969.
53. Lehmann, JF, Dundore, DE, and Esselman, PC: Microwave diathermy: Effects on experimental hematoma resolution. Arch Phys Med Rehabil 64:127, 1983.
54. LeBan, MM: Collagen tissue: Implications of its response to stress in vitro. Arch Phys Med Rehabil 43:461, 1962.
55. Wessling, KC, DeVane, DA, and Hylton, CR: Effects of static stretch and ultrasound combined on triceps surae muscle extensibility in healthy women. Phys Ther 67(5):674, 1987.
56. Feibel, A and Fast, A: Deep heating of joints: A reconsideration. Arch Phys Med Rehabil 57:513, 1976.
57. Barnes, L: Cryotherapy: Putting injury on ice. Physician Sports Med 7(6):130, 1979.
58. Wallace, L, et al: Immediate care of ankle injuries. J Orthop Sports Phys Ther 1:46, 1979.
59. Harris, ED and McCroskery, PA: The influence of temperature and fibril stability on degradation of cartilage collagen by rheumatoid synovial collagenase. N Engl J Med 290:1, 1974.
60. Hollander, JL: Collagenase, cartilage and cortisol. N Engl J Med 290:50, 1974.
61. Horvath, SM and Hollander, JL: Intra-articular temperature as a measure of joint reaction. J Clin Invest 28(3):469, 1949.
62. Dyson, M and Suckling, J: Stimulation of tissue repair by ultrasound: A survey of the mechanisms involved. Physiotherapy 64(4):105, 1978.
63. Dyson, M: Therapeutic applications of ultrasound. In Nyborg, WL and Ziskin, MC (eds): Biological Effects of Ultrasound. Churchill Livingstone, New York, 1985, p 121.
64. Dyson, M: Mechanisms involved in therapeutic ultrasound. Physiotherapy 73:116, 1987.
65. Enwemeka CS: The effects of therapeutic ultrasound on tendon healing: A biomechanical study. Am J Phys Med Rehabil 68(6):283, 1989.
66. Pilla, AA, et al: Noninvasive low intensity pulsed ultrasound accelerates bone healing in the rabbit. J Orthopaedic Trauma 4(3):246, 1990.
67. Gorkiewicz, R: Ultrasound for subacromial burtisis. Phys Ther 64:46, 1984.
68. Nussbaum, EL, Biemann, I, and Mustard, B: Comparison of ultrasound/ultraviolet-C and laser for treatment of pressure ulcers in patients with spinal cord injury. Phys Ther 74(9):812, 1994.
69. Edmonds, PD and Sancier, KM: Evidence for free radical production by ultrasonic cavitation in biological media. Ultrasound Med Biol 9:635, 1983.
70. Hogan, RD, Burke, KM, and Franklin, TD: The effect of ultrasound on hemodynamics in skeletal muscle: Effects during ischemia. Microvasc Res 23:370, 1982.
71. Fyfe, M and Chahl, LA: Mast cell degranulation and increased vascular permeability induced by therapeutic ultrasound in the rat ankle joint. Br J Exp Pathol 65:671, 1984.
72. Harvey, W, et al: The in vitro stimulation of protein synthesis in human fibroblasts by therapeutic levels of ultrasound. Proceedings of the 2nd European Congress on Ultrasonics in Medicine, Amsterdam, Excerpta Medica, 1975, p 10.
73. Maxwell L: Therapeutic ultrasound: Its effects on the cellular and molecular mechanisms of inflammation and repair. Physiotherapy 78(6):421, 1992.

CHAPTER 2

Anatomic and Functional Aspects of Pain: Evaluation and Management With Thermal Agents

Dennis M. DePace, PhD
Roberta Newton, PhD, PT

Pain is defined as an unpleasant sensory and emotional experience that is associated with actual or potential tissue damage.[1] It is a protective mechanism that alerts the individual to make an appropriate response to prevent further injury. Pain is a sensory experience described in terms different from other sensory modalities. Touch, for example, is a peripheral stimulus perceived as a particular touch sensation, whereas pain is a complex phenomenon encompassing sensory, emotional, motor, and cultural components.

Annually, one of every four people in the United States is affected by pain. When the pain state outlasts the initial trauma and subsequent recovery period, the multidimensional aspects of the pain experience are quite evident. The chronic pain state not only affects the individual experiencing pain, but it is also physiologically and psychologically draining to the individual's family and close associates. The total cost for treatment of the chronic pain patient and work days lost is tremendous.[2] Estimates in dollars and days lost at work pertain only to those individuals with chronic pain conditions and do not include the acute pain state—that is, headaches, injuries, or the postoperative period. With the increasing cost to remediate pain and the gap in the understanding of normal and chronic pain mechanisms, an Interagency Committee of the US Government was established to address these issues. Since 1978, the interdisciplinary investigation of pain mechanisms and its treatment has proliferated.

The ability of the clinician to treat a painful condition appropriately is dependent on a sound clinical problem-solving approach. Such an approach includes understanding the normal neurophysiologic mechanisms of pain; knowledge of mechanisms associated with acute, chronic, and referred pain; knowledge of appropriate assessment techniques; and understanding the rationale for selecting a particular therapy. Furthermore, the clinician needs to analyze the literature critically and use only those reports that have appropriate research design, good documentation of methodology, and corroboration of results. Caution should be taken when extrapolating data from laboratory animal research to direct patient care.

PERIPHERAL AND CENTRAL NERVOUS SYSTEM MECHANISMS SUBSERVING PAIN

When examining current concepts of pain, anatomic, physiologic, and neurochemical relationships need to be examined. The amount of knowledge gained in this area within the past two decades far exceeds the knowledge accumulated in other areas of neuroscience. This is witnessed by continuing changes in the current pain literature and in applications of pain theories to justify clinical procedures.

Peripheral Mechanisms

NOCICEPTORS

Receptors responsible for the transmission of pain impulses (nociceptors) are described morphologically as free nerve endings. The best-studied nociceptors are those located in the skin.[3-6] Nociceptors found in the viscera and in the cardiac and skeletal muscles are less well understood.[7] Stimuli adequate for excitation of a nociceptor include intense heat, intense cold, strong mechanical deformation, and chemical substances. Those receptors that respond to only one noxious stimulant are termed *specific nociceptors*, whereas those nociceptors that respond to several noxious stimuli are termed *polymodal nociceptors*. How the nociceptor changes the stimulus to action potentials is not completely understood.

In addition to mechanical activation of a nociceptor, tissue trauma results in the liberation of a number of chemical factors from the damaged tissue. When these substances accumulate in sufficient amount in the extracellular space, they can activate nociceptive endings.

Phospholipids that are liberated from damaged cells break down to form arachidonic acid, which subsequently forms prostaglandin E and bradykinin. This process can be modified by nonsteroidal anti-inflammatory drugs (NSAIDs) such as aspirin and ibuprofen. In addition, a number of substances released from traumatized tissues produce an inflammatory response that exacerbates the nociceptive response. Serotonin, released from platelets, produces vasoconstriction. This coupled with the release of histamine and heparin from mast cells results in localized edema.

Substance P, somatokinin, bradykinin, cholecystokinin, and vasoactive peptides have all been identified within the primary afferent neurons thought to mediate central pain transmission.[8,9]

PRIMARY AFFERENT NEURONS

The use of electrical stimulation with preferential blockade of peripheral nerves in humans has revealed two distinct populations of primary afferent neurons subserving pain.[6,10,11] One group, when preferentially stimulated, evokes a sharp and pricking pain sensation of short duration. This group of afferents is the lightly myelinated A-delta, or group III, primary afferents. Conduction velocities of these neurons range between 4 and 30 m/s; they constitute about 20% of primary pain afferents. When activated, the second group produces a longer-lasting, burning sensation, which is dull, aching, and more diffusely localized. These primary afferents are the unmyelinated C, or group IV, afferents. Conduction velocities of C afferents range between 0.5 and 2 m/s, and these contribute about 80% of primary pain afferents. The A-delta fibers mediate the "fast" component of pain, while the C fibers mediate the "slow" phase.

The A-delta and C afferent neurons are further subdivided according to the type of nociceptive stimuli that activate them. Three types of nociceptive afferents have been identified: noxious mechanical, mechanothermal, and polymodal (Table 2-1). The A-delta high-threshold mechanoreceptor afferent responds exclusively to noxious mechanical stimulation. The A-delta heat nociceptive afferent, called the *mechanothermal nociceptor*,[12] responds to both noxious mechanical and intense thermal stimuli. The C polymodal nociceptive afferent responds to noxious heat in the 45°C to 51°C range, to noxious mechanical stimulation, and to noxious chemical stimulation. Approximately one third of the C afferents respond to intense cold; however, their activation does not contribute to the perception of pain.[13] Approximately 85% to 90% of the C nociceptor afferents identified in primates are C polymodal afferents. To date, all identified C neurons in humans are C polymodal afferents. In humans, the relationship between activation of A-delta mechanothermal afferents and perception of "fast" pain and activation of C-polymodal afferents and perception of "slow" pain has been established.[14]

TABLE 2-1 Afferent Neuronal Types and Stimuli

Type	Stimulus
A-delta high-threshold mechanoreceptor	Intense mechanical stimulation
A-delta mechanothermal receptor	Noxious mechanical and intense thermal stimulation
C-polymodal nociceptor	Noxious mechanical, noxious thermal, and noxious chemical stimulation

TERMINATION OF NOCICEPTIVE AFFERENTS IN THE DORSAL HORN

Primary sensory neurons segregate into the dorsal root of the spinal nerve. Dorsal root fibers mediating epicritic sensibility (proprioception, kinesthesia) and two-point tactile discrimination enter the spinal cord in the medial division of the dorsal root. Those mediating nociceptive sensibility (A-delta and C fibers) enter the spinal cord in the lateral division of the dorsal root. Up to 30% of the C fibers are reported to enter the spinal cord via the ventral root of spinal nerves. This is a possible explanation for the return of pain following dorsal rhizotomy, a surgical procedure for pain control. Many of these so-called ventral root afferents actually curve back out of the ventral root to innervate the meninges or to re-enter the dorsal root.[15]

As the primary afferents for pain approach the spinal cord, they divide into short ascending and descending branches that enter the dorsolateral fasciculus (Lissauer's tract). These axons eventually terminate within the dorsal horn of spinal cord gray matter.

The dorsal horn of gray matter is divided into several laminae based on the morphology of their neurons and the types of afferent neurons terminating within each. A-delta and C fibers have been shown to terminate mainly within the dorsolateral parts of the dorsal horn within laminae I and II (substantia gelatinosa). The A-delta fibers also have a significant input to lamina V of the dorsal horn of gray matter. The afferents that terminate in lamina II are primarily those arising in nociceptive receptors of the skin, whereas those from viscera and muscle terminate largely in laminae I and V. Because lamina II is largely concerned with allowing the nervous system to localize painful stimuli, the fact that afferents from viscera and muscle do not project here may account for the diffuse and poorly localized quality of visceral and muscle pain (Fig. 2–1).

Central Mechanisms of Pain

SECOND-ORDER NEURONS

There are two major routes by which pain sensations ascend to higher brain centers. The first is the spinothalamic tract, which in general is associated with the central

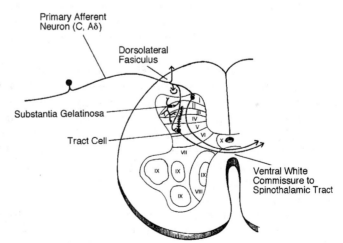

FIGURE 2-1. Transverse section of the spinal cord showing the terminations of incoming A-delta and C fibers that mediate pain. Tract cells located primarily in laminae I and V give rise to axons that transmit the sensation to higher brain centers. (Adapted from Barr, ML, and Kiernan, JA: The Human Nervous System: An Anatomical Viewpoint, ed 5. JB Lippincott, Philadelphia, 1988.)

Primary Afferent Neuron (C, Aδ)

Dorsolateral Fasiculus

Substantia Gelatinosa

Tract Cell

Ventral White Commissure to Spinothalamic Tract

conduction of pain impulses arising in the A-delta fibers, the fast component of pain. The second pathway is the spinoreticulothalamic tract, which is involved with the transmission of pain originating in the C-primary afferents, the slow component of pain.

The spinothalamic tract originates largely from neurons located in laminae I and V of the dorsal horn of spinal gray matter. These areas are a major point of termination for incoming A-delta nociceptive afferents. Axons arising from laminae I and V cross the midline in the ventral white commissure to ascend uninterrupted in the contralateral lateral funiculus as the lateral spinothalamic tract. This long ascending tract conducts pain information rostral through the spinal cord, medulla, pons, and midbrain with termination in the thalamus. Within the thalamus, the spinothalamic neurons terminate in the ventral posterolateral nucleus (VPL) as well as within the posterior complex and the intralaminar nuclei. It is these thalamic terminations that allow for the crude perception of painful stimuli. It is thought by some that the termination in the posterior nuclei is concerned with the immediate awareness of pain; those in the VPL allow for the ability to localize the origin of painful stimuli on the body surface and those to the intralaminar nuclei are concerned with the emotional and unpleasant aspects of pain. The pain impulses that terminate in VPL are projected to the somatosensory cortex of the precentral gyrus via the thalamocortical fibers. It is this projection that probably contributes to the ability to localize the original pain to the body surface. The spinothalamic tract is thought to represent a phylogenetically newer pathway and is called the *neospinothalamic tract*.

A second, and perhaps more important, ascending pathway for pain is the spinoreticulothalamic tract. The neurons that give rise to the spinoreticulothalamic pathways are located largely in laminae VII and VIII of the spinal cord dorsal horn of gray matter. Therefore, these neurons receive their nociceptive input via interneurons from the areas of gray matter where the A-delta and C fibers terminate. Unlike the spinothalamic tract, which consists of long ascending neurons, the spinoreticulothalamic tracts have short axons, thus requiring multiple neurons and synapses for the sensory information to be transmitted upward. The neurons of the spinoreticulothalamic tract are intermingled among the axons of the spinothalamic tract. Whereas the spinothalamic tract is a totally crossed pathway, the spinoreticulothalamic tract is bilateral. The fibers of the spinoreticulothalamic tract terminate predominantly in the intralaminar nuclei of the thalamus. This pathway is considered to be more concerned with the emotional and unpleasant aspects of pain perception. It is also believed that pain originating in diseased viscera is carried in the spinoreticulothalamic tracts, thereby providing explanation as to why visceral pain, though very compelling, is poorly localized (Fig. 2–2).

The spinothalamic tract cells (T cells) of the dorsal horn can be classified in their response properties into four basic categories: (1) low-threshold units, responding to light mechanical stimuli such as light touch; (2) wide-dynamic-range units reacting to high-intensity stimulation such as that which evokes pain as well as low-intensity stimulation; (3) high-threshold units responding to stimuli that are intense enough to inflict tissue damage and activate nociceptors; (4) thermosensitive units responding to warming or cooling of the skin. The wide-dynamic-range neurons and the high-threshold units are most important in the central conduction of pain.

The wide-dynamic-range neuron is considered to be the tract cell (T cell) described in the gate control theory. The cell body of this neuron is located in lamina V of the dorsal horn of the spinal gray matter. These neurons are termed *wide-dynamic range*

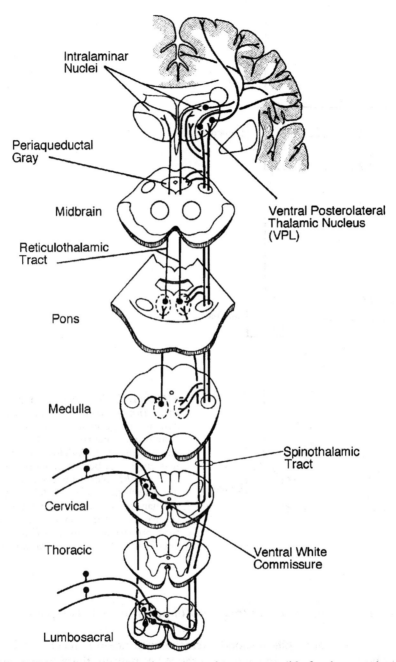

FIGURE 2–2. Diagram representing the major pathways responsible for the central projection of pain. The spinothalamic tract is a crossed, long ascending tract, whereas the reticulothalamic tract is a bilateral, multisynaptic pathway. (Adapted from Barr, ML, and Kiernan, JA: The Human Nervous System: An Anatomical Viewpoint, ed 5. JB Lippincott, Philadelphia, 1988, p 282.)

(WDR) because they receive input from multiple sources (Fig. 2–3A). A-beta mechanoreceptive, A-delta, and C nociceptive afferents impinge on the WDR neurons. Each neuron receives input from a large number of primary afferents. These second-order neurons code action potentials so that a low frequency of action potentials repre-

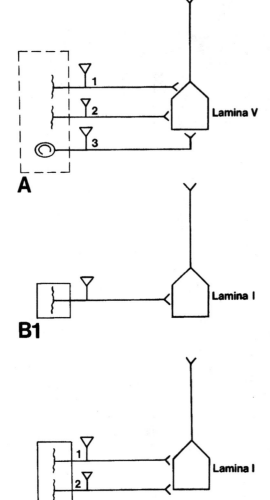

FIGURE 2–3. Schematic representation of categories of second-order neurons. (*A*) Wide-dynamic range neuron with convergent input from primary neurons: 1 = C polymodal afferent neuron; 2 = A-delta nociceptive afferent neuron; 3 = A-beta mechanoreceptive afferent neuron. (*B1*) Nociceptive-specific neuron with input exclusively from A-delta high threshold mechanoreceptive afferent neuron. (*B2*) Nociceptive-specific neuron with convergent input from primary neurons: 1 = C polymodal afferent; 2 = A-delta nociceptive afferent neuron.

sents a touch stimulus. A higher frequency of action potentials represents a noxious pinch.[16]

The high-threshold units respond exclusively to noxious mechanical or thermal stimuli, or both (Fig. 2–3*B*). In contrast to the WDR neuron, these neurons receive input from a small number of primary afferents. They are concentrated in lamina I, but some have been found in lamina V. As evidenced by their name, these neurons receive input from high-threshold A-delta mechanosensitive afferents and C polymodal nociceptive afferents. The nociceptive-specific neurons are further subdivided into a group that responds only to noxious mechanical stimulation carried exclusively by the A-delta high-threshold mechanosensitive afferents and a group that responds to intense, nonpainful pressure and to noxious stimuli.

The contributions of these second-order neurons to the perception of pain are well substantiated. The WDR neurons contribute to the localization aspect of pain, as well as modality discrimination (i.e., touch versus mechanical pinch). Furthermore, activation of these neurons in humans leads to reports of burning or needlelike sensations that are confined to a specific area of the body.[17] On the other hand, the nociceptive-specific neurons are more modality specific; that is, they provide information to the central nervous system about the specific type and location of the noxious stimuli.

Both the nociceptive-specific and the WDR neurons signal intensity of pain. Furthermore, a prolonged activation lasting several hundred milliseconds occurs in the cells.[7] The activation could be caused by the release of substance P from the endings of the WDR neurons.[18] This finding may provide one possible explanation for "slow" pain and one possible mechanism for continued pain perception following the removal of the primary stimulus.

ASCENDING PROJECTIONS AND HIGHER CENTERS SUBSERVING PAIN

In addition to the thalamic projections of the spinothalamic and spinoreticulothalamic tracts, each provides collateral branches to lower brainstem structures that modify the transmission of nociceptive stimuli.

Both laboratory and clinical evidence support the hypothesis that the WDR and the nociceptive-specific neurons are only two classes of neurons that compose the spinothalamic tract. Some second-order neurons activated by mechanical stimulation need to be considered in a modulatory role for pain control.[16] Thus, the spinothalamic tract participates in many of the components of pain, that is, affective, arousal, sensory-discriminative, as well as other functions. To classify this tract using the old terminology, that is, paleospinothalamic and neospinothalamic, is an oversimplification.[19] This classical pain pathway, located in the ventrolateral quadrant of the spinal cord, not only terminates in the ventroposterolateralis nucleus of the thalamus, but it also sends collaterals to the medial brainstem region.[20]

Many levels of the neuraxis have a role in the pain process. Data implicating higher-center processing of pain are derived from a variety of techniques performed on a variety of species, including humans.

MEDULLA AND PONS

Ascending fibers from the spinothalamic tracts send projections to (1) the medial portion of the reticular formation, particularly the nucleus gigantocellularis; (2) the lateral pons; and (3) the central gray area. These collaterals are termed the *spinoreticular projection*.

White and Sweet[21] noted that stimulation of structures in the medulla of conscious humans produces both the sensory-discriminative and the affective-motivational components of the pain response. The sensory component corresponds to observations of animals that show that many neurons in this area respond to noxious stimuli.[22] The affective-motivational component corresponds to the observation that electrical stimulation within the nucleus gigantocellularis (NGC) in animals produced escape behavior in cats,[23] whereas destruction of the NGC resulted in a deficit in escape behavior.[24]

The NGC is a relay in the spinoreticulothalamic system for pain transmission. Furthermore, the NGC connects with autonomic nuclei, which are also located in the reticular formation. These connections play a role in autonomic responses to intense and noxious stimuli.[25] Because reticular formation has connections with the autonomic centers, the limbic forebrain structures, and the hypothalamus, this area is more involved in the autonomic and affective components of pain than in subserving a discriminatory function.

MESENCEPHALON

Mesencephalic structures receive projections from a variety of areas, including the spinoreticular projection. Electrical stimulation of the medial periaqueductal gray region in humans elicits emotional responses such as an unpleasant sensation and fear. The pain tends to be deep and confined to midline structures.[26] Destruction of these mesencephalic structures does not alter localization of acute noxious stimuli.[27] The midline structures are more allied with the emotional aspects of the pain process, whereas the lateral structures are more closely associated with the sensory-discriminative aspect; however, this is not a mutually exclusive relationship.

THALAMUS

Considerable evidence demonstrates that WDR neurons and nociceptive-specific neurons of the spinal cord project to three main nuclei of the thalamus: the ventrobasal nuclei, the posterior nuclei, and the medial intralaminar nuclei. Few neurons of these groups respond exclusively to the nociceptive input.[28]   *VPL*

Noxious input to the ventrobasal complex (ventral posterolateral nucleus) arises from discrete areas of the contralateral side of the body. Approximately 6% to 10% of the cells in this region respond to noxious stimuli.[29] In humans, lesions in the ventrobasal complex produce deficits in somatosensory discrimination. Tingling in a specific location typically is described when these nuclei are stimulated.[26] This observation suggests a sensory-discriminative component of painful stimuli that is supported by studies in the cat. This observation is further supported by anatomic evidence that these neurons project to both the primary (SI) and secondary (SII) areas of the somatosensory cortex.[25]

Theories regarding the role of the posterior thalamic nuclei in pain are conflicting. This region lacks somatotopic organization and receives input from a wide sensory area.[28] The majority of somatosensory inputs arise from the contralateral side of the body. In humans, stimulation of this area elicits a pain sensation.

Cells of the medial and intralaminar thalamic nuclei have large receptive fields, lack somatotopic organization, and receive bilateral input. These nuclei respond to auditory, visual, and intense mechanical stimuli. They receive input from the ventrolateral quadrant of the spinal cord as well as indirect input from the NGC.

Electrical stimulation of part of the intralaminar complex in humans produces a burning or aching sensation referred primarily from contralateral regions of the body. Recordings from some neurons in these regions demonstrate that these cells respond to pinpricking.[30] Lesions in this area are marginally effective in relieving intractable pain. The nondiscriminative quality of pain is removed while preserving the sensory-discriminative aspect. This observation provides a clue that these diffuse thalamic nuclei are involved in the affective quality of pain. Further evidence is that these neurons project not only to the cerebral cortex but also to the limbic cortex and amygdala.

CORTEX

The role of the primary somatosensory (SI) area in pain perception is not clearly understood. Lesions in this area do not affect acute or chronic pain, and electrical stimulation does not produce pain.[21] Therefore, while serving an important function for spatiotemporal discrimination of sensation, the SI cortex is not an important region for perception of pain.

The secondary somatosensory (SII) area of the cerebral cortex has been more extensively studied. This area receives an extensive projection from the posterior thalamic nuclei. Furthermore, these neurons receive multisensory input. Although some researchers have reported no alteration in pain perception with lesions in this area,[21] others have reported hypalgesia.[17]

Researchers have recorded neuronal activity in this region following electrical stimulation of tooth-pulp afferents.[25,31] An increase in stimulus intensity produces an increase in activity recorded in the SII region.

The cortex, then, is involved with pain mechanisms at two levels. The first level is sensory discrimination, such as localization. The second level is a more complex system associated with complex behavioral responses that include affective and motivational responses and comparisons of pain sensation with past experiences.

In summary, the rostrad projections for pain involve many levels of the neuraxis. Table 2–2 summarizes components of the pain experience. The interconnections of these various systems are complex and not completely understood. The use of electrical stimulation or lesioning studies provides some information about the function of a particular system, but these studies may not be a true representation of what actually occurs in the intact, awake human.

Centrifugal Control of Pain

Several pathways have been identified within the nervous system that are able to regulate and inhibit the transmission of nociceptive stimuli. These systems primarily affect the activity of neurons in the spinal cord gray matter as well as higher brain centers concerned with pain transmission. The major interest in the existence of intrinsic brain centers for the regulation of pain began in 1969 when Reynolds[32] demonstrated that stimulation of the periaqueductal gray (PAG), an area of gray matter surrounding the cerebral aqueduct of the midbrain, produces analgesia in unanesthetized rats.

It has subsequently been found that the PAG works on the spinal cord indirectly through its connections to a nucleus in the center of the medulla, the nucleus raphe magnus (NRM). Stimulation of PAG activates NRM, which in turn projects to the dorsal horn of gray matter of the spinal cord.[33] The serotonergic neurons of the NRM ter-

TABLE 2–2 Components of
the Pain Experience

Aspect	Location
Discrimination	Cortex, thalamus
Affective	Limbic structures, thalamus
Autonomic responses	Reticular formation

minate largely in laminae I and II of the dorsal horn, the same areas in which large numbers of nociceptive afferents terminate. It is thought that serotonin is able to inhibit excitation of the spinothalamic neurons located in these laminae (Fig. 2–4).

A second major impetus was the isolation by Hughes[34] of an endogenous substance in neural tissues in 1974. This substance, enkephalin, fits the criteria for an endogenous substance that, when released, inhibits pain.

Correlative evidence for centrifugal control of pain is based on studies using stimulation-produced analgesia (SPA) and microinjections of exogenous opiates. Naloxone is used extensively in these studies. Naloxone is a morphine antagonist that competes for the same receptor site as the opiates (such as morphine), the enkephalins, and beta-endorphin (β-endorphin).

Location and density of the opiate receptors vary among species. The highest concentrations occur in the limbic cortex (most specifically, the anterior amygdala), the PAG, the hypothalamus, the thalamus, and, to a lesser degree, the cortex, the caudate nucleus, certain midbrain structures, and the gray matter of the spinal cord.[35] Although many brain structures have opiate receptor areas, the question arises as to the importance of the opiate receptor in a particular region subserving pain inhibition.

The two most-studied endogenous opiates are β-endorphin and methionine enkephalin (met-enkephalin). β-Endorphin is a 31-amino-acid chain with a half-life of approximately 4 hours. Half-life refers to the time needed for inactivation of one half of the amount of the substance by enzymes located in the tissue. β-Endorphin has potent effects, including catatonia with corresponding inhibition of neuronal cell activity in the caudate nucleus, cortex, brainstem, and thalamus; analgesia; and behavior disturbances. Since β-endorphin is found in the pituitary and is long lasting, it is involved with whole-animal responses associated with severe stress.[36]

The enkephalins—met-enkephalin and leucine enkephalin—are 5-amino-acid molecules with a half-life of 2 minutes. These peptides have been identified in many regions of the brain and in different concentrations. Areas that have a high concentration of enkephalin also have an increased density of neurons containing substance P or serotonin [5-hydroxylryptamine (5-HT)]. The postulated role of these neuropeptides in pain regulation is discussed subsequently.

SPINAL LEVEL

The neuronal activity for pain regulation at the spinal level is not completely understood. Wall[7] noted that electrical stimulation of cells in the substantia gelatinosa decreases primary afferent activity and inhibits neurons in lamina V that were activated by noxious stimuli. The neurochemical transmitter that mediates inhibition is gamma-aminobutyric acid (GABA). Microinjection of opiates into the spinal cord also inhibits the activity of dorsal-horn neurons elicited by noxious stimuli.[37] This observation is supported by the finding that neurons containing enkephalin exist in the substantia gelatinosa (Fig. 2–5).[38] These neurons are prominent in laminae I and II, but they are also found in laminae III and V. These neurons serve functions other than inhibitory ones and are activated independently of descending pain modulatory systems.

PAIN INHIBITION FROM SUPRASPINAL LEVELS

Control of pain transmission not only occurs at the spinal level, but also from supraspinal sites. These systems include both neural opiate and nonopiate projections.

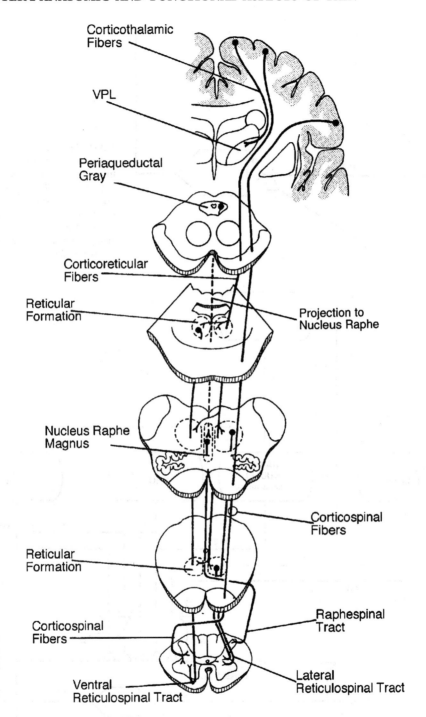

FIGURE 2-4. Diagram demonstrating the components of a pathway involved in the centrifugal control of pain. (Adapted from Barr, ML, and Kiernan, JA: The Human Nervous System: An Anatomical Viewpoint, ed 5. JB Lippincott, Philadelphia, 1988, p 290.)

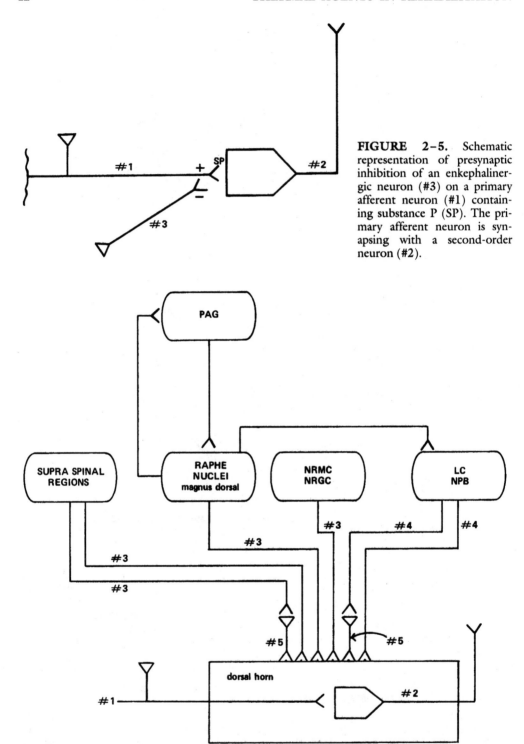

FIGURE 2-5. Schematic representation of presynaptic inhibition of an enkephalinergic neuron (#3) on a primary afferent neuron (#1) containing substance P (SP). The primary afferent neuron is synapsing with a second-order neuron (#2).

FIGURE 2-6. Schematic representation of centrifugal control of pain. Known and postulated pathways are drawn. PAG = periaqueductal gray; NRMA = nucleus reticularis magnocellularis; NRGC = nucleus reticularis gigantocellularis; LC = locus ceruleus; NPB = medial and lateral parabrachial nuclei; #1 = primary afferent neuron; #2 = second-order neuron; #3 = serotonin neuron; #4 = norepinephrine neuron; #5 = enkephalin neuron.

Furthermore, humoral opiate and nonopiate pain modulatory systems exist.[33] These latter systems are activated in response to very stressful situations and are involved in systemic responses.

Pain regulation by the PAG is mediated via indirect pathways. The PAG projects to the nucleus raphe magnus (Fig. 2–6), which in turn projects to the dorsal horn of the spinal cord.[39] When stimulated, the nucleus raphe magnus inhibits the A-delta afferent input more than the A-beta input. This nucleus also contains serotonin-carrying neurons.

Studies indicate that descending serotonergic neurons from the nucleus raphe magnus are heavily concentrated in lamina I and have a direct monosynaptic inhibitory effect on the second-order neuron (ascending tract neuron).[40]

A second system, originating in the pons, produces dorsal-horn inhibition and analgesia. This system is a norepinephrine-mediated system that originates in the region of the ventral locus ceruleus, nucleus subceruleus, and medial and lateral parabrachial nuclei. The descending inhibitory system terminates directly by second-order neurons, or indirectly by an enkephalinergic interneuron.

PAIN THEORIES: SPECIFICITY, PATTERN, AND GATE CONTROL

The phenomenon of pain can be divided into three major components. The sensory-discriminative component serves to analyze the noxious stimulus in terms of its location and intensity. The cognitive-evaluative component refers to the process by which the noxious sensation is examined, is compared with past experiences, and is given meaning in relation to the present and future implications of the pain experience. An individual's reaction to the noxious stimulus also is influenced by cultural connotations. Thus, the response to a noxious stimulus may range from a simple flexion response to more complex escape plans to a very complex psychophysiologic behavior pattern seen in the chronic pain patient.[41] The affective-motivational component includes the emotional responses, goals, desires, and expectations of the individual.

Early pain theories were based on simple neuroanatomic circuitry or a single neurophysiologic concept. As technology advanced and the complexity of the pain pathways became better understood, pain theory became more sophisticated. Since the articulation of the gate theory of pain put forth by Melzack and Wall[42] in 1965, neurophysiologic, neuroanatomic, and neurochemical approaches have begun to delineate the peripheral and central mechanisms of pain. Furthermore, several mechanisms involved in the centrifugal (descending) control of pain have also been identified.

Specificity and Pattern Theories

Two traditional and opposing theories for pain evolved during the late 1800s.[43,44] These theories are the specificity theory and the pattern theory, respectively. The specificity theory proposed that a specific pain system existed. When pain receptors located in the skin are stimulated, the impulses are transmitted via a direct pathway to the pain center located in the brain. Von Frey[43] used the Muller doctrine of specific nerve energies, anatomic evidence, and scientific deductive reasoning to develop his theory. The Muller principle states that a stimulus applied to a receptor produces the same sensation in the brain center regardless of the type of stimulus. Free nerve endings are located in skin throughout the entire body, and an intense stimulus applied anywhere on the skin results in a pain sensation; therefore, Muller logically reasoned that free nerve endings are pain receptors. Thus, the specificity theory states that any noxious or potentially tissue damaging stimulus applied to the surface of the skin results in a pain sensation.

The pattern theory denotes that the pattern or coding of sensory information is the key element. The coding is temporal, and spatial sequencing of action potentials are generated in the periphery. This theory negates the idea of a specific pain receptor, but rather considers the intense stimulation of nonspecific receptors as the adequate stimulus for eliciting the pain sensation. Figure 2–7 demonstrates this principle. A touch stimulus applied to a receptor produces a particular pattern of action potentials. The resultant sensation is touch. A potentially damaging touch stimulus applied to the receptor produces a different pattern of action potentials, and the resultant sensation is pain. One fallacy of this principle is that specific specialized receptors have been documented histologically.

Gate Control Theory

In 1965, Melzack and Wall[42] proposed a new theory relating to the pain experience. This theory represents a cornerstone in the development of neurophysiologic mechanisms that address the concept of peripheral and central gating. The gate theory incorporates the feature of receptor specialization from the specificity theory with spatiotemporal coding of action potentials from the pattern theory. To these two concepts, Wall[45] added the interaction of peripheral afferents with a modulation system proposed to be located in the substantia gelatinosa of the dorsal horn. Furthermore, they proposed a descending modulatory system. Figure 2–8 is a schematic representation of the gate control theory.

The neuroanatomic features of this circuit include large-diameter sensory neurons (A-beta); small-diameter sensory neurons (A-delta, C); the substantia gelatinosa that corresponds to Rexed's laminae II and III of the dorsal horn of the spinal gray matter; and a transmission cell (T cell), also known as a tract cell or second-order neuron. Both the large- (A-beta) and the small- (A-delta, C) diameter primary afferents impinge on

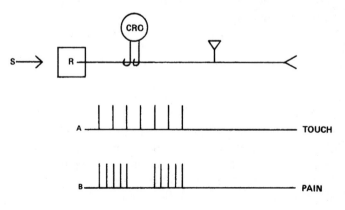

FIGURE 2–7. Schematic representation of pattern theory. (*A*) Action potentials resulting from a touch stimulus (stimuli) and recorded on a cathode ray oscilloscope (CRO). The resultant sensation is touch. (*B*) Action potentials resulting from a noxious stimulus and recorded on a cathode ray oscilloscope. The resultant sensation is pain. S = stimulus; R = receptor.

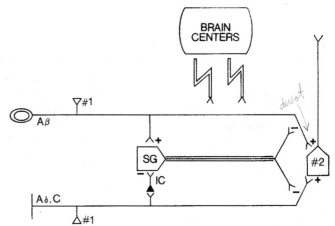

FIGURE 2-8. Schematic representations of the revised Melzack and Wall gate control theory. #1 = first-order neuron, either A-beta, A-delta, or C primary afferent neuron; #2 = second-order neuron (T cell); SG = substantia gelatinosa; IC = inhibitory interneuron.

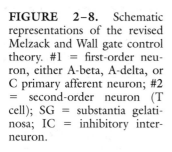

the substantia gelatinosa cells and on the second-order neuron. The substantia gelatinosa acts as a modulator (gate control) by terminating presynaptically on the large- and small-diameter afferent neurons just before their termination upon the second-order neuron. The control is postulated to occur by the neurophysiologic mechanism termed *presynaptic inhibition.*

When the substantia gelatinosa is active, an increase in presynaptic control on the first-order axons occurs and the "gate" is in the relatively closed position; that is, a decrease in the amount of sensory input to the second-order neuron cell occurs. On the other hand, a reduction in substantia gelatinosa activity results in a decrease in the amount of presynaptic control on the first-order neuron, and the "gate" is considered to be in a relatively open position; that is, the amount of sensory information reaching the second-order neuron is relatively unaltered. The balance of activity in the large- and small-diameter sensory neurons determines the relative position of the gate.

If large-diameter afferents are activated, an initial increase in the second-order neuron activity occurs and is followed by a reduction of activity. The initial increase is because of a direct activation of the second-order neuron by primary afferents. The reduction is an indirect result brought about by large-diameter afferents also activating substantia gelatinosa cells, which in turn leads to presynaptic inhibition of the primary afferents. This causes the gate to close.

If, however, the small-diameter afferents are activated, the initial increase in T-cell activity is caused by the primary afferents. The small-diameter primary afferents also activate inhibitory interneurons that inhibit activity of the substantia gelatinosa cells. This results in a decrease in the amount of presynaptic control on the large- and small-diameter sensory neurons and opens the gate.

Melzack and Wall[42] proposed that when the balance of small- to large-diameter neuronal input is no longer maintained and reaches a critical value, the second-order neurons are activated. The activation of this ascending system leads to the perception of pain and behavioral responses.

One component of the system that was briefly, but not fully, described was the descending control system. Wall[45] proposed that central events such as emotion and past experience evoke descending input, which impinges on the gating mechanism to block pain sensation at the spinal level.

As various hypotheses were tested, the theory was revised.[46,47] Revisions of the gate control theory led to the realization that a more complex neural circuitry exists in the dorsal horn. For example, postsynaptic connections play a modulatory role in the gating mechanism, and nonnociceptive (A-beta) and nociceptive (A-delta, C) neurons are the large- and small-diameter afferents, respectively. Furthermore, the hypothesis that A-beta afferents "close the gate" led to the use of transcutaneous electrical nerve stimulation (TENS) for pain modulation in humans.[48]

Extensive clinical testing of externally applied electrical stimulators for pain relief in the chronic-pain patient began in the early 1970s.[49] The Melzack and Wall gate control theory of pain provides a partial neurophysiologic explanation for the use of TENS to relieve acute and chronic pain.

PAIN CONDITIONS: ACUTE, CHRONIC, AND REFERRED

The neurophysiologic mechanisms underlying acute, chronic, and referred pain are not completely understood. Complexity arises in the chronic pain condition, because the pain state outlasts the initial trauma and involves complex psychologic and physiologic responses. Each pain state and proposed mechanisms associated with each will be explained. These are summarized in Table 2–3.

Acute Pain

The acute pain experience may last a few minutes or several days. It is defined as "pain of recent and sudden onset, usually, but not always, with demonstrable etiology and limited course."[50] Usually, the unpleasant experience is associated with autonomic and emotional responses. The primary function of acute pain is to alert the individual to actual or potential tissue damage so that appropriate measures may be taken—that is, withdrawal from the stimulus to prevent further injury. Pain is usually the reason most people seek medical assistance.

Generally, a noxious or potentially tissue damaging stimulus activates nociceptors, and the information is carried via A-delta or C afferents to the spinal cord. Upon reaching the spinal cord, several routes are available. The information is transmitted to the sympathetic preganglionic neuronal pool, whereby reflex responses in the periph-

**TABLE 2–3 Characteristics of
Pain Types**

Pain Experience	Characteristics
Acute	Short duration
	Usually demonstrable etiology
	May be localized
Chronic	Long duration
	Associated with negative affective qualities
	Often of vague etiology
Referred	May be acute or chronic
	Felt at site other than region of origin

eral vascular system and other visceral organs are elicited. Connections to the ventral horn, synapsing on the alpha and gamma motor neurons evoke reflex responses, including skeletal-muscle contraction to escape the stimulus or muscle spasm. Nociceptive information transmitted to higher centers results in autonomic and emotional responses, as well as pain perception.

Several mechanisms are proposed to explain the prolonged afterdischarge noted with acute pain. Sensitization of nociceptors causes a decrease in the threshold value of the receptor to additional stimuli or enhancement of the response. The increased insensitivity at the site of injury is termed *primary hyperalgesia*. The area surrounding the injury may also be sensitized, in which case the individual experiences secondary hyperalgesia. Secondary hyperalgesia is believed to be caused by antidromic activation of C primary afferents and release of substance P in the region.[12] A second postulate for afterdischarge is the release of substance P from small primary afferents upon the second-order neuron.

Similar mechanisms can explain the pain-spasm-pain cycle in skeletal muscle. Injury produces an initial contraction for splinting or immobilization of the injured part. Continued muscle contraction leads to muscle ischemia and release of chemical substances that sensitize A-delta and C pain afferents in the muscle. By-products of metabolism alone do not produce nociceptive activation,[51] but factors such as bradykinin, serotonin, and histamine are implicated.[52] The heightened sensitivity of the nociceptor leads to additional reflexive contraction in the muscle; the result is a positive feedback loop. A similar loop can be established in the sympathetic reflex arc. Re-establishment of inhibitory mechanisms stops the pain-spasm-pain cycle.

Chronic Pain

Chronic pain is defined as "pain of long duration, often associated with anguish, apprehension, depression, or hopelessness,"[50] and extends months to years beyond the recovery period or recurs intermittently for years. Some clinicians use 6 months posttrauma to postdisease onset as a basis to consider pain as chronic; others designate the length of time in accordance with a particular condition. Both environmental and psychologic factors are important considerations in the evolution of this type of pain.[53] Emotional, physiologic, and behavioral responses differ from acute pain.

Underlying neurophysiologic mechanisms include positive-feedback loops, as described previously; that is, an increase in the sensitivity of the nociceptor leads to a maintained pain-spasm-pain cycle. This results in semipermanent, or permanent, changes at the spinal level to maintain these loops. A second mechanism involves long-lasting peripheral nerve compression.[25] Compression results in the destruction of large primary afferent neurons. As a result, an imbalance of large (tactile) and small (pain) fiber input occurs, thereby keeping the gate open.

Chronic pain, however, extends beyond the neurophysiologic model, as is evidenced by Loser's schema.[54] The first level, nociception, is the application of a stimulus that activates A-delta and C primary afferents. The second level, pain, is the perception of the noxious stimulus. Suffering, the third level, is described as negative affective responses. This last level is activated by pain perception, stress, or anxiety. Suffering leads to the fourth level, pain behavior. The responses elicited by this level are evident in both verbal and nonverbal communication (i.e., posture, facial expressions, drug intake, continued seeking of medical attention, and becoming a nonfunctioning member of society). When treating these patients, observational analysis should be used to measure pain relief rather than relying exclusively on verbal reports. Although chronic pain has a physiologic component, a multidimensional view is needed to elucidate all components of this condition.

Referred Pain and Trigger Points

Referred pain is "pain felt at a site in the body elsewhere from the source of disease or injury."[50] It is considered an error in localization. Referred pain from the viscera to the body surface is projected on the same dermatome. For example, myocardial pain afferents arise from T-1 to T-5, and pain associated with a myocardial infarction is felt at the T-1 to T-5 dermatomes, radiating down the arm. Furthermore, referred pain is not exclusively unique to visceral afferents.[55]

Two theories explain the concept of referred pain. Both are based on the convergence of visceral and somatic terminations on higher-order neurons. Evidence is available for convergence on the same neuron in the deep layers of the dorsal horn.[56] The convergence-facilitation theory states that visceral afferents lower the threshold of the second-order neuron to incoming cutaneous input. Thus, only the cutaneous information reaches the higher centers of the nervous system.

The second theory, the convergence-projection theory, considers that the pain experienced at a particular site is learned by the association of multiple cues. This site, then, does not necessarily correspond to the site of injury.

Travell[57] identified irritable points in the muscle (trigger points) that referred pain. The term *trigger point* refers to a small, hypersensitive area in muscle or fascia. When a trigger point is stimulated by intense heat, cold, or pressure, pain is referred to a remote site. Other terms used to describe this hypersensitive area are fibrositis, myositis, myalgia, or myofascial pain. The cause of trigger points is unknown. Some researchers believe inflammation is a factor.[58] Others have examined fibrositic nodules taken from muscles and noted an increase in acid mucopolysaccharide in connective tissue.[59] It has been shown that prolonged muscle contraction results in local ischemia, causing chemical and morphologic changes in the muscle.[60,61] Morphologic changes include swelling of mitochondria and destruction of myofilament in the I-bands. In severe cases, contractile elements are destroyed. Further research is needed to determine the morphologic and neurophysiologic changes of trigger points.

Clinically, trigger points are identified primarily by palpation. Specific referred patterns elicited from trigger points are evidenced for each muscle. References are available that diagram muscles of the trunk and extremities with their referred pain profile.[62,63] In order to evaluate and select appropriate treatment for the pain patient, an understanding of the known and theorized mechanisms underlying various painful states is needed.

ASSESSMENT OF PAIN

A comprehensive assessment of the pain experience provides the clinician with an indication of the source(s) of pain, so that the cause of pain is treated rather than just the symptoms. Furthermore, the assessment helps in the selection of the appropriate thermal agent(s) and provides a baseline to document improvement. Not only verbal descriptions of pain, but nonverbal clues (including facial expressions and posture) also should be recorded. Components of pain assessment also should include the use of pain scales (to determine quantity), body diagrams (to delineate location), and word descriptors (to describe quality).

Pain Scales

The most commonly used pain assessment is a rating scale. A 10-cm scale is marked in several ways: (1) a series of numbers from 0 to 10 marked on the scale; (2) a verbal rating scale (VRS), with a series of descriptors; or (3) a visual analogue scale (VAS), with only the ends of the scale marked.[64] Depending on the word choice of the latter two scales, the intensity or the affective quality of pain is assessed. For example, the word choice of "strong" or "intense" is used to evaluate the intensity of pain, whereas phrases such as "bad as it can be" or "as unpleasant as it can be" are used to assess the affective quality.

When designing such a test, the following points should be considered. The scale should be drawn accurately. For example, if the horizontal line becomes thicker, then a cue concerning the intensity of pain is given to the patient. Only one pain scale is drawn on the page, so that an as-accurate-as-possible measure is obtained, not biased by previously marked pain scales. Another manipulation of the pain scale is the reversal of the scale so that the most intense measure is on the left, or so that the scale is presented vertically. Whether these reversals of scale provide a better documentation of pain has not been studied. Scott and Huskisson[65] examined a vertical versus horizontal VAS and noted that, although patients scored slightly lower using the horizontal scale, a significant difference was not noted between the two.

Both the VRS and VAS can be converted to a numeric format so that arithmetic manipulations can be performed. The scales correlate for pain measurement ($r = 0.84, P < .01$) and pain relief ($r = 0.81, P < .001$).[66] Many researchers believe the VAS is a more sensitive indicator.[67]

These scales are simple and quick to use, but they have limitations. First is the assumption that the categories of descriptors on the VRS or the numerical scale can be partitioned into equal psychologic units. Second is the assumption that a simple linear scale can assess one component in a very complex pain experience and that the patient can accurately remember pain intensity. These scales are also influenced by personal experience, culture, and expectations, including what the patient considers is expected of him or her by the therapist.

McGill Pain Questionnaire

In an attempt to assess the multidimensional aspects of pain, the McGill Pain Questionnaire (MPQ) was developed.[68,69] The researchers developed a pain assessment that included three classes of word choices to evaluate the sensory, evaluative, and affective components of pain. These descriptors were obtained with a high degree of agreement from subjects with different educational, socioeconomic, and cultural backgrounds. The questionnaire is also designed to quantify pain. The measures are the total number of words chosen (NWC), the pain-rating index (PRI), and the present-pain intensity (PPI).

The word descriptors are divided into 3 categories and 20 subcategories. Each subcategory contains up to six words that are qualitatively similar and are ranked in descending order according to intensity. Each word is assigned a numerical value. The sensory category contains 13 subcategories to describe the pain in terms of the spatiotemporal, pressure, thermal, and sharp-dull aspects of pain. Words such as "flickering" and "beating" describe the temporal aspect; "jumping" and "shooting" describe the spatial aspect; "stabbing," "cramping," and "tugging" describe the pressure aspect; and "burning" and "scalding" describe the thermal aspect of the pain experience. The affective category, divided into six subcategories, describes pain in terms of autonomic responses, fear, and tension. Pain descriptors such as "terrifying," "sickening," and "vicious" are included. The third category, evaluative, is a single category used to describe the intensity of the total pain experience. Words such as "annoying," "unbearable," and "troublesome" are used.

The patient is instructed to circle one word from each category that best describes his or her pain. If a category does not apply, it is left unmarked. Values for NWC and PRI are obtained from this list. NWC is the number of words (or categories) chosen. The PRI is obtained by assigning a numerical value to each word choice, then determining the mean. This value is an average measure of the pain experience and is a sensitive indicator in pain assessment.

Melzack[68,69] determined that the PRI correlated significantly with NWC ($P < .01$). Both the reliability and validity of the PRI scale have been tested on patients with a variety of painful conditions.[70-72] Unique profiles have been identified for chronic pain conditions, including, for instance, low back pain and arthritis.[73]

Another part of the pain questionnaire is the body diagram. Front and back views of a human are presented, and the patient marks the location of the pain on the diagram. The patient also marks "E" or "I" by the area where the pain is—"E" for external pain and "I" for internal pain.

Part three addresses pain in relation to duration and activities that influence the intensity. The patient describes the pain as being continuous, intermittent, or momentary, and then lists those activities that increase or decrease pain. The patient notes the time of day when the pain is better or worse, which can be correlated with the type of activities that cause or reduce pain.

The fourth part of the evaluation relates to pain intensity. A five-point scale is marked with the terms mild, discomforting, distressing, horrible, and excruciating. The patient is asked to describe pain intensity at that moment—at the time when the pain is at its worst, and at the time when the pain is at its least. This test is the present-pain index (PPI), which gives an indication of pain during the administration of the questionnaire.

Additional information gathered on the MPQ includes a medical history, drug intake, and present treatment (if further information is needed, the patient is given a standardized home recording card). The original questionnaire has been adapted to a shorter version (Fig. 2–9). The advantage of the MPQ is that it provides a greater sensitivity in assessing pain than the analogue scale does.

Other Assessments

Other testing methods have been used in the acute[74] and, most particularly, in the chronic-pain patient population. Two assessments deserve brief mention, but to provide details is beyond the scope of this text. The sensory decision, or signal detection theory (SDT), is designed to discriminate among sensory stimuli (pain sensations) and is not a measure of the intensity of pain experienced. Controversy exists as to the use of this test in pain measure. Another commonly used test to assess the chronic pain patient is the Minnesota Multiphasic Personality Inventory (MMPI). Specific chronic-pain-personality profiles have been determined from the MMPI. Additional information on assessment of pain is presented in Chapter 10.

APPLICATION OF THERMAL AGENTS FOR PAIN RELIEF

Clinical rationale for pain relief is based primarily on empiric observation and integration of information from basic and applied sciences. Although heat and cold are known to relieve pain in a variety of conditions, including tissue injuries and arthritis, the underlying mechanisms are unknown. Local neurologic and vascular changes in response to the thermal agent and the mechanism accounting for such changes await systematic testing and evaluation.

Heat

Muscle spasm secondary to some type of muscle, joint, or neurologic trauma is relieved by heat. To review, a pain-spasm-pain cycle arising from trauma excites nociceptors located in the skin or muscle. An increase in their activity causes pain perception and reflex muscle activation. With prolonged muscle activity, ischemia results, which activates muscle nociceptors and causes self-sustained muscle spasm. Trauma to the area releases algesic chemicals, such as substance P or bradykinin, in the area of the nociceptor. These chemicals sensitize the nociceptor. The sympathetic reflex arc also contributes to the pain-spasm cycle. For example, if vasoconstriction occurs, contraction of smooth muscle activates surrounding nociceptors. Inhibition of pain may result from nervous system changes or vascular changes (Fig. 2–10).

Cosentino and colleagues[75] reported a decrease in sensory nerve conduction velocity following the application of ultrasound. The decrease is similar to that reported for motor nerve conduction velocity. This observed phenomenon may be related to the frequency component of ultrasound and not the thermal effects. This mechanism, however, has yet to be elucidated.

Mense[76] noted that direct warming of the cat muscle spindle decreases neuronal activity of the secondary endings and increases the neuronal activity of the primary endings. Increases in primary afferent activity of the spindle closes the spinal gate. Mense also observed increased Golgi tendon organ (GTO) activity upon warming. GTOs inhibit the homonymous motor neuronal pool, which provides an inhibitory input to break up the pain-spasm-pain cycle. Caution should be used when extrapolating the data to clinical procedures, because the thermal agent in Mense's study was applied directly to exposed nerves of the cat.

The counterirritation theory is based on a gating mechanism[77] and can be used to explain thermal effects on the pain-spasm-pain cycle. Application of an external heat source produces a bombardment of activity from thermoreceptors. This increase in action potentials blocks pain input. Melzack and Wall's[78] gate theory provides the necessary circuitry for such blockage. Another central nervous system phenomenon is gen-

1. Where is your Pain?

Please mark, on the drawings below, the areas where you feel pain.
Put E if external, or I if internal, near the areas which you mark.
Put EI if both external and internal.

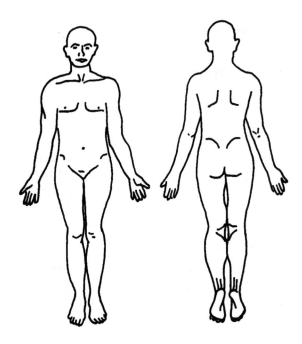

2. Please mark on the scale how much pain you have.

VISUAL ANALOGUE SCALE

PAIN AS
BAD AS IT _____ NO PAIN
COULD BE

FIGURE 2–9. Adapted from parts 1, 2, and 3 of the McGill Pain Questionnaire. Included are a body diagram to be marked by the patient (1) and a visual analogue scale (2) to quantify pain. Word descriptor to provide a quantitative description of pain are included in the Pain Rating Index (3).

eralized, or whole-body, relaxation. Relaxation produces pain relief, particularly if pain results from tension or skeletal muscle spasm. Activation of the descending pain inhibitory systems during thermal heating awaits justification.

Vascular changes in response to application of heat also can reduce pain. Vasodilatation and increase in blood flow up to 30 mL/100 g of tissue have been observed.[79] A greater blood flow increases the supply of nutrients to the area for the repair process

3. Pain Rating Index

There are many words that describe pain. From the list below, select only those words that describe your pain as it feels right now. Only select one word in each column, and only if it applies to your pain. YOU DO NOT NEED TO MARK A WORD IN EVERY COLUMN—ONLY MARK THOSE WORDS THAT DESCRIBE YOUR PAIN!

1.	2.	3.	4.
Flickering	Jumping	Pricking	Sharp
Quivering	Flashing	Boring	Cutting
Pulsing	Shooting	Drilling	Lacerating
Throbbing		Stabbing	
Beating			
Pounding			

5.	6.	7.	8.
Pinching	Tugging	Hot	Tingling
Pressing	Pulling	Burning	Itchy
Gnawing	Wrenching	Scalding	Smarting
Cramping		Searing	Stinging
Crushing			

9.	10.	11.	12.
Dull	Tender	Tiring	Sickening
Sore	Taut	Exhausting	Suffocating
Hurting	Rasping		
Aching			
Heavy			

13.	14.	15.	16.
Fearful	Punishing	Wretched	Annoying
Frightful	Grueling	Blinding	Troublesome
Terrifying	Cruel		Miserable
	Vicious		Intense
	Killing		Unbearable

17.	18.	19.	20.
Spreading	Tight	Cool	Nagging
Radiating	Numb	Cold	Nauseating
Penetrating	Drawing	Freezing	Agonizing
Piercing	Squeezing		Dreadful
	Tearing		Torturing

FIGURE 2–9 *Continued.*

and removes by-products from the injured tissue. By-products include prostaglandins, bradykinin, and histamine, all implicated in receptor and afferent fiber sensitization, which can cause a pain-spasm-pain cycle. Local heating also activates somatovisceral reflex arcs. Stimulation of cutaneous thermoreceptors decreases activity of the sympathetic nervous system and produces a vasodilatation in deeper blood vessels.

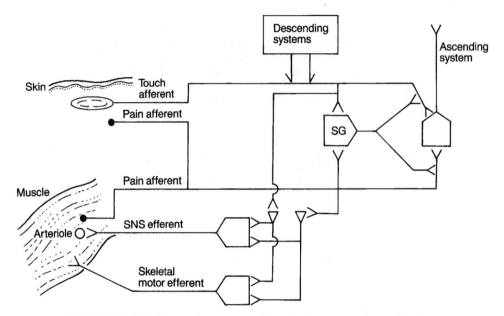

FIGURE 2–10. Schematic representation of pain-spasm-pain mechanism.

Cold

The use of cold to decrease pain is through brief intense or prolonged cold. Both local and central nervous system mechanisms are used to explain pain reduction.

Travell[80] identified three possible mechanisms underlying the effects of brief intense cold: receptor adaptation, a counterirritant effect, and a neurogenic effect. A decrease in skin temperature following the application of a vapocoolant spray produces cooling sufficient to cause receptor adaptation.[44] This idea was referenced to the findings of Cattell and Hoagland[81] whereby tactile receptors adapt to an intermittent stream of air. Whether or not the effects produced by these two dissimilar types of stimuli are equivalent is unknown at this time.

The counterirritant effect is based on the research by Gammon and Starr.[82] They observed that a 4°C to 10°C cold application to the skin relieves the pain induced by a topical application of capsaicin. This observation and the neurogenic effect can be based on the gate theory; that is, an irritant can block pain fibers by activation of receptors to close the gate. Furthermore, Yaksh and Hammond[25] noted that any intense stimuli that are noxious to the individual activate inhibitory processes, by a yet undefined mechanism. He does not advocate the use of noxious stimuli as a therapeutic means for pain reduction.

When cold is applied for a longer period of time, both local and central changes occur. One central nervous system model, the gate mechanism, has been described. Cooling the skin (35°C to 24°C during a 7- to 10-second period) results in a rapid increase in the frequency of the action potentials recorded on the afferent fiber.[83] This activity blocks pain input. To date, no evidence supports activation of the endorphin system by cold thermal agents.

Metabolic changes occur in both the receptor and afferent axons. Nerve conduction velocities have been examined in response to cooling longer than 5 minutes. For every 1°C decrease in intramuscular temperature, a decrease of 1.2 m/s in motor conduction occurs,[79] and a corresponding 2-m/s decrease is noted for sensory nerve conduction in velocities.[84] Smaller-diameter afferents are more sensitive to cold than larger-diameter afferents. These observations, then, would decrease the probability of pain input to continue.

The local vasomotor response to cold is immediate vasoconstriction. This would result in an initial decrease in the amount of vasodilator substances released into the surrounding tissue, which would decrease the degree of sensitization of nociceptor.

SUMMARY

As is shown in this chapter, pain theories are dynamic and changing. What is postulated to date will be successfully defended or refuted. Current review articles are available to keep the clinician abreast of these changes. As the theories advance, so must the rationale for clinical treatment using thermal modalities.

Study Objectives

Having completed this chapter, the reader should now be able to:

1. Describe the various neurons that are responsible for transmitting pain impulses from the periphery.
2. Discuss the processing of pain information in the spinal cord.
3. Describe the major pathways for the central transmission of pain stimuli.
4. Differentiate between the fast and slow components of the pain experience.
5. Discuss how the perception of pain is modified by various parts of the central nervous system.
6. Describe the anatomic pathways involved in the mitigation of pain by higher brain centers.
7. Discuss the specificity, pattern, and gate control theories of pain.
8. Differentiate among acute, chronic, and referred pain.
9. Discuss the concept of "trigger points."
10. Describe methods that are used to make clinical assessments of pain.
11. Describe the usefulness of thermal agents in the relief of pain.

REFERENCES

1. Merskey, H and Able-Fessard, DG: Pain terms: A list with definitions and notes on usage. Pain 6:249, 1979.
2. Bonica, JJ: Pain research and therapy: Past and current status and future needs. In Ng, KY and Bonica, JJ (eds): Pain, Discomfort and Humanitarian Care. Elsevier, New York, 1979, p 1.
3. Georgopopulos, AP: Functional properties of primary afferent units probably related to pain mechanisms in primate glabrous skin. J Neurophysiol 39:79, 1976.
4. Burgess, PR and Perl, ER: Myelinated afferent fibers responding specifically to noxious stimulation of the skin. J Physiol (Lond) 190:541, 1967.
5. LaMotte, RH and Campbell, NJ: Comparison of responses of warm and nociceptive C-fiber afferents in monkey with human judgments of thermal pain. J Neurophysiol 41:509, 1978.

6. Bonica, JJ: The Management of Pain. Lea & Febiger, Philadelphia, 1990.
7. Wall, PD: Textbook of Pain. Churchill Livingstone, New York, 1994.
8. Kerr, FWC: Neuroanatomical substrates of nociception in the spinal cord (review). Pain 1:325, 1975.
9. Sladek, JR and Walker, P: Serotonin-containing neuronal parikarya in the primate locus coeruleus and subcoeruleus. Brain Res 134:359, 1977.
10. Torebjork, HE and Hallin, RG: Perceptual changes accompanying controlled preferential blocking of A and C fibre responses in intact human skin nerves. Exp Brain Res 16:321, 1973.
11. Kerr, FWL: An overview of neural mechanisms of pain. Neurosci Res Program Bull 16:30, 1978.
12. Dubner, R and Bennett, GJ: Spinal and trigeminal mechanisms of nociception. Annu Rev Neurosci 6:381, 1983.
13. LaMotte, RH, et al: Peripheral neural mechanisms of cutaneous hyperalgesia following mild injury by heat. J Neurosci 2:765, 1982.
14. Price, DD, et al: Peripheral suppression of first pain and central summation of second pain evoked by noxious heat pulses. Pain 3:57, 1977.
15. Brodal, P. The Central Nervous System. Oxford University Press, New York, 1992.
16. Price, DD and Dubner, R: Neurons that subserve the sensory-discriminative aspects of pain. Pain 3:307, 1977.
17. Mayer, DJ, Price, DD, and Becker, DP: Neurophysiological characterization of the anterolateral spinal cord neurons contributing to pain perception in man. Pain 1:59, 1975.
18. Hokfelt, T, et al: Experimental immunohistochemical studies on the localization and distribution of substance P in cat primary sensory neurons. Brain Res 100:235, 1975.
19. Melzack, R: The Puzzle of Pain. Basic Books, New York, 1973.
20. Price, DD, et al: Spatial and temporal transformation of input to spinothalamic tract neurons and their relation to somatic sensation. J Neurophysiol 41:933, 1978.
21. White, JC and Sweet, WH: Pain and the Neurosurgeon: A Forty-Year Experience. Charles C Thomas, Springfield, 1969.
22. Pearl, GS and Anderson, KV: Response patterns of cells in the feline caudal nucleus reticularis gigantocellularis after noxious trigeminal and spinal stimulation. Exp Neurol 58:231, 1978.
23. Casey, KL: Somatosensory responses of bulboreticular units in awake cat: Relation to escape-producing stimuli. Science 173:77, 1971.
24. Anderson, KV and Parl, GS: Long term increases in nociceptive threshold following lesions in feline nucleus reticularis gigantocellularis (abstr). 1st World Congress on Pain 1:70, 1975.
25. Yaksh, TL and Hammond, DL: Peripheral and central substances involved in rostrad (ascending) transmission of nociceptive information. Pain 13:1, 1982.
26. Nashold, BS, Jr, Wilson, WP, and Slaughter, G: The midbrain and pain. In Bonica, JJ (ed): Advances in Neurology, Vol 4. Raven Press, New York, 1979, p 69.
27. Schwarcz, JR: Periaqueductal mesencephalotomy for facial central pain. In Sweet, HW, Labrador, R, and Martin-Rodriguez, JG (eds): Neurosurgical Treatment in Psychiatry, Pain, and Epilepsy. University Park Press, Baltimore, 1977, pp 661–667.
28. Casey, KL and Jones, EG: Suprasegmental mechanisms: An overview of ascending pathways: Brain-stem and thalamus. Neurosci Res Program Bull 16:103, 1978.
29. Nyquist, JK: Somatosensory properties of neurons of thalamic nucleus ventralis lateralis. Exp Neurol 48:123, 1975.
30. Inshijima, B, et al: Nociceptive neurons in the human thalamus. Confin Neurol 37:99, 1975.
31. Andersson, SA, Keller, O, and Vyklicky, I: Cortical activity evoked from tooth pulp afferents. Brain Res 50:473, 1973.
32. Reynolds, DV: Surgery in the rat during electrical analgesia induced by focal brain stimulation. Science 164:444, 1969.
33. Mayer, DJ: The centrifugal control of pain. In Ng, L and Bonica, JJ (eds): Pain, Discomfort, and Humanitarian Care. Elsevier, Amsterdam, 1980, p 83.
34. Hughes, J: Search for the endogenous legend of the opiate receptor. Neurosci Res Program Bull 13:55, 1975.
35. Basbaum, A and Fields, HL: Endogenous pain control systems: Brainstem spinal pathways and endorphin circuitry. Annu Rev Neurosci 7:309, 1984.
36. Hughes, J: Intrinsic factors and the opiate receptor system. Neurosci Res Program Bull 16:141, 1978.
37. Duggan, AW: The differential sensitivity to L-glutamate and L-aspartate of spinal interneurons and Renshaw cells. Exp Brain Res 19:522, 1974.
38. Elde, R, et al: Immunohistochemical studies using antibodies to leucine-enkephalin: Initial observations on the nervous system of the rat. Neuroscience 1:349, 1976.
39. Basbaum, AI, Clanton, CH, and Fields, HL: Three bulbospinal pathways from the rostral medulla of the cat. J Comp Neurol 178:209, 1978.
40. Hoffert, MS, et al: Immunocytochemical identification of serotonergic axonal contacts on characterized neurons in cat spinal dorsal horn. Anat Rec 202:83A, 1982.
41. Mayer, DJ and Price, DD: A physiological and psychological analysis of pain: A potential model of motivation. In Pfaff, D: Physiological Mechanisms of Motivation. Springer-Verlag, New York, 1982, p 433.
42. Melzack, R and Wall, PD: Pain mechanism: A new theory. Science 150:971, 1965.
43. Von Frey, J: Beitrage zur physiologica des schmerzsinns. Ber Kgl Sachs Ges Wiss 46:185, 1894.

44. Goldscheider, A: Veber den Schmertz in Physiologischer and Klinischer Hensicht. Berlin, Hirschwald, 1894.
45. Wall, PD: The role of substantia gelatinosa as a gate control. In Bonica, JJ (ed): Pain. Raven Press, New York, 1980, p 205.
46. Nathan, PW: The gate-control theory of pain: A critical review. Brain 99:123, 1976.
47. Wall, PD: The gate control theory of pain mechanisms: A re-examination and re-statement. Brain 101:1, 1978.
48. Wall, PD and Sweet, WH: Temporary abolition of pain in man. Science 155:108, 1967.
49. Long, DM: External electrical simulation as a treatment of chronic pain. Minn Med 57:195, 1974.
50. Report of the Panel on Pain to the National Advisory Neurological and Communicative Disorders and Stroke Council. HEW, NIH Pub #79-11912, Bethesda, MD, 1979, p 201.
51. Kniffki, KD, et al: Responses of group Ia afferent units from skeletal muscle to stretch, contraction, and chemical stimulation. Exp Brain Res 31:511, 1978.
52. Fock, S and Mense, S: Excitatory effects of 5-hydroxytryptamine, histamine and potassium ions on muscular Ia afferent units: A comparison with bradykinin. Brain Res 105:459, 1976.
53. Fordyce, WE: Behavior Methods for Chronic Pain and Illness. CV Mosby, St Louis, 1976.
54. Fordyce, WE: A behavioral perspective on chronic pain. In Ng, KLY and Bonica, JJ (eds): Pain, Discomfort, and Humanitarian Care. Elsevier, New York, 1980, p 233.
55. Pracci, P and Zoppi, M: Pathophysiology and clinical aspects of visceral and referred pain. In Bonica, JJ, et al: Advances in Pain Research and Therapy, Vol 5. Raven Press, New York, p 643.
56. Hancock, MD, et al: Convergence of visceral and cutaneous input onto spinothalamic tract cells in the thoracic spinal cord of the cat. Exp Neurol 47:240, 1975.
57. Travell, J: Temporomandibular joint dysfunction. J Prosthet Dent 10:745, 1960.
58. Frost, A: Diclofenac versus lidocaine as injection therapy in myofascial pain. Scand Rheumatol 15:153, 1986.
59. Brendstrip, P, Jespersen, K, and Asboe-Hansen, G: Morphological and chemical connective tissue changes in fibrositic muscles. Ann Rheumatol 16:438, 1957.
60. Begtsson, A, Henriksson, K-G, and Larsson, J. Muscle biopsy in primary fibromyalgia. Light microscope and histochemical findings. Scand Rheumatol 15:1, 1986.
61. Lund, N, Begtsson, A, and Thornborg, P: Muscle tissue oxygen pressure in primary fibromyalgia. Scand Rheumatol 15:165, 1986.
62. Travell, JG and Simons, DG: Myofascial Trigger Point Manual. Williams & Wilkins, Baltimore, 1982.
63. Simons, DG and Travell, JG: Myofascial origins of low back pain. Postgrad Med 73:66, 1983.
64. Cracely, RH: Psychophysical assessment of human pain. In Bonica, JJ, et al: Advances in Pain Research and Therapy, Vol 5. Raven Press, New York, p 805.
65. Scott, J. and Huskisson, EC: Vertical and horizontal analogue scales. Ann Rheum Dis 38:560, 1979.
66. Ohnhaus, EE and Adler, R: Methodological problems in the measurement of pain: A comparison between the verbal rating scale and the visual analogue scale. Pain 1:379, 1975.
67. Price, DD and Harkins, SW: Combined use of experimental pain and visual analogue scales in providing standardized measurements of clinical pain. Clin J Pain 3:1, 1987.
68. Melzack, R and Torgerson, WS: On the language of pain. Anesthesiology 34:50, 1971.
69. Melzack, R: The McGill Pain Questionnaire: Major properties and scoring methods. Pain 1:277, 1975.
70. Klepac, RK, et al: Sensitivity of the McGill Pain Questionnaire to intensity and quality of laboratory pain. Pain 10:199, 1981.
71. Bryne, M, et al: Cross validation of the factor structure of MPQ. Pain 13:193, 1982.
72. Reding, AE: A comparison of MPQ in chronic and acute pain. Pain 13:185, 1982.
73. Gracely, RH: Pain measurement in man. In Ng, KLY and Bonica, JJ (eds): Pain, Discomfort, and Humanitarian Care. Elsevier, New York, 1980, p 111.
74. Reeves, JL, Jaeger, B, and Graff-Radford, SB: Reliability of the pressure algometer as a measure to trigger point sensitivity. Pain 24:313, 1986.
75. Cosentino, AB, et al: Ultrasound effects on electroneuromyographic measures in sensory fibers of the median nerve. Phys Ther 63:1789, 1983.
76. Mense, S: Effects of temperature on the discharges of muscle spindles and tendon organs. Flugers Arch 374:159, 1978.
77. Parsons, CM and Goetzl, FR: Effect of induced pain on pain threshold. Proc Soc Exp Bio Med 60:327, 1945.
78. Melzack, R and Wall, P: The Challenge of Pain. Penguin Books, New York, 1982.
79. Lehmann, JF and DeLateur, B: Therapeutic heat. In Lehmann, JF (ed): Therapeutic Heat and Cold, ed 4. Williams & Wilkins, Baltimore, 1990, p 429.
80. Travell, J: Myofascial trigger points: Clinical view. In Bonica, JJ and Able-Fessard, DG (eds): Advances in Pain Research and Therapy, Vol 1. Raven Press, New York, 1976, p 919.
81. Cattell, M and Hoagland, H: Response of tactile receptors to intermittent stimulation. J Physiol 72:392, 1931.
82. Gammon, DG and Starr, I: Studies on the relief of pain by counter-irritation. J Clin Invest 20:13, 1941.
83. Hensel, H: Thermoreception and Temperature Regulation. Academic Press, New York, 1981.
84. Buchthal, F and Rosenfalck, A: Evoked action potentials and conduction velocity in human sensory nerves. Brain Res 3:1, 1966.

Instrumentation: Methods and Application

CHAPTER 3

Instrumentation Considerations: Operating Principles, Purchase, Management, and Safety

H.T.M. Ritter III, BA, CBET

Electromagnetic Energy
Power Supply: 115 Volts AC-60
  Hz
Transformers
Power Distribution at the User's
  End
Ground Fault Circuit Interrupters
Isolation Transformers
One to Six Thousand Milliamperes
Oscillators

Prepurchase Evaluation and
  Acquisition of Equipment
Operator Manuals
Equipment Care and Service
Device-Specific Inspections
Superficial Heat and Cold
Hydrotherapy
Ultrasound
Diathermy
Electrical Safety

    In opening this chapter, it is significant to note that most of the earliest applications of electricity in medicine were intended as physical therapy devices. Experiments with electrotherapy are on record from the eighteenth century.[1] Diathermy was first described late in the nineteenth century, and ultrasound was under investigation shortly thereafter.[2] Today, there is perhaps a greater variety of instrumentation to be found in hospital physical therapy departments than in any other patient care area. Outpatient physical therapy centers also can have a large variety of equipment.

A basic knowledge of electrical principles is essential for safety in the physical therapy clinic and for an understanding of devices such as ground fault circuit interrupters, diathermy units, and ultrasound generators. The author assumes that the reader has had previous exposure to these basic principles, including electron flow, Ohm's law, capacitance, and inductance. For a comprehensive review of electrical terminology and theory, the reader may refer either to Cromwell[3] or to Spooner.[4]

ELECTROMAGNETIC ENERGY

The entire range of radiation, or electromagnetic spectrum, includes heat, radio, and light waves, as well as ultraviolet, x-rays, and cosmic rays. It is important to know, however, that ultrasound energy is not electromagnetic, but rather is a mechanical/pressure waveform that cannot be transmitted by air. Notice from careful study of Figure 3–1 that shortwave (SWD) and microwave (MWD) diathermy are both safely in the nonionizing section. Their energies are not capable of stripping electrons from atoms and their radiation effects are thought to be purely thermal.

The electromagnetic spectrum also reveals that each form of radiation can be described by a frequency (f) and a wavelength (λ). All forms of radiant energy are self-propagating and travel in a vacuum at the speed of light (c), which is 300 million m/s. The reader should be aware of the formula that interrelates these three quantities: $c = f\lambda$. Because c is a constant, frequency or wavelength can be derived even when just one of them is known. For instance, given that the wavelength of shortwave diathermy is 11.062 m, calculate its frequency.

$$f = c/\lambda = \frac{3 \times 10^8 \text{ m/s}}{11.062 \text{ m}} = 27.12 \times 10^6 \text{ cycles/s} = 27.12 \text{ MHz}$$

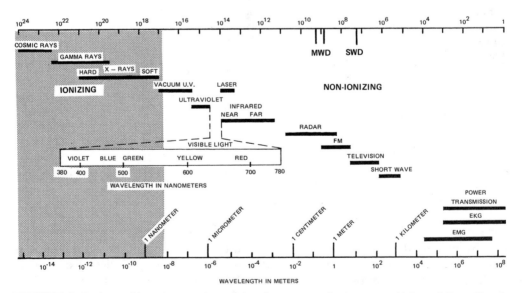

FIGURE 3–1. A graphic representation of the electromagnetic spectrum. (Adapted from Illuminating Engineering Society of North America Lighting Handbook, New York, ed 8, 1993.)

Radiation energy is directly proportional to frequency. Therefore, cosmic rays are far more penetrating than is infrared radiation. Within the infrared spectrum, the higher-frequency radiation, near visible light, is more penetrating than "far" infrared. The biologic effects of electromagnetic radiation depend on frequency, exposure duration, tissue characteristics, and power density.

In dealing with instrumentation for thermal therapy, there is no need to be concerned with direct current (DC). The domain of relevant alternating current (AC) frequencies ranges from the 60-Hz power-line supply through the megahertz region for diathermy up to infrared radiation.

POWER SUPPLY: 115 VOLTS AC-60 Hz

Conventional power-line voltage in North America alternates at the very regulated frequency of 60 Hertz (abbreviated Hz and denoting cycles per second). The accuracy of electric clocks, for instance, depends on this constant, because "line" voltage frequently varies between 110 and 125 V. Every electrical device intended for operation on line voltage will bear a label that typically lists 110, 115, 117 or 120 V—alternating current (volts AC), as distinguished from direct-current voltage (volts DC). (Some heavy-duty devices, such as treadmills, may require a 230-V source.) The label will also indicate the line frequency (60 Hz) and either a current or a power rating. For instance, a new solid-state ultrasound unit specifies "120 volts AC 60 Hz, 0.5 amp maximum." The same information could have been conveyed by indicating 60 W instead of listing current:

$$\text{Power} = \text{voltage } (E) \times \text{current } (I) = 120 \times 0.5$$

Voltages and their frequencies can be seen and measured with an oscilloscope. A comparison of symbols and waveforms for DC and AC is illustrated in Figure 3–2.

TRANSFORMERS

Electricity is transmitted from generating stations over long distances at very high voltages (e.g., 230,000 V). Before commercial distribution, voltage must be dropped to the 115-V range. Whereas whirlpool motors, paraffin baths, and infrared lamps operate

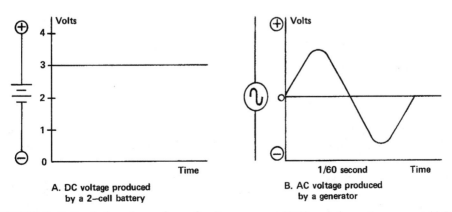

FIGURE 3–2. Symbols and waveforms for direct current (DC) and alternating current (AC).

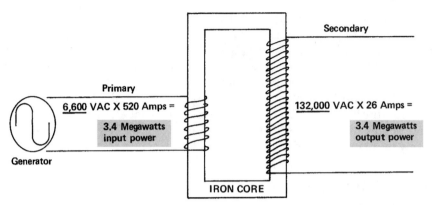

FIGURE 3–3. A step-up transformer used for electrical power transmission. Lowered secondary current greatly reduces losses due to heating of the power distribution wires. Step-up or step-down refers to secondary voltage.

directly off this line voltage, some instruments have power supplies that require a lower AC voltage. Others may require a boosting of voltage at some point.

Transformers accomplish these necessary voltage manipulations. Typically, they are composed of two adjacent coils on an iron core and operate on the principle of electrical induction. When alternating current flows through the input or primary winding of a transformer, it creates a surrounding magnetic field. This field, in turn, cuts through the secondary winding and induces an output current. Note that there is no electron flow between primary and secondary windings. Output voltage and current are determined by the ratio of primary to secondary winding turns. When transformer windings have approximately the same number of turns, output voltage will equal input voltage, and the unit is referred to as an isolation transformer. This type of transformer, which can be used as a safety device, will be discussed later.

The concept of input power equaling output power (assuming no coupling losses) is fundamental to understanding step-up and step-down transformers. Again reviewing the power formula $P = E \times I$, it can be seen that, for a given input power to the primary, a stepped-up voltage is associated with a proportional reduction in secondary current (Fig. 3–3).

If a transformer secondary has fewer turns than its primary winding, output voltage will be reduced. For example, an ultrasound generator has a step-down transformer that drops line voltage to approximately 24 V, which is then fed to the unit's power supply.

POWER DISTRIBUTION AT THE USER'S END

Figure 3–4 illustrates the terminology and mechanism of power distribution to the familiar point of an electrical receptacle. It also depicts a simplified current flow to, from, and within a representative ultrasound unit.

As previously described, electrical power is commercially supplied in a range of 110 to 125 V, alternating at the frequency of 60 Hz. Although only two conductors (referred to as "hot" and "neutral") are actually required for a voltage source, a third conductor can be employed to enhance electrical safety. This line is referred to as "ground" and, most often, is actually connected to a rod in the earth either in, or just outside, a building. As a rule, the plumbing system of a building is also considered to

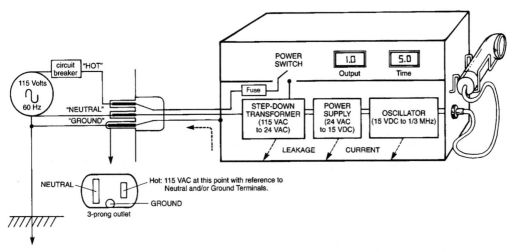

FIGURE 3–4. A device is powered by the voltage between the hot and neutral conductors. Normal leakage current is conducted away from metal housing (chassis) by the ground wire.

be "grounded." Ground is a universal electrical reference point that is at a zero-voltage potential.

Current circulates to and from the ultrasound unit through wires designated as hot and neutral. In spite of careful design and proper insulation, minute currents will nevertheless stray (much of it capacitively) from the hot circuit to adjacent conductive surfaces. Then, if a path exists, these so-called leakage currents will flow to any object that is grounded, completing their return back into the power system. (Note carefully in Fig. 3–4 that the neutral side of the electrical service is also connected to ground.)

If an electrical device loses its line cord/receptacle grounding, a patient or therapist, or both, can become a substitute path for leakage current from its conductive exterior, for instance, to any grounded surface. Most people have experienced leakage current as a mild tingling or buzzing sensation in touching certain electrical devices that are powered by two-wire line cords. Because resistance of the human body is in a range of 100 to 1,000,000 ohms (depending, for instance, on how much tissue is between the contact sites, and if they are damp or dry), the normally intact ground wire in three-wire line cords, with resistance less than 1 ohm, will divert any nontherapeutic current before it can cause electrical shock. Such current is simply dumped into the receptacle's ground terminal.

Users of line-powered instruments should know that leakage current is a normal phenomenon. Widely recognized standards[5,6] recommend a maximum of 300 μA for exterior surface (chassis) leakage. This amount is approximately one third the current believed necessary to stimulate sensory perception. Leakage from an applicator (or electrode) intended for direct patient connection should not exceed 50 μA.

In the event of a major degradation of electrical insulation (for example, water seepage into the unit's electronic circuits), an unintended path to ground, or "ground fault," is likely to result. This would produce excessive leakage current, commonly termed "fault current." As with normal leakage current, the fault current would be conducted away from the unit by its ground wire. The fuse, with a typical current rating of 1 to 2 A, should then melt open when fault current exceeds that limit.

At this point, visualize the hazard that would exist in the absence of a low-resistance grounding connection. The 1 to 2 A could end up flowing to ground through someone's body, with possibly fatal consequences. Ground-wire integrity, therefore, must be inspected routinely to verify low resistance between conductive chassis surfaces and the grounding pin of the power plug.

Double insulation is a design technique that introduces a second layer of insulation between the "live" internal components of a device and the operator. Many manufacturers are turning to plastic and other nonconductive materials for chassis fabrication as an alternative method of minimizing risks from stray currents. This usually makes chassis grounding unnecessary, and a two-wire line cord would therefore be acceptable. The device should be labeled, preferably on its nameplate, as being double-insulated. Hydrotherapy devices, however, are an exception; these always require grounding.[7]

Ground Fault Circuit Interrupters

The equipment used in hydrotherapy areas presents a major potential for electrical hazards arising from ground faults. Installation of ground fault circuit interrupter (GFCI) protection for all receptacles that serve these locations can effectively eliminate such hazards. In general, GFCIs are required for all receptacles within 1.5 m of therapeutic tubs.[7]

Note that the name for this device is nearly descriptive: the (power) circuit is interrupted when a ground fault is sensed. The same device is frequently referred to as a ground fault interrupter, or GFI. This terminology is misleading, because it suggests that the fault itself is eliminated.

A sensor within the GFCI constantly monitors the currents in the hot and neutral lines that feed a given receptacle. The assumption is that input current in the hot line of a device should very nearly equal current in its neutral line. A substantial difference of 5 mA between hot and neutral suggests that a ground fault exists and is diverting current return from neutral to ground (Fig. 3–5). Because the maximum safe transthoracic current (through intact skin) is deemed to be 5 mA, GFCI activation is set to occur at this level.

Tripping time is almost instantaneous; a button labeled RESET extends out of its channel when the circuit is interrupted. Once the ground fault is identified and eliminated, this same button is depressed to reactivate the GFCI. Depressing the TEST button generates a low-level internal ground fault, causing the unit to trip. This test should be exercised monthly to verify operation. Annual inspection of GFCIs, using a calibrated external test device, is also advocated.[6]

A GFCI can be integrated within a power receptacle or as part of the circuit breaker for that receptacle. Figure 3–6 illustrates both configurations.

Isolation Transformers

As older equipment is being replaced, external isolation transformers are fading into history. Isolation transformers are used to lower the leakage current of some older devices that generate chassis leakage far in excess of 300 µA, but that are otherwise safe and functional.

As previously discussed, output voltage of an isolation transformer is of the same

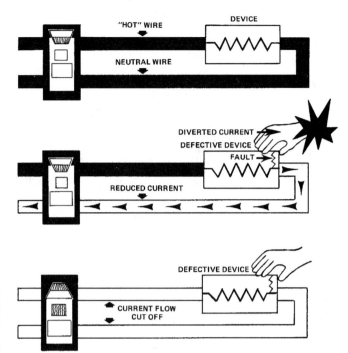

FIGURE 3–5. Operation of a ground fault circuit interrupter (GFCI). (Adapted from Square D Company product information literature, Lexington, KY.)

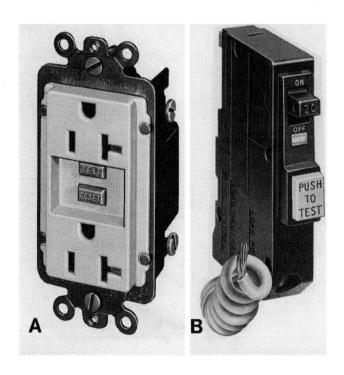

FIGURE 3–6. Ground fault circuit interrupters. (*A*) Receptacle style. (*B*) Circuit breaker style. (Courtesy of Square D Company, Lexington, KY.)

magnitude as line voltage. The difference is that the secondary voltage is not referenced to ground. Therefore, the leakage current from a device plugged into the transformer will not seek or flow to ground.

One to Six Thousand Milliamperes

The effects of 1-second exposures to 60-Hz currents are summarized in Table 3–1. The current levels listed are average figures; actual effects would vary as a function of many factors, including body size, physical condition, and age. Wet skin also would greatly increase resultant risk current. For perspective in reviewing Table 3–1, it is helpful to know that the current that flows through a 100-W bulb is almost 1 A.

As current frequency increases, its physiologic shock hazards diminish. At frequencies greater than 10 kHz, current of sufficient intensity produces tissue heating with no other apparent effect on the neuromuscular system. High-frequency electromagnetic current is the active mechanism of shortwave diathermy and is most commonly delivered with capacitive air-gap applicators or inductance drum applicators.

Oscillators

As is commonly known, AC signals in radio frequency range can be directed and transmitted through air. A shortwave diathermy unit, for instance, with a frequency of 27.12 MHz, is just a step removed from a citizens' band (CB) radio transmitter. An electronic circuit known as an oscillator is used to develop an alternating or oscillating output from a DC source. Any specific (resonant) frequency can be obtained as a function of the associated timing circuit's capacitance and inductance. Waveforms produced can be sinusoidal, square, sawtoothed, or unidirectional pulses, as illustrated in Figure 3–7.

In physical therapy instrumentation, oscillators are integral to ultrasound, shortwave diathermy, and electric stimulator units. For patient treatment, the waveform can be either continuous or cyclically interrupted (pulsed).

TABLE 3–1 Effects of 60-Hz AC Current Flowing Arm to Arm
through the Chest

Current in Milliamperes	Physiologic Effect
1	Threshold of perception; tingling
5	Maximum current considered to be harmless (Typical GFCI tripping level is 4–6 mA)
10–20	Sustained muscular contractions
50	Pain, exhaustion; possible fainting
100–300	Ventricular fibrillation
1000–6000 (1–6 amps)	Body muscle system contracts violently; probable respiratory paralysis and burns

Adapted from Bruner, JMR: Hazards of electrical apparatus. Anesthesiology 28:400, 1967.

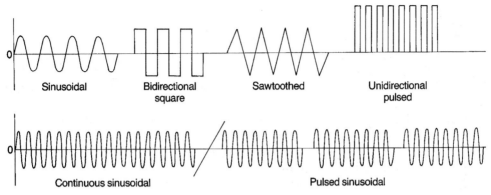

FIGURE 3-7. Oscillator waveforms.

PREPURCHASE EVALUATION AND ACQUISITION OF EQUIPMENT

Considering equipment costs, and the fact that most devices have a reasonable life expectancy of 8 to 10 years, it is essential that a thorough prepurchase investigation be conducted. Information should be sought and assembled from every possible source. ECRI (formerly, Emergency Care Research Institute) is an independent nonprofit health services research agency and a collaborating center of the World Health Organization. It provides independent, objective judgment for selecting, purchasing, managing, and using medical devices, equipment, and systems. *Health Devices* is a monthly journal that features brand-name evaluations and ratings based on ECRI's testing. *The Healthcare Product Comparison System* presents background information on a large number of device categories coupled with a listing of manufacturers and a tabulation of specifications and features for each model. *The Health Devices Sourcebook* is a directory of medical devices, trade names, manufacturers, and service organizations, which is updated annually.

It would be additionally advisable to solicit the experiences of therapist colleagues who have used specific devices in various clinics and departments. Review the following questions:

1. Have there been any major defects or failures? If so, was warranty service readily available?
2. Have there been any problems in obtaining accessories or product support?
3. Does the device have any operational difficulties?
4. Is operation of the equipment adequately described/prompted/labeled?
5. Has clinical effectiveness been assessed?

After limiting the field to perhaps three models, the next step is to arrange for a minimum 1-week trial period for each unit under a normal patient load. The salesperson or a technical representative should perform an in-service presentation for all staff members who will be evaluating the equipment.

During the test period, difficulties are likely to arise under the varying circumstances of patient treatment. A log should be maintained to record all such problems and relevant patient comments so that they can be reviewed with the representative. Careful documentation will help to distinguish genuine deficiencies in the equipment or accessories from operator error.

When available, consult with the biomedical instrumentation department (may also be referred to as biomedical or clinical engineering), a biomedical equipment technician (BMET), or whoever is responsible for maintaining existing equipment. They should be asked to perform an electrical safety inspection on the loaned equipment and to examine its service manual. Review their experience with the product and manufacturer, and establish whether any specialized test equipment would be required for inspection, repair, or calibration. Consider together whether there would be any unusual assembly or installation requirements and estimate associated costs. If accessories are needed for routine operation of the device, their annual cost should be estimated.

Finally, analyze the terms of the warranty; most are for 1 year. Verify that the warranty will not start until the equipment is installed and functional. Ascertain how this service would be performed: Is it available locally or must the user package and ship the defective unit back to the manufacturer?

The end result of the decision process will be a purchase order (PO) for the selected device. In addition to quantity, description, and shipping address, a PO should specify:

1. Operator and service manuals (two each: one for the physical therapy department, and one for the biomedical instrumentation department).
2. All applicators and accessories agreed upon.
3. An introductory in-service presentation.
4. How and where warranty service will be performed and, possibly, a maximum "down" time limit.
5. Payment will be made after successful completion of an acceptance inspection.

It may be desirable to notify the sales representative upon delivery of the equipment so that this person can do the unpacking and assembly. If shipping damage has occurred, the representative can handle any necessary adjustments. Otherwise, an in-service orientation can then be performed for the entire staff.

In an institution with a biomedical instrumentation department, the new equipment generally will be tagged with a control number to facilitate documentation of inspection and repair. Manufacturer performance specifications should be selectively verified. (For instance, ultrasound and diathermy output frequencies would not normally be checked.) When the unit passes its acceptance inspection, final authorization for payment can be made.

Operator Manuals

Under ideal circumstances, a therapist should be very familiar with a newly acquired device by the time it is put into service. Many manufacturers provide a checklist in their operator or service manuals (Table 3–2) for troubleshooting anticipated problems.

In addition, operator manuals typically include the following information: indications, contraindications, and precautions for using the device; function and location of controls; serial procedures for treatment. Accessories and methods of application are generally illustrated and described. The stocking of certain spare items may also be recommended. A careful review of all operator manuals, therefore, should be a definite part of orientation for employees new to a clinic.

TABLE 3–2 A Checklist for Troubleshooting for
a Hot Pack Unit (Hydrocollator M-2)

Problem	Cause	Remedy
Unit plugged in, water does not get hot with switch on	Breaker for electric circuit off	Turn breaker on
	Thermostat not functioning	Replace thermostat
	Heating element burned out	Replace element
	On-off switch broken	Replace switch
Cloudiness of water	Seepage from packs (worn out)	Replace packs
	Too long a period between cleanings	Drain and clean
Packs too hot	Thermostat set too high	Adjust thermostat
	Thermostat failure	Replace thermostat
Unit boils	Thermostat failure	Replace thermostat
Packs too cool	Thermostat set too low	Adjust thermostat
	Power failure	Check electric circuit

From Chattanooga Corporation, Chattanooga, TN, with permission.

Equipment Care and Service

Instrumentation service personnel generally estimate that 30% to 60% of reported equipment problems turn out to be attributable to operator error of some sort. Therefore, before initiating a request for service, recheck the entire setup and, if necessary, review the operator manual.

In the absence of a pilot light or output power, first test the electrical receptacle with another device. When either the circuit breaker for the receptacle or the breaker on the instrument is tripped (and the institution does not have a policy requiring an electrician or equipment technician to reset breakers), the therapist can attempt the reset. Circuit breakers do occasionally trip for no apparent reason. If, however, a reset breaker immediately trips again, do not attempt to reset it a second time. Remember also to check for a tripped GFCI in situations of interrupted power.

There are three cases of equipment malfunction that should cause a device to be instantly removed from operation. Whenever anyone experiences an electrical shock, smells an unusual odor (chemical or burning), or actually sees smoke, the device in question should be unplugged and prominently labeled "DEFECTIVE–DO NOT USE." Request an immediate investigation by the biomedical instrumentation department. Decide whether an incident report is necessary. Communicate the experience to ECRI directly by phone or with a copy of the ECRI Problem Reporting Form (Fig. 3–8).

Accidental damage will occur: transducers are inevitably bumped and dropped, and fluids have a way of finding chassis ventilation openings. Repeated operator abuse, on the other hand, is inexcusable. Never roll a device over its line cord or pull a power plug by yanking the cord. Avoid wrapping cables and cords too tightly; it is likely to make them intermittent or degrade their insulation. Do not force controls that are stuck, or connectors improperly mated. Significantly, the experience of biomedical instrumentation personnel indicates that the majority of legitimate equipment defects are mechanical rather than electrical. Loose knobs and hardware, broken casters, and damaged strain reliefs are very common defects.

Whenever a nonemergency problem cannot be resolved by the user, it should be

ECRI Problem Reporting Form
User Experience Network™

Mail or fax this form to report a hazard or problem related to the use of medical devices or equipment. Telephone reports are also acceptable, but should be followed by a completed form.

Your personal and institutional identities will not be revealed in any way without your permission.

Name: _____   Date: _____
            (Please type or write legibly.)

Title: _____

Department: _____

Institution: _____

Address: _____

_____

Telephone: _____   Ext.: _____

May we identify you to the manufacturer and/or supplier of the device(s) involved?   ☐ Yes   ☐ No

DEVICE IDENTIFICATION

Please be as specific as possible in identifying the devices involved. Please add any other information that might be helpful, and omit any items that are not known or that appear to be irrelevant to this particular problem.

Type(s) of Device(s) Involved: _____

_____

Manufacturer: _____   Model: _____

Serial/Lot No.: _____   Expiration/Use Before Date: _____

How Long in Use? _____   Condition: _____

Date Last Inspected or Serviced: _____   Date Problem Occurred: _____

If requested, will you send the affected device to ECRI for examination?   ☐ Yes   ☐ No

Were other devices involved?   ☐ Yes   ☐ No   If yes, please identify all other units on the reverse side of this form, including the information listed above.

Are other units of the same model similarly affected?   ☐ Yes   ☐ No

PROBLEM DESCRIPTION

Could (or did) the described problem result in injury?   ☐ Yes   ☐ No   ☐ Unknown

Please use the reverse side of this form or separate sheets to describe the hazard or problem in detail. Include how it was discovered, any action you took, and the response of any vendors or manufacturers. Attach copies of any related correspondence, when possible. Sketches, photographs, or copies of portions of operating manuals are often helpful in describing the problem, especially if the affected device is not available for examination at ECRI. Retain all disposable accessories involved in an incident. Please do not send any device to ECRI until requested.

SIGNATURE: _____

Please mail completed form to ECRI at the address below.

ECRI
A NONPROFIT AGENCY

5200 Butler Pike, Plymouth Meeting, PA 19462-1298, U.S.A. • Telephone (610) 825-6000 • Fax (610) 834-1275   V460UL3A
This form may be reproduced without prior permission.

FIGURE 3–8. Problem Reporting Form.

reported with ample detail to the appropriate service group. Unless this happens to be the manufacturer, it may be necessary for the therapist first to explain the function or demonstrate the operation of the equipment to the service individual. In most cases, the training of biomedical equipment technicians and even clinical engineers tends to focus on operating room and intensive care unit instrumentation. As a result, their inspections of physical therapy equipment are frequently limited to electrical safety checks, with little or no attention to actual performance. Be prepared, therefore, to review jointly each device in the department and to develop protocols for functional inspections. The next section of this chapter offers suggestions relevant to this task.

DEVICE-SPECIFIC INSPECTIONS

Superficial Heat and Cold

Most devices employed to deliver superficial heat or cold therapy incorporate thermostats to maintain defined temperature ranges. For instance, paraffin bath and hot pack conditioner unit temperatures are usually maintained between 49°C and 54°C and 71°C and 82°C, respectively. Cold pack conditioner units typically operate between -5°C and -12°C.

Thermostats are mechanical switches that may actually turn on and off many times an hour to achieve temperature regulation. They do fail periodically and require replacement. More commonly, however, control settings are tampered with, both inadvertently and intentionally. Calibration, therefore, may be required at any time. The internal thermometers of therapy appliances must also be monitored during inspections.

Some units may have integral timers for terminating treatment after a prescribed interval. Timer accuracy and actual power deactivation or alarm functions must be verified on such devices.

Hydrotherapy

Again, with whirlpool baths and Hubbard tanks, thermometer precision must be routinely checked. In fact, it is probably advisable that a therapy department or clinic have its own calibrated electronic thermometer with both air and submersible sensors. This will prove useful for occasional spot-checking of any of its device thermometers.

A whirlpool turbine must never be operated without water fully covering its impeller. Impellers should be checked to ensure free rotation. Often impellers are partially wrapped with bandage material that restricts flow and turbulence.

Experience of some therapists suggests the wisdom of securing a turbine to its bath tank with an additional set screw or bolt.[8] This precaution eliminates the hazard of an energized motor falling into a filled tank during adjustment of turbine ejector height.

Inspections of hydrotherapy locations should additionally test the secureness of hand rails, stools, and overhead patient lifts. If a tank is mobile, the condition of its casters and drain hose should be assessed.

Ultrasound

To date, of all physical therapy devices, Federal Performance Standards exist only for ultrasonic products.[9] (A 1980 proposed standard for microwave diathermy[10] was withdrawn in 1983.) Specifically, in terms of performance, ultrasound units sold since 1979 are required to:

1. Indicate the magnitudes of ultrasonic power and intensity with an accuracy of ±20% (both for continuous and amplitude-modulated waveform operation).
2. Control treatment time: 0 to 5 minutes, ±0.5 minutes; 5 to 10 minutes, ±10%; > 10 minutes, ±1 minute.

Although some generators manufactured before 1979 may still be in use, most, with proper calibration, should be able to meet these specifications.

An ultrasound power meter, pictured in Figure 3–9, should be a standard piece of test equipment in a biomedical instrumentation department. Transducer output power is radiated into distilled, degassed water at 30°C. Verification of output power accuracy is advisable on at least an annual basis, and recalibration is always necessary when a transducer is replaced.

For more detailed information about transducer beam patterns and intensities, a device known as a hydrophone would be required. Principles of hydrophone operation are illustrated in Figure 3–10. The use of this test instrument by therapists is generally limited to ultrasound research applications. A manufacturer uses a hydrophone to establish and specify the beam nonuniformity ratio (BNR) of a transducer. BNR is the ratio of the maximum intensity on the transducer to the average intensity of the transducer's effective radiating area (refer to the discussion of BNR in Chapter 7).

Most problems with ultrasound units are traceable to either the transducer or its cable assembly. A therapist can quickly check for ultrasonic output by wrapping a ring

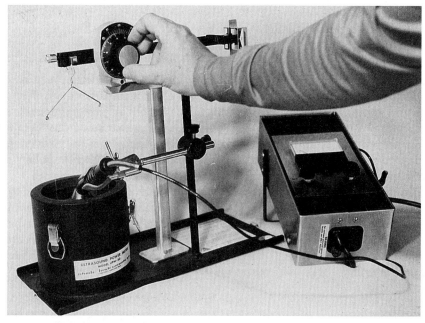

FIGURE 3–9. Testing of an ultrasound unit using a power meter. (Courtesy of Ohmic Instruments, Easton, MD.)

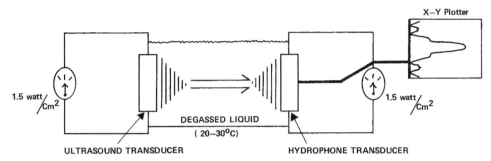

FIGURE 3-10. Piezoelectric materials can convert AC voltage to mechanical vibrations. which can then be converted back to voltage of the original frequency. Using a hydrophone and recorder, a transducer's spatial characteristics can be depicted.

of 1-inch tape around the front edge of the transducer and pouring a half inch of water into this cavity. At a power setting of 10 to 15 W, boiling agitation and possibly a cone will be observed. During this test, the transducer cable should be flexed, especially at the transducer and chassis connector strain reliefs. If an intermittency exists, it will be manifested by a sudden decrease or interruption of output power, causing the water agitation to diminish or disappear. Defective transducer assemblies are usually returned to the manufacturer for rebuilding.

Diathermy

An accurate, standardized method for verifying output power actually delivered to a patient has not been developed for shortwave diathermy.[11] The electromagnetic energy actually coupled to a patient and the resultant amount of heating produced are functions of operator technique, exposure time, the anatomy and electrical properties of the treatment location, as well as spatial distribution and temporal characteristics (continuous versus pulsed output) of the radiated energy. At present, commercially available diathermy power meters are of little use other than for gathering baseline data on output, beginning with the acceptance inspection. They merely indicate power delivered to a fixed resistance in a test device.

A simple and inexpensive neon light bulb taped to a tongue blade is generally sufficient to indicate the presence of diathermy output. The bulb will have an orange glow if held near the applicator(s), or next to their cables (unless they are shielded).

Cables should always be kept spaced apart and several inches away from anything that is conductive (mattress covers of springs) or that may be grounded (including other energized devices and their line cords and plumbing fixtures). Also be cautious of some plastics and synthetics (e.g., nylon) which, although nonconductive, possibly may be heated by electromagnetic diathermy.[12]

Timers can be tested against manufacturer's specifications. Observe that output power is, in fact, deactivated when a set time expires. Operation of patient emergency cut-off switches and their pull cords should also be verified.

ELECTRICAL SAFETY

As discussed previously, electrical safety depends greatly on maintaining the integrity of device grounding, and periodically verifying that chassis leakage currents do not exceed 300 μA. For physical therapy equipment, a minimal testing interval of 12 months is advisable. The National Fire Protection Association (NFPA), along with organizations such as AAMI, ANSI, ECRI, and JCAHO (Table 3–3), have developed a variety of guidelines, protocols, and standards for an extensive range of medical instrumentation and facilities.[5,6,13,14] In some cases, legislative bodies have adopted certain standards and made them binding regulations. Hospitals generally comply with standards, however, to reduce potential equipment-related liabilities and to obtain institutional accreditations.

Appropriate documentation for every inspection (and repair) must be generated and kept for each piece of equipment. An inspection interval of less than 12 months may be indicated if a device has an extensive repair history or if use is especially heavy.

Equipment that is either portable or mobile tends to be repeatedly plugged in and out of receptacles. For this reason, all AC power receptacles and plugs should be hospital-grade quality (usually signified by a green dot). Annual testing of receptacles is also recommended.[6] Such inspections verify correct voltage, as well as the physical integrity of the outlet (e.g., grounding tension ≥ 4 oz).

Generally, documented inspection of devices, receptacles, and GFCIs is performed by the hospital's biomedical instrumentation department or an outside service contractor. Although standards do not specifically apply to private clinics or offices, these locations should nevertheless have grounded power receptacles throughout and GFCIs in hydrotherapy areas. So-called cheater plugs, which adapt three-blade power plugs

TABLE 3–3 Organizations Dealing with Medical
Device Information, Standards, and Regulations

AAMI	Association for the Advancement of Medical Instrumentation 3330 Washington Boulevard, Suite 400 Arlington, VA 22201 (703) 525-4890
ANSI	American National Standards Institute 11 West 42nd Street, 13th Floor New York, NY 10036 (212) 642-4900
ECRI	5200 Butler Pike Plymouth Meeting, PA 19462 (610) 825-6000
FDA	Center for Devices and Radiological Health Food and Drug Administration 1390 Piccard Drive HFZ1 Rockville, MD 20850 (301) 443-4690
JCAHO	Joint Commission on Accreditation of Healthcare Organizations One Renaissance Boulevard Oakbrook Terrace, IL 60181 (708) 916-5600
NFPA	National Fire Protection Association Batterymarch Park Quincy, MA 02269 (617) 770-3000

to two-blade receptacles (thus defeating grounding), and extension cords are never to be used.

SUMMARY

Effective and safe use of thermal instrumentation requires a thorough familiarity with each device, as well as a general understanding of electrical principles. A therapy department or clinic should establish and maintain a file of clinical and technical information for every piece of equipment in use.

Therapists should develop a close working relationship with biomedical instrumentation personnel, using their resources to help evaluate new devices and to perform regular inspection and preventive maintenance of existing equipment. Inspections should verify both electrical safety and performance. Appropriate documentation of all inspection and repair activities must be kept for each device. Electrical receptacles and ground fault circuit interrupters require annual testing.

Study Objectives

Having completed this chapter, the reader should now be able to:

1. Discuss the basic principles and physiologic effects of 60 Hz alternating current.
2. Discuss the reasons for grounding electrical devices and for installing ground fault circuit interrupters in hydrotherapy areas.
3. Explain guidelines for prepurchase evaluation, acquisition, and knowledgeable management of equipment.
4. Describe general and device-specific inspection procedures, including calibration methods and electrical safety verification.

REFERENCES

1. Licht, SH: History of electrotherapy. In Stillwell, GK (ed): Therapeutic Electricity and Ultraviolet Radiation, ed 4. Williams & Wilkins, Baltimore, 1983.
2. Dunn, D and Frizzell, LA: Bioeffects of ultrasound. In Lehmann, JF (ed): Therapeutic Heat and Cold, ed 4. Williams & Wilkins, Baltimore, 1990.
3. Cromwell, L, et al: Medical Instrumentation for Health Care. Prentice-Hall, Englewood Cliffs, NJ, 1976.
4. Spooner, RB: Hospital Electrical Safety Simplified. Instrument Society of America/Prentice-Hall, Englewood Cliffs, NJ, 1983.
5. Safe Current Limits for Electromedical Apparatus. ANSI/AAMI:ES1, 1993.
6. Safe use of electricity in patient care areas of hospitals. In Standard for Health Care Facilities. National Fire Protection Association 99, Quincy, MA, 1993.
7. Therapeutic pools and tubs in health care facilities. In National Electrical Code. National Fire Protection Association 70, Quincy, MA, 1993.
8. Gieck, JH: Precautions for hydrotherapeutic devices. Clinical Management 3:44, 1983.
9. Performance Standards for Sonic, Infrasonic, and Ultrasonic Radiation Emitting Products: 21 CFR 1050:10. Federal Register 43:7166, 1978.
10. Performance Standard for Microwave Diathermy Products: 21 CFR 1030. Federal Register 45:50359, 1980.
11. Evaluation: Shortwave diathermy units. Health Devices 8:175, 1979.
12. Shortwave or microwave diathermy: A fire hazard? Health Devices 12:197, 1983.
13. Health Devices Inspection and Preventive Maintenance System (ed 3). ECRI, Plymouth Meeting, PA, 1995.
14. Accreditation Manual for Hospitals. Joint Commission on Accreditation of Healthcare Organizations, Chicago, 1995.

CHAPTER 4

Cryotherapy

Kristin von Nieda, MEd, PT
Susan L. Michlovitz, MS, PT, CHT

Cold agents are used as first-aid measures after trauma and as adjunctive tools in rehabilitation of musculoskeletal and neuromuscular dysfunctions. *Cryotherapy* is an age-old remedy for pain relief, fever reduction, and control of bleeding; more recently, it has been applied to prevent or reduce edema of traumatic origin and inflammation, decrease muscle-guarding spasms, and temporarily diminish spasticity before exercise.

A number of agents are available to achieve the common goal of reducing tissue temperature. These agents include cold or ice packs, ice cubes or ice massage, vapocoolant sprays, cold baths, and controlled cold-compression units.

PHYSICAL PRINCIPLES

Heat removed or lost from an object is referred to as *heat abstraction,* or *cooling.* Therefore, when cold is applied, it lowers the temperature of the skin and underlying tissues by abstracting, or removing, heat from the body. The principal modes of energy transfer used for therapeutic cooling include conduction and evaporation.

Conduction

The most common methods of cooling are placing ice or cold packs over an area or immersing a distal extremity in cool or cold water. The body part comes in direct contact with the cold agent. Energy transfer in these cases is by conduction. Conduction is the transfer of heat by the direct interaction of the molecules in the warmer area with those in the cooler area. Internal energy is gained by the slower-moving, cooler particles from the more rapidly moving, hotter particles.[1]

The magnitude of the temperature change and secondary biophysical alterations will depend on several factors, including: (1) the temperature difference between the cold object and the tissue; (2) the time of exposure; (3) the thermal conductivity of the area being cooled; and (4) the type of cooling agent (for example, ice versus water).

The rate of heat transfer by conduction can be summarized by the following equation:

$$D = \frac{\text{area} \times k \times (T_1 - T_2)}{\text{thickness of tissue}}$$

where D equals rate of heat loss (cal/s); area equals amount of body surface area cooled or heated (cm²); k equals thermal conductivity of tissues (cal/s/cm² × °C/cm²) (Table 4–1); and T_1 and T_2 equal temperatures of warm and cool surfaces (°C).

The greater the temperature gradient between the skin and the cooling source, the greater will be the resulting tissue temperature change. For example, following a 15-minute immersion of the forearm in a water bath of 1°C, subcutaneous tissue temperature dropped by 24°C.[2] With the same duration and area of exposure at 17°C, the decrease in temperature in the subcutaneous tissue was only 6°C.[3]

When considering the ability of cold to lower the temperature of subcutaneous tissues, muscle, and joints, the time of exposure is important. The deeper the tissue, the

TABLE 4–1 Thermal Conductivities
(cal/s)/(cm² × °C/cm)

Material/Tissue	Thermal Conductivity (k)
Silver	1.01
Aluminum	0.50
Ice	0.005
Water at 20°C	0.0014
Bone	0.0011
Muscle	0.0011
Fat	0.0005
Air at 0°C	0.000057

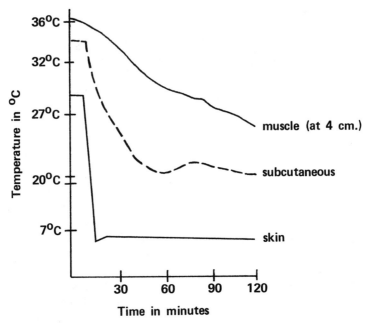

FIGURE 4-1. Temperature changes during ice pack application of the calf. (Adapted from Bierman and Friedlander.[5])

longer the time required to lower the temperature (Fig. 4–1). Changes in skin temperature will occur very rapidly (within a minute or less) upon exposure to cold. Subcutaneous tissue and muscle temperature can also be reduced by topical cold application, but additional time is required to allow for conduction of energy. Muscle temperature at a depth of 4.3 cm can be lowered by an average of 1.2°C when cooled with an agent at 10°C.[4] It can take as long as 30 minutes, though, to lower muscle temperature at a depth of 4 cm by 3.5°C using ice packs.[5]

Thermal conductivity (Table 4–1) is a measure of the efficiency of a material or tissue to conduct heat. For example, metals are better heat conductors than are nonmetals. Tissues with a high water content, such as muscle, have better thermal conductivity than does adipose tissue. Adipose tissue acts as an insulator, providing resistance to heat transfer (for example, gain or loss). The amount of fat may influence the degree and rate at which muscle can be cooled[6,7] and, conversely, can be returned to its precooled temperature.

In addition to the consideration of thermal conductivity, the effects of cold on blood flow to the area are important in order to understand why a cooled area can take such a long time to return to the precooled temperature. In fact, it can take a cooled area longer than a heated area to return to resting values. Arterial blood coming from the body core is warmer than the cooler venous blood returning from the periphery. Arteries and veins course through the body in juxtaposition to each other. Normally, as warm blood flows toward the periphery, it passes by the cooler blood in veins, which are in juxtaposition to the arteries. There is a countercurrent heat exchange between the warmer arterial blood and the cooler venous blood. After an area is heated, the vasodilation of arterioles allows cooler blood to rush into the area and carry away the heat. Cold causes a vasoconstriction of arterioles, decreasing the amount of warm blood flowing into the area. Thus, countercurrent heat exchange is reduced, and the area may not rewarm very rapidly. When ice packs were applied around the knee of a dog for 1 hour, it took longer than 60 minutes after removal of the cold source before tissue temperature returned to resting values.[8] When hot packs were applied for the same duration, temperature rose to peak within 15 minutes, and then began to decline. The hot packs caused a vasodilation, allowing cooler blood to flow into the area, dissipating heat. As long as the heat being added was greater than that being carried away, the temperature remained elevated. After the heat source was removed, heat was rapidly lost by convection and radiation.

Intramuscular temperature of the gastrocnemius muscle remained lowered for at least 3 hours following 20 minutes of cold baths at 10°C for at least 4 hours following a 30-minute cold bath at 10°C[10] and for at least 1.5 hours following 20 minutes of ice packs.[11] The level of activity can also influence the return of temperature to precooling levels. If exercise is performed following cooling, this will facilitate an increase of blood flow to the area, resulting in a faster rate of rewarming.

The form in which cold therapy is applied (e.g., ice or cold-water baths) may contribute to the degree of cooling. The magnitude of temperature change would be expected to be greater when ice packs are used, compared with cold-water baths or frozen gel packs. Quadriceps muscle temperature in dogs was reduced by 11.3°C following 1 hour of chipped ice, compared with a decrease of 8.4°C when gel packs were applied for the same amount of time.[12] The ice may be more effective in cooling an area because of the amount of internal energy required to melt the ice, that is, to break apart the solid bonding forces of the ice molecules. The internal energy is used first to change the ice to water before raising its temperature.[1]

Evaporation

Vapocoolant sprays use evaporation as a means of energy transfer. Vapocoolant sprays, such as Fluori-Methane and Ethyl Chloride (Gebauer Company, Cleveland, OH) are volatile liquids that are bottled under pressure and are emitted in fine sprays when the bottles are inverted. As the liquid comes out of the bottle, it begins to evaporate. When this transition occurs, the steam cools and, upon contact with the skin, extracts heat. The vapocoolant spray feels colder than room-temperature water sprayed on the skin because, like alcohol, it evaporates more quickly than water. The spray is applied for only a few sweeps across the skin. Skin temperature can drop to about 15°C, with negligible changes in subcutaneous tissue and muscle temperatures.[13] The use of fluorocarbons was banned by the Clean Air Act of 1990. However, in accordance with an exception to the ban on chlorofluorocarbons, granted by the U. S. Environmental Protection Agency to Gebauer, Fluori-Methane may continue to be sold and distributed by Gebauer for use in clinical practice. [40 CFR Ch. 1 # 82.66(d)(2)(iv)(7-1-95)]

BIOPHYSICAL PRINCIPLES OF TISSUE COOLING

Many of the clinical uses of cold are predicated on the physiologic changes resulting from tissue-temperature reduction. Cold is used in the management of acute trauma, because (1) the resulting arteriolar vasoconstriction reduces bleeding; (2) the decrease in metabolism and vasoactive agents (e.g., histamine) reduces inflammation and outward fluid filtration; and (3) elevation of the pain threshold affords the patient more comfort. A reduction in skeletal muscle spasm can be postulated to be an interplay of factors, including a decrease in pain and a decrease in sensitivity of muscle-spindle–afferent fibers to discharge. Spasticity can be temporarily diminished owing to a decrease in the sensitivity of the muscle spindle to stretch. Muscle performance may be temporarily enhanced following short-duration cold. Pain, and perhaps joint inflammation in certain inflammatory rheumatic diseases, can be decreased. But some patients may experience an increase in joint stiffness secondary to the effect of cold on increasing tissue viscosity and decreasing tissue elasticity. When tissue viscosity is increased, and elasticity is decreased, the resistance to motion increases.

Hemodynamic Effects

When cold is applied, the immediate response is vasoconstriction of cutaneous blood vessels and reduction in blood flow. The amount of blood flow to an area is inversely proportional to the resistance factors impeding flow. Vessel diameter is the most significant factor relating to blood flow. Any influence that will cause vascular smooth muscle to contract will reduce vessel diameter (i.e., vasoconstriction). Conversely, when smooth muscle tone decreases, as happens with heating, vessel diameter increases (i.e., vasodilation).

Generally, exposure to cold for a short time (15 minutes or less) results in vasoconstriction of arterioles and venules. The mechanism of action causing vasoconstriction involves an interplay of factors, including the direct action of cold on smooth muscle[15] and a reflex cutaneous vasoconstriction.[16] Figure 4–2 summarizes how flow microcirculation is affected by cold application.

The blood flow to skin is primarily under neural control and plays an important role in thermoregulation.[16] Vasoconstriction of cutaneous vessels occurs as part of the heat-retention mechanisms of the body. When skin temperature is lowered, cold thermal sensors (free nerve endings) in the skin are stimulated, causing a reflex excitation of sympathetic adrenergic fibers. Increased activity of these fibers causes vasoconstriction. This reflex vasoconstriction can also result in a generalized cutaneous vasoconstriction. The blood-flow decrease is greatest in the area that is directly cooled. For example, blood flow in a hand cooled in ice water changed from a resting value of 16 mL/100 mL/min down to 2 mL/100 mL/min (Fig. 4–3).[17] Contralateral changes resulting from generalized cutaneous vasoconstriction were less pronounced.

As cooled blood returns to the general circulation, it stimulates the heat-conserva-

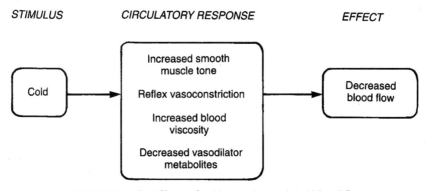

FIGURE 4–2. Effects of cold stimulus on local blood flow.

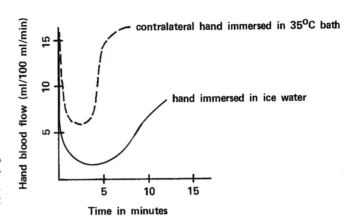

FIGURE 4–3. Blood flow to the hands following ice water immersion of one hand. (Adapted from Folkow, et al.[16])

tion area in the preoptic region of the anterior hypothalamus. Stimulation of this area will result in further reflex cutaneous vasoconstriction. If a large area of the body is cooled, shivering will occur as a heat-retaining mechanism.

Decreases in joint blood flow have also been demonstrated following cold application.[18] Ten minutes of ice packs at 0°C to the knee joints of dogs resulted in decreases in resting blood flow averaging 56%. The flow returned to precooled values approximately 25 minutes after the cold was removed.

In part, the viscosity of blood determines resistance to blood flow. If viscosity increases, so does resistance to blood flow. The increase in blood viscosity resulting from cold exposure contributes to the decrease in blood flow (Fig. 4–2).

When tissue temperature reduction is maintained for a long time, or when temperature is reduced below 10°C, a cold-induced vasodilation can follow the initial period of vasoconstriction. This phenomenon was first recognized and reported by Lewis[18] in 1930. He found that when fingers were immersed in an ice bath, skin temperature decreased during the first 15 minutes. This reduction was followed by cyclic periods of increasing and decreasing temperature, which Lewis correlated with vasodilation and vasoconstriction, respectively. During the cycling periods, temperatures never returned to near-preimmersion values. This cycling was termed the "hunting response" and was felt by Lewis to be mediated by activity within an axon reflex. As skin was cooled to less than 10°C, pain would result, causing afferent sensory impulses to be carried antidromically toward skin arterioles. An unidentified neurotransmitter, termed substance "H," similar in action to histamine, was hypothesized to be released, resulting in arteriolar vasodilation. As warm blood came into the area and elevated temperature above 10°C, the ice bath was again effective in causing a vasoconstriction. The "hunting response" appears to occur predominantly in apical areas, where arteriovenous (AV) anastomoses are located in the skin.[19,20]

Cold vasodilation can also occur without the hunting (cycling) component. Clarke and associates[2] cooled human forearms at a temperature of 1°C. A marked increase in blood flow to three to four times the precooled values occurred after 15 minutes of immersion. Only a slight increase in blood flow was noted with temperatures at 10°C. This cold vasodilation was thought to be a deep response, probably in skeletal muscles, and was assumed to be local, because no reflex changes were noted in the contralateral extremity.

TABLE 4–2 Effects of Cryotherapy on Microcirculation in Rats

	⊖ Contusion ⊖ Cryotherapy	⊕ Contusion ⊖ Cryotherapy	⊖ Contusion ⊕ Cryotherapy	⊕ Contusion ⊕ Cryotherapy
Diameter of arteriole	Unchanged	Increased	Unchanged	Increased
Diameter of venule	Unchanged	Unchanged	Increased	Increased

Source: Adapted from Smith et al.[21]

Alterations in the microcirculation of rats in response to cryotherapy was studied by Smith and associates.[21] Ice cubes were placed against the skin of rats for 20 minutes; this treatment was initiated 24 hours after contusion. The authors found that there was an increase in the diameter of the arterioles following the contusion, but that there was no further change in arteriolar size in response to cryotherapy. Conversely, there was no change in the diameter of the venules following injury, but there was a significant increase in the size of the venules in response to cryotherapy (Table 4–2). The results of the study suggest that the increase in the diameter of the venules allows for greater fluid reabsorption, thus providing an additional mechanism to reduce edema.

There has been much speculation and investigation over the ensuing years to clarify the causes of cold vasodilation. In addition to activation of an axon reflex, some researchers feel that cooling to less than 10°C can inhibit myogenic activity of smooth muscle[2,22] or reduce the sensitivity of blood vessels to catecholamines,[16] thus causing vasodilation.

Post-traumatic Edema and Inflammation

For the first 24 to 48 hours following injury, cold is usually the thermal agent of choice. The rationale for its use includes: (1) less fluid filtration into the interstitium, owing to vasoconstriction; (2) less inflammation and less pain; and (3) a decrease in metabolic rate. Knight[23] hypothesizes that the efficacy of cold for the care of acute injuries is because of the reduction in metabolism and, thus, a decrease in secondary hypoxic injury. The choice of cold has largely been based on empiric evidence. The length of cold exposure and the temperature can have significant effects on tissue swelling. (Some animal laboratory studies are discussed in this section, while clinical reports will be presented subsequently under "Clinical Indications for Cryotherapy.")

In most of the animal experiments, trauma was induced through some type of crushing force, resulting in soft-tissue damage or fracture. Cold was then applied for varying lengths of time. Matsen and colleagues[24] used ice bags following tibial fractures in rabbits. Animals treated with ice, at temperatures ranging from 5°C to 15°C for 24 hours and at 10°C for 6 hours, had more swelling than control limbs. The swelling in a group cooled at 20°C to 25°C did not differ from that of the control group. This study suggests that application of more intense cold immediately postinjury resulted in greater edema formation when compared to the control group and to the group exposed to less intense cold. Although the study failed to show the beneficial effects of cold postinjury, it did show that less intense cold had no deleterious effects.

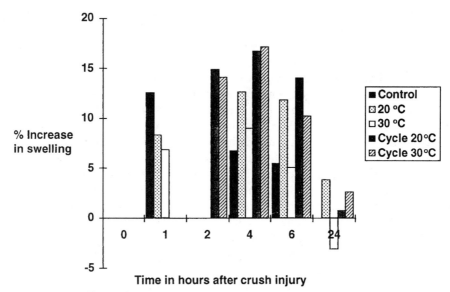

FIGURE 4–4. The effects of cold immersion on postcrush injury swelling in rabbits. Cycling consisted of three consecutive cycles of 1-hour immersion, 1-hour no immersion, 1-hour immersion. (Adapted from McMaster and Liddle.[24])

Four different protocols were given by McMaster and Liddle[25] to treat crush injuries to rabbit forelimbs. The protocols included limb immersion in: (1) 20°C water bath for 1 hour; (2) 30°C water bath for 1 hour; (3) 20°C water bath for 1 hour in, 1 hour out, 1 hour in; and (4) 30°C water bath for 1 hour in, 1 hour out, 1 hour in. Results are detailed in Figure 4–4. It is interesting to note that both groups treated at 20°C had greater residual edema at 24 hours postinjury than did the control group. It would have been interesting to see the results if compression wraps had been applied to all groups after immersion in the baths. Results supported Matsen and colleagues'[24] findings that more intense cold increased the amount of swelling. Cycling also appeared to result in greater edema formation. In this study less intense cold (immersion at 30°C) generally resulted in less swelling compared to that of the control group.

Jezdinsky and associates[26] also gave prolonged cold for 2, 5, 7, and 10 hours, with a constantly maintained temperature of 11.5°C to 12.5°C for postcrush edema in the rat. They reported a slight tendency for increased edema in the cold-treated animals. In a later group of experiments from the same laboratory,[27] the degree of cooling was less. Cold compresses at an initial temperature of 15°C to 18°C were applied to traumatized rat paws and were changed at 30-minute intervals. Tissue cooling was probably not as great as with the first set of experiments,[26] because the compresses increased in temperature during each 30-minute period. There was no apparent reactive hyperemia after the compresses, as was reported after constant cold of 11.5°C to 12.5°C. Also, there was less tendency for edema formation if cold was applied at 2 hours posttrauma rather than immediately postinjury.

Tissue cooling was probably not as great as with the first set of experiments, as evidenced by the absence of reactive hyperemia when using cold compresses. In the first experiment, constant temperature was maintained throughout the cold application, whereas in the latter experiment, the temperature of the compresses increased during the 30-minute interval.

Postapplication edema was also measured in each of the Jezdinsky experiments. When used 1 hour after injury, the cold compresses showed a reduction in edema formation when applied for a period of 4 hours. In all other cases there was an increase in edema formation after the removal of the cold stimulus.[26,27] It is important to note that the edema formation was less pronounced with less intense cold (cold compresses) and occurred later when the treatment was given 2 hours postinjury.

No attempt was made by the investigators previously described to correlate changes in tissue swelling with inflammatory exudates. Farry and Prentice[28] applied crushed-ice packs to treat experimentally induced radiocarpal ligament sprains in pigs. Cold was given for 20 minutes, followed by a 1-hour rest period, followed by another 20 minutes of cold. This protocol was probably similar to actual clinical practice. Even though the cold produced an increased swelling in subcutaneous tissues, there was histologic evidence of decreased inflammation. Only 1 of the 20 treated limbs had signs of a pronounced inflammatory response (that is, numerous polymorphonuclear leukocytes, plasma cells, lymphocytes, and fibrinous exudate). All others had either no inflammatory cells or occasional to moderate amounts of polymorphs and lymphocytes.

For the most part, the animal studies showed an increase or no change in the amount of swelling after cold application. The increase in edema could have been caused by cold-induced vasodilation or thermal damage as a result of prolonged or intense cold exposures. Although these studies did not appear to support the theory that cold prevents or reduces edema, there was some evidence to suggest that the extent of the injury and application parameters, such as temperature, type of application, duration and timing of the initiation of treatment, have some bearing on the outcomes of the studies. Further research is warranted regarding these parameters, as well as use of cold in conjunction with compression and elevation.

Effects on Peripheral Nerves

Cold can alter the conduction velocity and synaptic activity of peripheral nerves. If the temperature of the nerve is decreased, there will be a corresponding decrease in sensory and motor-conduction velocities, or even a failure of the nerve to conduct impulses. Synaptic transmission can be impeded or blocked. The quantity of the change elicited depends on the duration and the degree of the temperature alteration.

Isolated cat nerves of various diameters and degrees of myelination were found to have different thresholds or sensitivities to cold stimuli.[29] Changes in nerve conduction velocity were observed first in small-diameter myelinated fibers. The fibers least sensitive to cold were small-diameter unmyelinated fibers. In the cat saphenous nerve (afferent) cooling blocked conduction in A fibers, and additional cooling was necessary before conduction in C fibers was blocked. Further examination showed that conduction in smaller diameter A fibers (A delta fibers) was affected, while conduction in those with the largest diameter (A alpha fibers) was affected last. When the motor fibers of the sciatic nerve of cats were isolated and cooled, conduction was eliminated in the gamma fibers before the alpha fibers.

Cold can decrease nerve-conduction velocity. Motor-conduction velocity of the ulnar nerve after cold application has been investigated by two groups of researchers.[30,31] Following his study of 5 minutes of cold to the elbow, Zankel[30] recorded an average of a 6% decrease in motor-conduction velocity in eight out of ten subjects. In those eight, conduction velocity returned to precooled values within 15 minutes. Zankel[30] postulated that cold can alter the rate of transmembrane ionic flow.

With longer durations of cold, a greater decrease in temperature and conduction velocity was predicted. Ice packs over the ulnar nerve for 20 minutes resulted in an average decrease in motor-conduction velocity of 29.4% from precooling values.[29] Thirty minutes after the ice packs were removed, the conduction velocity was still 8.3% lower than before ice application, suggesting a long-lasting effect when ice is given for a longer duration than in the experiment of Zankel.[30] One group of investigators could find no direct correlation between percentage of body fat and velocity or temperature changes.[31] Lee et al.[31] predicted that a greater decrease in temperature and in conduction velocity occurred with longer durations of cold.

Li[32] demonstrated in the rat that neuromuscular synaptic transmission was impeded when temperature dropped as low as 15°C, and that it was blocked at 5°C. The peripheral nerve stopped conducting impulses at 4°C.

Cryotherapy resulted in four cases of neurapraxia and one of axonotmesis, in young athletes.[33] The ice packs were applied either over a major nerve branch that was superficially located (for example, over the peroneal nerve at the lateral border of the knee) or around the thigh for up to two hours (as in the case of axonotmesis). One hour of cryotherapy (on two occasions) around the knee of a male patient following a hamstring strain was reported as causing an axonotmesis of the peroneal nerve.[34]

Muscle Strength

Thermal agents can affect the ability of a muscle to generate tension. The effects of cold applied prior to muscle contraction and applied after muscle fatigue have been examined. Most studies were limited to addressing only isometric strength.

McGown[35] measured isometric strength of the quadriceps before and after 5 minutes of ice massage to the entire anterior thigh of normal subjects. After icing, there was an increase in strength compared with pretest values and with changes in the control group. There was no reported follow-up to examine further whether strength changed over time. Because muscle temperature was not expected to be lowered with such a short period of ice massage over the large muscle mass, the author felt the increase in strength may have been brought about by increased muscle blood flow via sympathetic nerve activity changes. In addition, those who received ice could have been psychologically motivated to perform better posttest.

One other possible explanation for the observed increases could have been a result of the effect of short-duration cold on motor nerve excitability.[36] Facilitation of a single motor unit was seen after 1 to 2 minutes of icing over the biceps brachii muscle of healthy human subjects.[37]

When the duration of cold exposure is lengthened, muscle temperature can be expected to decrease. Following cold immersion of normal legs for 30 minutes at 10°C to 12°C, Oliver and associates[9] found that muscle temperature and plantarflexion strength decreased. This decrease could have been the result of reduced muscle blood flow at these lowered temperatures or of an increase in the viscous properties of the muscle. At 45 minutes postimmersion, plantarflexion strength began to increase over pretreatment values and continued to do so for the next 3 hours (Fig. 4–5).

The findings of Johnson and Leider[38] were similar to those of Oliver.[9] Following 30 minutes of immersion of the hand and forearm in a bath of 10°C to 15°C, grip

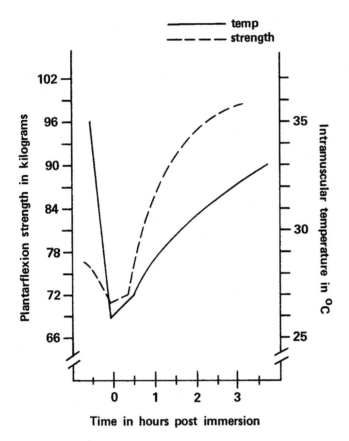

FIGURE 4–5. Plantarflexion strength and intramuscular temperature measurements postcold immersion at 10°C. (Adapted from Oliver, et al.[9])

strength was decreased for up to 1 hour, then increased over the pretest values for the next 2 hours.

Neither Johnson and Leider[38] nor Oliver[9] carried out posttest measurements past 3 hours. Therefore, time to recovery of the pretest values is not known. Also, both groups only tested one repetition of isometric strength at each interval. This paradigm is not representative of a therapy setting in which a patient often is expected to perform multiple repetitions within a few minutes. On the other hand, Clarke[39] reported that cold baths at 10°C following fatiguing isometric exercise did not alter the period of recovery.

The fact that cold can change muscle strength can have important implications when evaluating patients and carrying out treatment plans. Short-duration cold could perhaps be used to enhance muscle performance during a therapy program, thus maximizing muscle performance. Because cold can change muscle strength, caution should be taken when performing initial and follow-up evaluations on patients during a therapy program. Strength evaluation should be done before cold application to that muscle and not for at least a few hours after cooling.

Neuromuscular Effects

Spasticity limits a person's ability to carry out purposeful movements at the varying speeds required to perform activities of daily living. Spasticity is associated with an increased resistance to passive stretch, increased deep-tendon reflexes, and clonus. Many therapeutic agents and regimens are used to reduce spasticity. Cryotherapy can temporarily reduce spasticity. Although the mechanisms responsible for the changes seen have not been fully elucidated, many animal and human studies have been designed to clarify and provide a rationale for these observed responses.

Eldred and associates[40] directly cooled the gastrocnemius muscle in cats and recorded the discharge of muscle spindle primary (Ia) and secondary (II) sensory endings and Golgi-tendon organs (GTOs). The muscle spindles were de-efferented in these experiments. As the muscle temperature dropped from 38°C to 28°C, there was a linear decrease in the frequency of discharge of Ia and II afferents. GTO discharge decreased by approximately 50%. Between temperatures of 25°C and 20°C, firing became irregular and, in some instances, ceased altogether.

Newton and Lehmkuhl[41] also directly cooled cat gastrocnemius muscles. Recordings from dorsal-root filaments revealed a decrease in action-potential firing when muscle was cooled to 25°C. This finding indicated a decrease in muscle-spindle–afferent fiber discharge secondary to cooling. The method of cold application may have an effect on axonal discharge in cutaneous sensory afferents. Differences may occur with direct cooling of an isolated muscle rather than with transcutaneous cold application. Cold packs were applied for 20 minutes to the calves of healthy humans by Knuttson and Mattsson.[36] Skin temperature dropped abruptly (by as much as 25°C) within the first few minutes, and the H response increased in amplitude. This increase in H amplitude suggested facilitation of alpha motoneuron activity by short-duration cold. The amplitude of the Achilles tendon reflex (ATR) decreased shortly after the cold was started and continued to do so during the 20-minute period. Because the ATR amplitude decreased before the intramuscular temperature fell, the changes in muscular activity could be explained by a reflex reaction to the activation of cutaneous afferent nerve fibers. The amplitude of the ATR continued to decrease as the muscle temperature dropped. Therefore, changes in the muscle-spindle sensitivity after cooling also could have contributed to the overall response of the ATR.

Another finding by Eldred and associates[40] was a decrease in monosynaptic reflexes following cooling of the gastrocnemius muscle in cats. Wolf and Letbetter[42] also examined the effects of short-duration cold stimulus on spontaneous electromyogram (EMG) activity of decerebrate cats. Cold was applied to the skin overlying the gastrocnemius muscle. EMG activity and subcutaneous and muscle temperature were recorded. Rigidity, as measured by integrated EMG activity, decreased within 1 to 5 seconds after the skin was cooled. The decrease in muscle temperature was not as great as that predicted to change muscle-spindle-afferent activity. Therefore, Wolf and Letbetter[42] concluded that a change in cutaneous afferent firing through reflex mechanisms produced a decrease in skeletal muscle activity.

Ten patients with spasticity were studied by Hartvikksen.[11] Iced towels placed over the calf for 20 minutes resulted in the elimination of both the ATR and clonus. A decrease in ATR activity was seen after 3 to 5 minutes, too soon for these changes to be attributed to a drop in intramuscular temperature. This suggested that early activation of skin receptors in response to cold produced a reflex decrease in gamma motoneuron activity. These findings were supported by those of Mecomber and Herman,[43] who also reported a decreased tendon jerk response before a drop in intramuscular temperature.

Hartvikksen[11] recorded a decrease in muscle temperature after 10 minutes of cooling. After removal of the cold stimulus, no ATR was observed for approximately 1 hour, and no return of clonus was observed for 2 hours. The initial elimination of the ATR and clonus was attributed to stimulation of skin receptors, while the more prolonged effects were attributed to the sensitivity of muscle spindles to cold.

Two studies by Miglietta[44,45] investigated the effects of cold on sustained ankle clonus in neurologically involved patients. Cold whirlpool baths at 18.3°C were given to 15 patients with ankle clonus. After 15 minutes the clonus was either decreased or abolished and remained so for 4 to 5 hours.[44]

In the second study both clonus and muscle twitch time in 40 patients with spasticity were examined.[45] Cold baths at 7°C were given for 10, 20, or 30 minutes, and clonus frequency and twitch contractions were recorded before and after each exposure. In contrast to previously stated findings, the majority of the subjects (87%) did not demonstrate the absence of clonus until 30 minutes of cold immersion, well after the demonstrated decrease in intramuscular temperature. A prolonged muscle twitch time appeared after 10 minutes and continued to increase with longer durations of cold exposure. Because the onset of the prolonged muscle contraction time occurred prior to a decrease in intramuscular temperature, the author concluded that the duration of muscle twitch and the frequency of clonus in response to cold were not related.

Knuttsson[46] used 15 minutes of cold packs to the upper extremity, or 20 minutes to the lower extremity, of patients with spasticity. Ten out of 15 patients had a decrease in resistance to passive motion, two had no change, and three had an increase. Clonus decreased in frequency, duration, and threshold in all patients who had displayed it initially. Voluntary range of motion improved in two thirds of those who had reduced range of motion.

Urbscheit and associates[47] reported inconsistent findings following cooling of the calf of patients with hemiplegia for 12 to 20 minutes. H responses and ATRs were measured. In addition to having no consistent changes among the patients in H response and ATR, the patients' uninvolved side often responded differently than the involved side. This finding points out that the change in spasticity following cold cannot always be accurately predicted. The underlying pathophysiology of the spasticity must be considered in predicting the responses to cold.

In many patients with spasticity, cold application can temporarily decrease the amplitude of deep-tendon reflexes (DTR) and the frequency of clonus and can improve the patient's ability to participate in therapy programs. Cold facilitates alpha-motoneuron activity and decreases gamma-motoneuron firing. In order for spasticity to be reduced, the reduction in gamma activity should be proportionally greater than the increase in alpha activity. In summary, spasticity reduction with cold may occur through at least two mechanisms: (1) a reflex decrease in gamma-motoneuron activity through stimulation of cutaneous afferents and (2) a decrease in afferent-spindle discharge by direct cooling of the muscle.

CLINICAL INDICATIONS FOR CRYOTHERAPY

Most clinicians will agree that in the acute states (24 to 48 hours) following trauma, cold should be the thermal agent of choice. Even though cold may be uncomfortable for the patient during the first few minutes, pain will ultimately be reduced, and edema, inflammation, and muscle spasm will most likely be lessened. Beyond the acute phase of injury, heat may be the first agent for treatment. But in many cases, cold has been a successful part of a therapeutic regimen to reduce spasticity, facilitate muscle contractions, reduce joint pain caused by arthritis, and lessen muscle spasm.

Musculoskeletal Trauma

One of the most common applications of cryotherapy is for musculoskeletal trauma or postorthopedic surgical swelling and pain. One of the earliest clinical reports supporting cold therapy for edema control and pain management appeared in 1946.[48] A comparison was made between two groups of patients who had undergone a variety of orthopedic procedures. One group ($n = 479$) had no ice packs, while the other ($n = 345$) had ice bags over their soft casts for a 48-hour period. Even though the cooling period was prolonged, the decrease in tissue temperature was probably minimal, owing to the cast interference between the ice pack and the skin.

The group treated with ice packs required less splitting of casts (5.31%) compared with that of the noniced group (41.3%). In addition to the benefit of less swelling, the ice-treated group had less inflammation, as evidenced by a lower white blood cell count, and fewer elevated temperatures. None of the experimental group had apparent hematomas or hemarthrosis, compared with 16 of those in the group receiving no ice. Fewer narcotics were taken by those who were ice treated, indicating that their pain was less. Reduction of analgesic intake following cold also has been reported by others.[49]

For acute trauma, cold is most often used in conjunction with compression and elevation. Most of the animal studies discussed under the heading of "Biophysical Effects" failed to show edema reduction or prevention in response to cryotherapy. However, these studies did not incorporate the use of either compression or elevation. Basur and associates[50] looked at a more common clinical model by comparing cold and compression with compression alone in patients with ankle sprains. One group of patients received cold packs once every 4 hours followed by application of a compression wrap bandage. The mean period of disability for patients treated with cold and compression was 9.7 days, compared with 14.8 days for those who received compression only, and swelling was better controlled in the group receiving cold.

Two groups of researchers investigated cold and compression for the postoperative management of patients with total knee arthroplasty (TKA).[51,52] Levy and Marmar[51] measured pain relief, swelling, blood loss, and range of motion (ROM) in 80 patients who underwent unilateral or bilateral TKA. The patients received either compression alone or combined cold and compression, provided by a commercially manufactured inflatable cuff filled with ice water. Those patients who received cold and compression had less pain, less swelling, and a lesser degree of blood loss, while demonstrating a greater increase in ROM. These findings supported those of Basur and associates,[50] in that a greater reduction in swelling was seen in groups receiving some type of cryotherapy.

Healy and associates[52] compared types of cold compressive dressings applied to 105 knees of 76 patients after TKA. A commercially available cuff, consisting of an inflatable bladder filled with ice water, was used for one group of subjects; the control group was treated with elastic bandage wraps and ice packs. Knee ROM, swelling, narcotic requirements, and wound drainage were measured. There were no significant differences between the groups for any of the variables. Both studies advocated the use of cold-compressive dressings for the postoperative treatment of TKA, but the type of cold-compressive dressing did not appear to make any significant difference.

The duration of cold and the extent of the resultant temperature drop are important in the final outcome. To lessen risk of thermal damage or an increase in limb volume during acute or postoperative phases, the nature of the cold treatment must be taken into consideration. Less intense cold applied for durations of 20 to 30 minutes several times a day, in conjunction with elevation and compression, appears to be a logical choice.

If cold is applied for edema or pain control over casts or bandages, the application time is usually longer than when cold is applied on the bare extremity. Kaempffe[53] recorded a reduction of 3.5°C when cold gel packs were applied for 60 minutes to upper extremities casted with plaster and with fiberglass. Maximal temperature reduction occurred by 12 minutes over the plaster cast and by 40 minutes over the fiberglass. It should be noted, however, that in Kaempffe's work the casts were allowed to dry for 72 hours before the study. Temperature changes may be different during the initial hours after cast application, particularly over plaster, when an exothermic reaction of the plaster may occur.

Although intuition might lead us to believe that cold rather than heat, during the early phases postinjury, would lead to a faster recovery, this comparison was not reported until 1982 by Hocutt and associates.[54] One group of patients with ankle sprains was treated with superficial heating agents 1 to 3 times a day for 15 minutes and wore elastic bandage wraps within the first 36 hours postinjury. Other ankle-sprain patients had cold whirlpools of 7°C to 10°C or ice packs for the same duration and frequency as the heat-treated group. A third group of patients was seen after 36 hours and treated with cold. Treatment was continued for a minimum of 3 days among all patients. The patients treated with early cold (within the first 36 hours) returned to full activity (running and jumping without pain) an average of 8 days before the other two groups. Therefore, the time at which thermotherapy is initiated following trauma can be expected to influence the time course for functional outcome.

As sequelae to trauma, skeletal-muscle spasm and pain limit mobility and function. Many therapeutic techniques, including thermal agents, electrical stimulation, and massage, are given with the common goals of reducing pain and muscle spasm, thus facilitating a more expedient recovery to normal function. In addition, many of these agents could be given in lieu of pain medication. Patients easily can be instructed in the use of cold packs or ice massage at home for control of pain and muscle spasm.

Cooling the skin can elevate the pain threshold[55] and reduce pain by acting as a counterirritant.[56] The proposed mechanism by which counterirritation influences pain perception is based on the gate control theory.[57] Stimulation of thermal receptors in the skin by either heat or cold results in a lessening of pain sensation by hypothetically overriding or bypassing pain signals. During acute episodes of tendinitis or bursitis, severe pain can limit motion and ultimately lead to joint stiffness, if there are no interventions. Therapeutic interventions are aimed at reducing pain and inflammation and maintaining or increasing ROM. Lane[58] reported on a patient with bicipital tendinitis who regained full, pain-free ROM after four treatments with ice massage.

Cryokinetics (cold and exercise) was a technique popularized in the 1960s by Hayden[59] and Grant.[60] Hayden wrote about a group of 1000 military patients who sustained sprains, strains, and contusions during training. Ice massage or ice-water immersion was used to provide analgesia before ROM exercises. All but three of the patients returned to active duty within 2 days; most of them required only one physical therapy treatment. Of the 700 patients reported by Grant,[60] 80% had no more than three formal treatments with ice massage. Both Grant[60] and Hayden[59] cite that ice massage and exercise have the additional advantage of allowing patients to be more easily instructed in self-treatment.

Cold in combination with static stretch or contract-relax techniques has been recommended for reducing muscle spasm or decreasing exercise-induced muscle soreness, thus increasing ROM. Cold is applied over the painful muscle using ice massage, ice packs, or iced towels. Either during or immediately following the cold application, the exercise is carried out with the idea of returning the muscle to its normal resting length. Knight[23] suggests that, when cold is used in conjunction with exercise, the area is first cooled, followed by exercise (active or passive stretch). This cycle is then repeated.

Prentice[61] induced muscle soreness in normal subjects through fatiguing concentric and eccentric contraction of the hamstrings. The following day, EMG activity of the exercised muscle was increased from the preexercise measurement. EMG activity was measured as an indicator of muscle pain and spasm.[62] Following 20 minutes of cold packs and static stretch to the hamstrings, EMG activity was reduced, suggesting a decrease in muscle soreness and spasm. Cold application, followed by a proprioceptive neuromuscular facilitation (PNF) technique, slow-reversal-hold, was done with another group. This technique was also successful in reducing EMG activity. These techniques were compared with an untreated control group and two groups who were given hot packs and static stretch or PNF. Those who received cold had less measured EMG activity.

With 15 minutes of ice massage only, pain and ROM did not improve in subjects with exercise-induced soreness in the biceps.[63] No stretching or other form of exercise was given. The combination of ice and exercise may successfully decrease muscle soreness. The cold may be used to reduce the pain, thus permitting stretching to be carried out. In addition, cooling of 10 or more minutes may reduce muscle temperature and decrease the sensitivity of the muscle spindle to stretch.

A series of patients with low back pain was studied by Landen.[64] Patients with chronic pain (an onset of greater than 2 weeks' pretreatment) received ice massage or hot packs followed by flexion exercises. Those patients who were treated with ice had a significantly shorter hospitalization period than did those treated with heat—an average of 6.27 days compared with 9.29 days, respectively. Interestingly enough, however, those patients classified as acute had a shorter hospitalization when given hot packs instead of ice massage, an average of 4.08 days compared with 5.53 days, respectively.

CASE STUDY 1

A 55-year-old man sustained a severe left ankle sprain while jogging 5 weeks ago. He was immobilized in an ankle stirrup brace splint for 4 weeks and used crutches to reduce weight bearing. He progressed to using a cane but is not yet bearing full weight on the left. There was no evidence of bony abnormalities or neurological involvement. He would like to be able to walk without an assistive device and eventually return to jogging.

PROBLEMS

1. Swelling on the anterior and lateral aspects of the ankle.
2. Pain with weight bearing and with active and passive motion.
3. Limited ankle motion.
4. Abnormal gait.

ASSESSMENT TECHNIQUES

1. Volume measurement of left foot and ankle.
2. Pain quantity, quality, and location.
3. ROM measurements.
4. Strength measurements of muscles of ankle.
5. Functional activities assessment, including gait.

GOALS

1. Decrease swelling and maintain the reduction.
2. Reduce pain.
3. Increase range of motion of the ankle.
4. Increase strength of the ankle musculature.
5. Improve gait to normal.
6. Increase functional activities.

SELECTION OF TREATMENT MODALITY

Cryotherapy—Cold Whirlpool

Whirlpool at 65°F for a duration of 15 minutes was used for four treatments. This allowed for active ankle exercise, while the immersion in cold water decreased pain. Although the treatment was issued with the extremity in a dependent position, swelling did not increase, perhaps because of simultaneous cold and exercise.

Following the whirlpool treatment, the patient was given an elastic compressive garment for the ankle and proceeded with stretching exercises, active exercises, and isometric strengthening exercises. With reduction in pain and swelling, the patient was able to progress to ambulation without an assistive device, but he required an ankle stirrup brace to increase stability and maintain pain reduction with extended distances.

Cold whirlpool was no longer necessary after the initial four treatments. For occasional exacerbations of pain after prolonged exercise, the patient was instructed to use a cold pack to decrease the pain and prevent an increase in swelling.

HOME PROGRAM

This patient should be instructed to use a cold pack at home, as needed, whenever he notes increased swelling or pain. Active exercises and passive stretching should be carried out on a daily basis. In order to prepare for jogging, a gradual increase in the amount of weight-bearing exercises and activities is advisable. The written home program should include clear, concise instructions regarding the number of repetitions, frequency and method for safely increasing activities.

RATIONALE FOR CLINICAL DECISION MAKING

Because pain and swelling appeared to be the primary problems initially, these areas need to be addressed first. A decrease in ROM and strength is expected following immobilization. ROM is further affected by pain and swelling. Cold whirlpool addresses the pain and allows concurrent motion. The only disadvantage is the dependent position of the ankle during treatment, which potentially could promote increased edema, but in this case the potential swelling was offset by active exercise during treatment. The decrease in strength was primarily caused by disuse, and regaining strength is not expected to be a problem, although progress may be limited by pain.

Myofascial Pain Syndrome

Myofascial pain syndrome is defined as "pain and/or autonomic phenomena referred from active myofascial trigger points with associated dysfunction."[13] The dysfunction can be manifested as decreased ROM in the area of the myofascial trigger point or area of referred pain. A trigger point in muscle may result from muscular strain and may be associated with sensitized nerves, increased metabolism, and decreased circulation. Trigger points also are thought to be present in skin, ligaments, and fascia.

The pioneering work in trigger-point localization and therapy was done by Janet Travell, MD. She had designated active and latent trigger points. Active points are associated with a decrease in motion and moderate to severe pain. With latent trigger points, the person may have restricted ROM, but pain is present only on palpation. Trigger points can be located by digital pressure and electronic point locators such as the Neuroprobe (Physio Technology, Inc., Topeka, KS). Trigger points can be treated using a variety of techniques, including stretch and spray, ice massage, deep pressure, ultrasound, electrical stimulation, and low-power laser. The choice of treatment seems to be based upon empiricism.

Common areas of trigger points can be around the cervical spine, shoulder girdle, and low back. Poor body mechanics and faulty posture are probably contributing forces. Therefore, in addition to cryotherapy techniques, a complete therapeutic program should include postural exercises and instruction in proper body mechanics.

CASE STUDY 2

A 32-year-old graduate student reports to physical therapy with complaints of right-sided scapular pain, neck pain, and occasional radiating pain to the right arm. There was no history of injury or previous pain in the area. Over the past 4 months the pain has worsened to such a degree that it is interfering with studying, working on the computer, and, most recently, sleeping. The student is concerned about falling behind in her studies.

PROBLEMS

1. Pain with prolonged sitting (more than 30 minutes) and when carrying books.
2. Exquisite tenderness to palpation over the levator scapulae on the right.
3. Decreased ROM of neck motions, primarily rotation and side bending.
4. Forward head posture with rounded shoulders in sitting.
5. Limited functional activities and increased difficulty sleeping.

ASSESSMENT TECHNIQUES

1. Pain quantity, quality, and location.
2. ROM measurements.
3. Strength measurements of scapular muscles.
4. Postural assessment.
5. Functional daily activities assessment.

GOALS

1. Reduce pain.
2. No abnormal tenderness to palpation.
3. Increase ROM of the neck.
4. Increase strength of the scapular muscles.
5. Improve sitting posture.
6. Increase functional activities.

SELECTION OF TREATMENT MODALITY

Cryotherapy—Ice Massage

Ice is applied over the levator scapulae trigger point in circular motions for 3 to 5 minutes (Fig. 4–6). The duration of the ice application should be sufficient to produce analgesia and allow for deep pressure massage over the trigger point and stretching of the neck muscles.

Ice massage is used for the first treatments to reduce symptoms and allow for stretching and strengthening. After pain has subsided, the patient can continue with self-stretching, postural exercises, and strengthening.

HOME PROGRAM

This patient should be instructed in self-stretching, active exercises, and postural awareness, especially during sitting. Modifications of chair height and work table height may be necessary to reduce strain of neck and shoulder girdle musculature. If pain recurs, she could use a cold pack at home to reduce the symp-

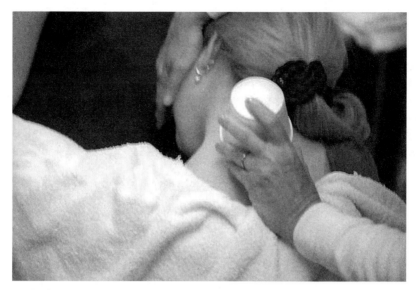

FIGURE 4–6. Ice massage to trigger point in levator scapulae muscle.

toms, since self-applied ice massage to the scapular region is not convenient. The home program should be written in clear and concise terms with appropriate illustrations for exercises and posture. Periodic reassessments may be necessary to revise the program.

RATIONALE FOR CLINICAL DECISION MAKING

The pain associated with the levator scapulae trigger point resulted from overuse and cumulative trauma from extensive studying, computer work, and carrying books. Ice massage was necessary initially to deactivate the trigger point, so that stretching and active exercise could occur. Instruction in proper sitting posture, especially during computer work and study, is essential to prevent recurrence.

Reduction of Spasticity

Spasticity associated with upper motoneuron lesions often interferes with the performance of activities of daily living and gait. Cryotherapy can be used as an adjunct in the total treatment plan of the patient with spasticity to reduce temporarily the hypertonicity, thus permitting instruction in purposeful movements and activities. Levine and associates[65] suggested cryotherapy as part of the treatment regimen. Cold is applied over the hypertonic muscle for 10 to 30 minutes. The method of application (for example, cold baths and cold packs) depends on accessibility, size, and contour of the body area to be treated. Once the area has been cooled, and the spasticity reduced, an exercise program is carried out. The effects of the cold can be expected to last about 1 to 1.5 hours.

As discussed previously in the chapter, many researchers have documented decreases in ATR and clonus following cold. These measures, though, were not directly related to an ability to perform skillful and purposeful activities. Hedenberg[66] reported on a series of hemiplegic patients with onset of their disability from 3 months to 10 years. All patients had hypertonia and hyperreflexia in the involved arm. The study was designed to measure upper extremity function, using a standardized test to evaluate if cryotherapy contributed to improvement of function. The hemiplegic upper extremities of the patients were immersed in a 12°C water bath for 15 minutes. Following immersion, all patients improved test scores. Seventeen of the 24 had significant improvements. The greatest improvements in skill were with precision movements involving the thumb and the index and middle fingers.

More clinical documentation on the use of cryotherapy for patients with spasticity should be encouraged. This technique may be appropriate prior to exercise or activities of daily living in nonclinical settings, because application by patients, family members, and care providers is safe and uncomplicated.

GUIDELINES FOR METHODS OF CRYOTHERAPY

Cold is administered by a variety of means. The methods discussed include cold packs, ice massage, cold baths or whirlpools, vapocoolant sprays, and controlled cold-compression units. The choice of which agent to use depends on accessibility, body part to be treated, and size of the area to be cooled. The foot may be best covered by a cold immersion bath, for example, and the knee by a cold pack wrapped around the entire joint (Fig. 4–7). Treating the ankle and leg can be done more efficiently with cold packs than with ice massage.

When considering cryotherapy, the therapist must be familiar with the patients' medical status (precautions for cryotherapy are discussed in a later section). Before actual treatment, particularly before ice massage or cold immersion bath, a small area of skin should be tested for hypersensitivity.[67] If hypersensitivity is apparent, this should be documented and the cold discontinued. Generally speaking, conductive cooling is administered for 10 to 30 minutes, with the longer time periods recommended for obese patients.[6]

Often, the skin underlying the cooling agent will redden. This may occur for one of two reasons. First, oxygen does not dissociate as freely from hemoglobin at lowered temperatures; therefore, the blood passing through the venous system is highly oxygenated, giving a red color to the skin. Second, after a 10- to 15-minute period of chilling, or upon removal of the cold stimulus, a reactive hyperemia may occur, bringing a greater amount of blood to the area.

For an hour or two after cryotherapy, patients should avoid stresses that could potentially reinjure or aggravate the pathologies for which they were treated. The analgesia produced by the cold could mask exercise-induced pain, thus giving patients false senses of security. Lowering of joint temperature can increase stiffness,[68] thereby decreasing reaction time and velocity of motion.[69] This fact, in combination with analgesia, predisposes patients to further injury.

Cold Packs

Cold packs can be inexpensively purchased or easily made. The commercial brands usually contain a silica gel or sand-slurry mixture encased in vinyl and are

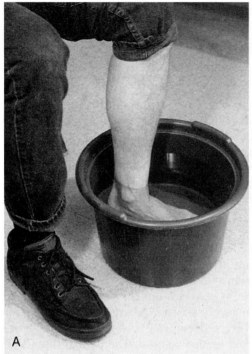

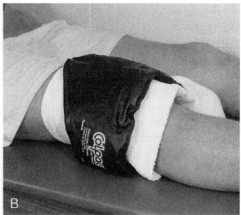

FIGURE 4-7. (*A*) Cold immersion bath for the foot and ankle. (*B*) Cold pack wrapped around the knee.

available in a variety of sizes and shapes to contour the area to be treated. The packs can be stored in a special refrigeration unit or in a household freezer. Storage temperature should be approximately $-5°C$ for at least 2 hours before use. For hygienic reasons, a layer of towel should be placed between the pack and the skin surface. Air is a poor thermal conductor; therefore, a moist towel will facilitate energy transfer by eliminating as much air interference as possible. If the towel is wet with room-temperature or lukewarm water, the initial contact will be more comfortable for the patient. The packs can be secured by a strap, with the patient positioned so that the area is well supported.

There are some cold packs that are chemically activated by squeezing or hitting them against a hard surface. These packs are usually marketed for first aid and designed for one-time use only. The chemical reaction inside some of the packs is at an alkaline pH and can cause skin burns if the package splits open and the contents spill out.

Commercial gel packs are suitable for home use. Cold packs remain at a sufficiently low temperature for 15 to 20 minutes. If longer treatment time is desired, the pack should be replaced with another.

Ice Massage

Ice massage is usually done over a small area—over a muscle belly, tendon, or bursa, for instance, or over trigger points—before deep-pressure massage. The technique is simple and can be taught to reliable patients for home use.

Water is frozen in paper cups to make handling of the ice by the therapist easier. The cup is peeled back as the ice melts. As an alternative, ice "lollipops" can be made by putting a wooden tongue depressor in the cup with the water. The ice pop can be taken out of the cup and held by the tongue depressor for application. An area 10 cm by 15 cm can be covered in 5 to 10 minutes.[70] The ice is rubbed over the skin using small overlapping circles or strokes.

During ice massage, the patient will most likely experience four distinct sensations, including intense cold, burning, aching, then analgesia. The stages of burning and aching should pass rapidly within about 1 to 2 minutes. A prolonged phase of aching or burning may result if the area covered is too large, or if a hypersensitive response is imminent (see "Precautions for Cryotherapy"). Skin temperature will usually not drop below 15°C when this technique is employed; therefore, the risk of damaging tissue is minimal.

Cold Baths

When cooling the distal extremities, immersion of those parts in a cold bath is most practical (unless simultaneous elevation is desired). This approach ensures circumferential contact of the cooling agent. Water temperatures for immersion vary from 13°C to 18°C. The lower the temperature range, the shorter the duration of immersion. In fact, immersion at 13°C often will be very uncomfortable. A basin of water or a small whirlpool filled with water and crushed ice can be used. The patient can also be instructed to use this technique at home.

Vapocoolant Spray

Historically two types of vapocoolant sprays are used in the treatment of trigger points. Fluori-Methane is nonflammable and nontoxic. It contains the class of chlorofluorocarbons that were banned by the Clean Air Act of 1990[14], but the product received a medical exemption and is available for use.

Ethyl Chloride is not affected by the Clean Air Act. It is a local anesthetic that was originally used for trigger point treatment. Its use was discontinued, because it was volatile and flammable and could freeze the skin on contact. Ethyl Chloride continues to be used in some instances for immediate treatment of athletic injuries.

Vapocoolant sprays are used in the treatment of trigger points. A brief summary of application techniques may be useful. After locating the treatment area, the patient is positioned comfortably and the muscle is maintained on passive stretch. Spraying is done in unidirectional sweeps along the muscle over the trigger point areas and over the areas of referred pain, while maintaining the passive stretch. When using the spray to increase ROM without identified trigger points, the muscle is sprayed along its length from the proximal to the distal attachments. Repeated treatments during the same session are done only after the skin has been rewarmed to avoid frosting the skin.

Controlled Cold-Compression Units

Controlled cold-compression units like the Cryotemp (Jobst Corporation, Toledo, OH) can be adjusted to selected temperatures (ranging from approximately 10°C to

25°C) and can be maintained during the time the unit is turned on. Cooled water is circulated through a sleeve that is applied over an extremity. The sleeve is inflated intermittently to pump edema fluid from the extremity. These units are probably most commonly seen in centers, such as sports medicine facilities, that treat a number of acute musculoskeletal injuries.

SELECTING A COOLING AGENT

When selecting a cooling agent, the clinician should consider which body area, and how much of the body surface, is to be cooled. For small areas (such as over a tendon, bursa, or small muscle belly), ice massage may effectively produce the cooling desired. If a distal extremity is to be cooled, as mentioned previously, a cool bath will most efficiently cover all surfaces.

When cooling around a joint such as the knee, elbow, or shoulder, or a larger muscle mass, such as lumbar or cervical paravetebral muscles, a cold pack or chipped ice wrapped in a terry cloth towel may be the best choice. Belitsky and colleagues[71] compared the abilities of three cooling agents—wet ice, dry ice, and a commercial gel pack—in reducing skin temperature over the gastrocnemius muscle. Average skin temperature before cooling was 29.5°C to 30°C. The greatest temperature reduction, 12°C, was recorded after wet ice (chipped ice in a terry cloth towel) was applied for 15 minutes, while cold gel packs applied for the same amount of time reduced skin temperature by 7.3°C. These authors emphasize the importance of accurate placement of a cold agent over, and completely covering, the area to be treated. Skin temperatures proximal and distal to the ice or other cooling agent were not significantly lowered.

DOCUMENTATION OF TREATMENT

As with any therapeutic technique, the use of cold in a therapy program is based on the goals of the treatment. The goals are determined by the patient and the therapist after thorough evaluation of the patient, including the history of the present problem and subjective and objective measures of impairments and current functional status. Documentation includes an accurate recording of the treatment parameters, changes in patient response to treatment during and between sessions and any modifications of the goals or treatment program. Specific parameters for cold applications are the type of cold agent, treatment duration, site of application, and position of the patient. Treatment outcomes may include volume or girth measurements, pain status measures, ROMs, and strength grades. Further descriptions of changes in skin temperature or appearance, quality of edema, and sensation are also documented. Clinical notes include periodic reassessments of the patient's overall functional level, especially in relationship to those impairments directly affected by treatment.

PRECAUTIONS FOR CRYOTHERAPY

Contraindications

Cryotherapy should not be used when treating patients with specific cold-sensitivity symptoms. These conditions include, but are not limited to, cold urticaria, cryoglobulinemia, Raynaud's phenomenon, and paroxysmal cold hemoglobinuria.[72] Cold urticaria can include both local and systemic reactions. In response to local cold application, patients develop wheals, which are characterized by erythematous, raised borders and blanched centers.[73,74] Mast-cell degranulation causes histamine to be released into the area, markedly increasing capillary permeability and leading to redness, swelling, and wheal formation.[75] In severe cases patients develop generalized swelling involving mucous membranes and viscera. Systemic reactions include flushing of the face, a sharp drop in blood pressure, an increase heart rate, and syncope.[76]

Cryoglobulinemia is a disorder characterized by the presence of an abnormal blood protein that forms a gel when exposed to low temperatures. This gel formation can lead to ischemia or gangrene. Cryoglobulinemia is associated with multiple myeloma, certain types of viral and bacterial infections, chronic liver disease, systemic lupus erythematosus, and other rheumatic diseases.[77]

Raynaud's phenomenon is a vasospastic disorder, which can be either idiopathic or associated with other disorders, such as systemic scleroderma, systemic lupus erythematosus, thoracic outlet syndrome, and trauma. Approximately 50% of patients with thromboangiitis obliterans (Buerger's disease) also display Raynaud's phenomenon.[78] Cycles of pallor, cyanosis, rubor, and normal color of the digits may be accompanied by numbness, tingling, or burning. Attacks are precipitated by exposure to cold or by emotional stress.[73]

Paroxysmal cold hemoglobinuria can occur following local or general exposure to cold. Hemoglobin, which is normally found within red blood cells, is released from lysed red cells and appears in the urine.

Cold should not be applied over areas of compromised circulation. For patients with peripheral vascular disease affecting arterial circulation, the vasoconstrictive effects of cold could potentially compromise an already nutritionally deprived area.

Precautions

Because cold can cause a transient increase in systolic and diastolic blood pressures,[79,80] careful monitoring should take place when using cryotherapy for hypertensive patients. Blood pressure should be monitored prior to and throughout treatment. Treatment should be discontinued if an elevation of blood pressure occurs.

Cold should be applied with caution for individuals with hypersensitivity to cold, impaired circulation, and thermoregulatory disorders.[81] If, after careful consideration, cryotherapy is the treatment of choice for these patients, close monitoring of the response to treatment and appropriate adjustments of treatment parameters are necessary. Decreasing the duration and adjusting the intensity of the cold application may produce the desired effects without eliciting adverse reactions.

Wound healing may be impaired by cold temperatures. Lundgren and associates[82] demonstrated a 20% reduction in wound tensile strength in rabbits kept at environmental temperatures of 12°C, compared with those kept at 20°C. The decreased healing might be caused by a decreased blood supply to the area. Only innervated animals showed this impaired healing response, suggesting a reflex cutaneous vasoconstriction. Until demonstrated otherwise, it is probably a prudent decision to avoid vigorous cold application directly over a wound during the initial 2- to 3-week period of healing.

As mentioned earlier, prolonged cold application, from 1 to more than 2 hours, over an area containing a superficial peripheral nerve (e.g., around the medial epicondyle of the elbow or fibular head) can lead to neuropraxia or axonotmesis.[33,34]

In addition to certain physiologic reasons contraindicating use of cryotherapy, the psychologic response of the patient to this form of treatment should be taken into account. Some people have an aversion to cold and thus would not tolerate this thermal agent. This consideration is particularly important if cold is being used to decrease pain and promote skeletal-muscle relaxation.

SUMMARY

The use of cryotherapy is based on the physiologic responses to a decrease in tissue temperature. Cold decreased blood flow and tissue metabolism, thus decreasing bleeding and acute inflammation. Spasticity and muscle-guarding spasms can be diminished, allowing for a greater ease of motion. Pain threshold is elevated, allowing exercises to be carried out with increased comfort.

Cold can be easily applied through a variety of means, including cold packs, ice massage, cool baths, vapocoolant sprays, or controlled cold/compression devices. Caution should be taken, though, to avoid undue exposure to cold in persons with cold-hypersensitivity syndromes, impaired circulation, and hypertension.

Study Objectives

Having completed this chapter, the reader should now be able to:

1. Describe the effects of local cold application on blood flow.
2. Describe the relationship between the duration, temperature, and mode of cold application and the resultant change in tissue temperature.
3. Distinguish the effects of prolonged (intense) and brief (less intense) local cold application on edema.
4. Describe the rationale for clinical use of cryotherapy for edema management.
5. Describe the effects of local cold application on peripheral nerves.
6. Describe the effects and clinical implications of local cold application on muscle strength.
7. Discuss the clinical implications of the effects of local cold application on muscle tone.
8. Discuss the advantages and disadvantages of various methods of cold applications.
9. Describe the treatment parameters and their rationale for various cryotherapy techniques.
10. Discuss possible outcome measures to determine the effectiveness of the cryotherapy treatment.
11. Differentiate contraindications and precautions for cryotherapy treatments.

REFERENCES

1. Nave, CR and Nave, BC: Physics for the Health Sciences, ed 2. WB Saunders, Philadelphia, 1980, p 178.
2. Clarke, RSJ, Hellon, RF, and Lind, AR: Vascular reactions of the human forearm to cold. Clin Sci 17:165, 1958.

3. Abramson, DI: Physiologic basis for the use of physical agents in peripheral vascular disorders. Arch Phys Med Rehabil 46:216, 1965.
4. Wolf, SL and Basmajian, JV: Intramuscular temperature changes deep to localized cutaneous cold stimulation. Phys Ther 53:1284, 1973.
5. Bierman, W and Friedlander, M: The penetrative effect of cold. Arch Phys Ther 21:585, 1940.
6. Lehmann, JF and DeLateur BJ: Cryotherapy. In Lehmann, JF (ed): Therapeutic Heat and Cold, ed 4. Williams & Wilkins, Baltimore, 1990, p 590.
7. Lowdon, BJ and Moore, RJ: Determinants and nature of intramuscular temperature changes during cold therapy. Am J Phys Med 54:223, 1975.
8. Wakim, KG, Porter, AN, and Krusen, KH: Influence of physical agents of certain drugs on intra-articular temperature. Arch Phys Med 32:714, 1951.
9. Oliver, RA, et al: Isometric muscle contraction response during recovery from reduced intramuscular temperature. Arch Phys Med Rehabil 60:126, 1979.
10. Johnson, DJ, et al: Effect of cold submersion on intramuscular temperature of the gastrocnemius muscle. Phys Ther 59:1238, 1979.
11. Hartvikksen, K: Ice therapy in spasticity. Acta Neurol Scan 38:79, 1962.
12. McMaster, WC, Liddle, S, and Waugh, TR: Laboratory evaluation of various cold therapy modalities. Am J Sports Med 6:291, 1978.
13. Travell, JG and Simons, DG: Myofascial Pain and Dysfunction. The Trigger Point Manual. Williams & Wilkins, Baltimore, 1983.
14. Clean Air Act of 1991, Federal Register, effective January 1, 1996.
15. Perkins, J, et al: Cooling and contraction of smooth muscle. Am J Physiol 163:14, 1950.
16. Guyton, AC: Textbook of Medical Physiology, ed 8. WB Saunders, Philadelphia, 1991, p 798.
17. Folkow, B, et al: Studies on the reaction of the cutaneous vessels to cold exposure. Acta Physiol Scan 58:342, 1963.
18. Cobbold, AF and Lewis, OJ: Blood flow to the knee joint of the dog: Effect of heating, cooling and adrenaline. J Physiol 132:379, 1956.
19. Lewis, T: Observations upon the reactions of the vessels of the human skin to cold. Heart 15:177, 1930.
20. Fox, RH and Wyatt, HT: Cold-induced vasodilation in various areas of the body surface in man. J Physiol 162:289, 1962.
21. Smith, TL, et al: New skeletal muscle model for the longitudinal study of alterations in microcirculation following contusion and cryotherapy. Microsurgery 14:487, 1993.
22. Major, TC, Schwainghamer, JM, and Winston, S: Cutaneous and skeletal muscle vascular responses to hypothermia. Am J Physiol 240 (Heart Circ Physiol 9): H868, 1981.
23. Knight, KL: Cryotherapy: Theory, Technique, Physiology. Chattanooga Corp., Chattanooga, TN, 1985, p 154.
24. Matsen, FA, Questd, K, and Matsen, AL: The effect of local cooling on post fracture swelling. Clin Orthop 109:201, 1975.
25. McMaster, WC and Liddle, S: Cryotherapy influence on post traumatic limb edema. Clin Orthop 150:283, 1980.
26. Jezdinsky, J, Marek, J, and Ochonsky, P: Effects of local cold and heat therapy on traumatic oedema of the rat hind paw. I: Effects of cooling on the course of traumatic oedema. Acta Universitatis Palackianae Olomucensis Facultatis Medicae 66:185, 1973.
27. Marek, J, Jezdinsky, J, and Ochonsky, P: Effects of local cold and heat therapy on traumatic oedema of the rat hind paw. II: Effects of cooling on the course of traumatic oedema. Acta Universitatis Palackianae Olomucensis Facultatis Medicae 66:203, 1973.
28. Farry, PJ and Prentice, NG: Ice treatment of injured ligaments: An experimental model. NZ Med J 9:12, 1980.
29. Douglas, WW and Malcolm, JL: The effect of localized cooling on conduction in cat nerves. J Physiol 130:53, 1955.
30. Zankel, HT: Effect of physical agents on motor conduction velocity of the ulnar nerve. Arch Phys Med Rehabil 47:787, 1966.
31. Lee, JM, Warren, MP, and Mason, SM: Effects of ice on nerve conduction velocity. Physiotherapy 64:2, 1978.
32. Li, C-L: Effect of cooling on neuromuscular transmission in the rat. Am J Physiol 194:200, 1958.
33. Drez, D, Faust, DC, and Evans, JP: Cryotherapy and nerve palsy. Am J Sports Med 9:256, 1981.
34. Collins, K, Storey, M, and Peterson, K: Peroneal nerve palsy after cryotherapy. The Physician and Sports Medicine 14:105, 1986.
35. McGown, HL: Effects of cold application on maximal isometric contraction. Phys Ther 47:185, 1967.
36. Knuttsson, E and Mattsson, E: Effects of local cooling on monosynaptic reflexes in man. Scand J Rehabil Med 1:126, 1969.
37. Clendenin, MA and Szumski, AJ: Influence of cutaneous ice application on single motor units in human. Phys Ther 51:166, 1971.
38. Johnson, J and Leider, FE: Influence of cold bath on maximum handgrip strength. Percept Mot Skills 44:323, 1977.

39. Clarke, DH: Effects of immersion in hot and cold water upon recovery of muscular strength following fatiguing isometric exercise. Arch Phys Med Rehabil 44:565, 1963.
40. Eldred, E, Lindsley, DF, and Buchwald, JS: The effect of cooling on mammalian muscle spindles. Exp Neurol 2:144, 1960.
41. Newton, M and Lehmkuhl, D: Muscle spindle response to body heating and localized muscle cooling: Implications for relief of spasticity. J Am Phys Ther Assoc 45:91, 1965.
42. Wolf, SL and Letbetter, WD: Effect of skin cooling on spontaneous EMG activity in triceps surae of the decerebrate cat. Brain Res 91:151, 1975.
43. Mecomber, SA and Herman, RM: Effects of local hypothermia on reflex and voluntary activity. Phys Ther 51:271, 1971.
44. Miglietta, O: Electromyographic characteristics of clonus and influence of cold. Arch Phys Med Rehabil 45:502, 1964.
45. Miglietta, O: Action of cold on spasticity. Am J Phys Med 52:198, 1973.
46. Knuttsson, E: Topical cryotherapy in spasticity. Scand J Rehabil Med 2:159, 1970.
47. Urbscheit, N, Johnston, R, and Bishop, B: Effects of cooling on the ankle jerk and H-response in hemiplegic patients. Phys Ther 51:983, 1971.
48. Schaubel, HH: Local use of ice after orthopedic procedures. Am J Surg 72:711, 1946.
49. Conolly, WB, Paltos, N, and Tooth, RM: Cold therapy—An improved method. Med J Aust 2:42, 1972.
50. Basur, R, Shephard, E, and Mouzos, G: A cooling method in the treatment of ankle sprains. Practitioner 216:708, 1976.
51. Levy, AS and Marmar, E: The role of cold compression dressings in the postoperative treatment of total knee arthroplasty. Clin Orthop 297:174, 1993.
52. Healy, WL, et al: Cold compressive dressing after total knee arthroplasty. Clin Orthop 299:143, 1994.
53. Kaempffe, FA: Skin surface temperature reduction after cryotherapy to a casted extremity. Sports Phys Ther 10:448, 1989.
54. Hocutt, JE, et al: Cryotherapy in ankle sprains. Am J Sports Med 10:316, 1982.
55. Benson, TB and Copp, EP: The effects of therapeutic forms of heat and ice on the pain threshold of normal shoulder. Rheumatol Rehabil 13:101, 1974.
56. Gammon, GD and Starr, I: Studies on the relief of pain by counterirritation. J Clin Invest 2:13, 1941.
57. Melzack, R and Wall, PD: Pain mechanisms: A new theory. Science 150:971, 1965.
58. Lane, LE: Localized hypothermia for the relief of pain in musculoskeletal injuries. Phys Ther 51:182, 1971.
59. Hayden, CA: Cryokinetics in an early treatment program. J Am Phys Ther Assoc 44:990, 1964.
60. Grant, AE: Massage with ice (cryokinetics) in the treatment of painful conditions of the musculoskeletal system. Arch Phys Med Rehabil 45:233, 1964.
61. Prentice, WE: An electromyographic analysis of the effectiveness of heat or cold and stretching for inducing relaxation in injured muscle. J Orthop Sports Phys Ther 3:133, 1982.
62. Cobb, CR, et al: Electrical activity in muscle pain. Am J Phys Med 54:80, 1975.
63. Yackszn, L, Adams, C, and Francis, KT: The effects of ice massage on delayed muscle soreness. Am J Sports Med 12:159, 1984.
64. Landen, BR: Heat or cold for the relief of low back pain? Phys Ther 47:1126, 1967.
65. Levine, MG, et al: Relaxation of spasticity by physiological techniques. Arch Phys Med Rehabil 35:214, 1954.
66. Hedenberg, L: Functional improvement of the spastic hemiplegic arm after cooling. Scand J Rehabil Med 2:154, 1970.
67. Olson, JE and Stravino, VD: A review of cryotherapy. Phys Ther 52:840, 1972.
68. Wright, V and Johns, RJ: Physical factors concerned with the stiffness of normal and diseased joints. Bull Johns Hopkins Hosp 106:215, 1960.
69. Fox, RH: Local cooling in man. Br Med Bull 17:14, 1961.
70. Waylonis, GW: The physiologic effect of ice massage. Arch Phys Med Rehabil 48:37, 1967.
71. Belitsky, RB, Odam, SJ, and Hubley-Kozey, C: Evaluation of the effectiveness of wet ice, dry ice, and Cryogen packs in reducing skin temperature. Phys Ther 67:1080, 1987.
72. Ritzmann, SE and Levin, WC: Cryopathies: A review. Arch Intern Med 107:186, 1961.
73. Austin, KD: Diseases of immediate type hypersensitivity. In Isselbacher, KJ, et al (eds): Harrison's Principles of Internal Medicine, ed 9. McGraw-Hill, New York, 1980.
74. Day, MJ: Hypersensitive response to ice massage: Report of a case. Phys Ther 54:592, 1974.
75. Shelley, WB and Crao, WA: Cold erythema: A new hypersensitivity syndrome. JAMA 180:639, 1962.
76. Horton, BT, Brown, GE, and Roth, GM: Hypersensitiveness to cold with local and systemic manifestation of a histamine-like character: Its amenability to treatment. JAMA 107:1263, 1936.
77. Schumacher, HR (ed): Cryoglobulinemia. In Primer on Rheumatic Diseases, ed 9. Arthritis Foundation, Atlanta, 1988, p 82.
78. Creager, MA and Dzau, VJ: Vascular diseases of the extremities. In Isselbacher, KJ, et al (eds): Harrison's Principles of Internal Medicine, ed 13. McGraw-Hill, New York, 1994.
79. Boyer, JT, Fraser, JRE, and Doyle, AE: The haemodynamic effects of cold immersion. Clin Sci 19:539, 1980.

80. Claus-Walker, J, et al: Physiological responses to cold stress in healthy subjects and in subjects with cervical cord injuries. Arch Phys Med Rehabil 55:485, 1974.
81. Harchelroad, F: Acute thermoregulatory disorders. Clin in Geriatr Med 9:621, 1993.
82. Lundgren, C, Muren, A, and Zederfeldt, B: Effect of cold vasoconstriction on wound healing in the rabbit. Acta Chir Scand 118:1, 1959.

CHAPTER 5

Biophysical Principles of Heating and Superficial Heating Agents

G.A. (Sandy) Rennie, MSc, BPT
Susan L. Michlovitz, MS, PT

Warmth is associated with tranquility and relaxation. Heating of injured tissue has been used for centuries for pain relief and reduction of muscle spasm. In physical therapy, locally applied heating agents are used not only to promote relaxation and provide pain relief, but they are also used to increase blood flow, to facilitate tissue heal-ing, and to prepare stiff joints and tight muscles for exercise.[1-5] The physiologic effects that occur as a result of tissue temperature elevation are included in the rationale for selecting these agents as part of a therapy program. Elevation of collagen tissue tem-perature, for example, can alter viscoelastic properties, thus enhancing the effects of passive stretch for increasing range of motion.[6,7]

There are many thermal agents available for tissue heating. These generally fall within one of two broad categories: superficial and deep-heating agents. Superficial heating agents primarily cause an increase in skin and superficial subcutaneous tissue temperature. Superficial heating agents such as hot packs, paraffin wax, and Flu-idotherapy are used: (1) to heat superficial joints, such as the hand, which has little soft tissue covering; (2) to cause a heating effect in deeper structures such as muscle, through reflex mechanisms; or (3) to heat collagen tissue in order to increase its exten-sibility. If the goal of treatment is to increase the temperature of deeper tissues, such as the knee joint, or the muscle belly of the quadriceps muscle, then a deep-heating agent is logically selected. Deep-heating agents, including shortwave diathermy and contin-uous-wave ultrasound, can increase tissue temperature at depths ranging from 3 to 5 cm without overheating the skin and subcutaneous tissues. Deep-heating agents are discussed in Chapters 7 and 8.

BIOPHYSICAL EFFECTS OF TEMPERATURE ELEVATION

Many sequelae can occur as a result of an increase in temperature of body tis-sues. The occurrence and magnitude of these physiologic changes are dependent upon several factors, including: (1) the extent of the temperature rise; (2) the rate at which energy is being added to the tissue; and (3) the volume of tissue exposed. In order to meet therapeutic levels of vigorous heating, Lehmann and deLateur[1] state that tissue temperature must be elevated to between 40°C and 45°C (104°F to 113°F). Within these temperatures, hyperemia, which is indicative of increased blood flow, will occur. Above this range, there is potential for tissue damage. Below 40°C (104°F), heating is considered to be only mild.[1,6] Behavioral regulation and subjec-tive responses associated with surface temperatures are illustrated in Table 5-1.

The rate of temperature rise in response to the addition of thermal energy can influence physiologic responses. Temperature elevation increases local blood flow,[2,3,8-14] thus cooler blood comes into the area and acts to remove some of the heat produced. If the rate of temperature increase is very slow, the amount of heat added could be balanced out by the convective effect of cooler blood so that thera-peutically effective heating levels may not be obtained. On the other hand, if tem-perature rises faster than excess heat can be dissipated, heat may build up to a point that stimulates pain receptors, and may cause tissue damage. The goal of heating is to achieve a therapeutic level of temperature elevation without causing adverse re-sponses.

Physiologic alteration can occur at the site of local temperature rise and in areas remote from the area of heat absorption. Usually, the larger the tissue volume affected by the addition of thermal energy, the greater the likelihood for reflex, or consensual, changes in other areas and for systematic alterations. An increase in forearm tempera-ture as a result of hot pack application could be expected to cause an increase in local

TABLE 5–1 Temperature Ranges

Temperature (°C)	Body and Environmental Temperatures		Subjective Feeling Associated with Surface Temperatures
60		Behavioral regulation	
55			
50			
45			Tissue damage, burning pain
40			Very hot
35	Normal range of of resting temperature of body 36.3–37.3°C	Approximate region of physiologic temperature regulation	Hot
30			Warm
			Neutral
25	Region of thermal environmental comfort		Cool
20			Cold
15			
10			Very cold
5		Behavioral regulation	Very cold + pain → tissue damage
0			

blood flow, with minimal or no alterations in overall peripheral vascular resistance. On the other hand, immersion of a person in a water bath of 40°C (104°F) could result in systemic changes, such as a decrease in mean blood pressure, an increase in heart rate, and an increase in pulmonary minute ventilation.[1]

Several physiologic responses to temperature elevation are important to understand when considering a heating agent for therapeutic purposes. The most relevant changes to address include alterations in metabolic activity, hemodynamic function, neural response, skeletal muscle activity, and collagen tissue physical properties. These changes, in part, serve as a foundation for the use of heat as an effective therapeutic agent. As well, an understanding of the adverse reactions to the addition of thermal energy is imperative for the delivery of a safe treatment.

Metabolic Reactions

Chemical reactions in cells of the body are influenced by temperature. Generally speaking, chemical activity in cells and metabolic rate will increase twofold to threefold for each 10°C (50°F) rise in temperature.[11,15] Therefore, energy expenditure will increase with increasing temperature. As temperature rises past a certain point, usually 45°C to 50°C (113°F to 122°F), human tissues will burn because the metabolic activity required to repair tissue is not capable of keeping up with thermally induced protein denaturation.

An increase in chemical reaction rate can also have positive effects on human function. Oxygen uptake by tissues will increase.[8] Theoretically, therefore, more nutrients will be available to promote tissue healing.[5]

Vascular Effects

Increasing tissue temperature is usually associated with vasodilation, and thus with an increase in blood flow to the area.[1,2,8–14,16,17] This blanket statement, however, can be misleading. It is important to know which regions have increased blood flow. The control mechanisms are different for blood flow to different structures — for example, skin compared with skeletal muscle. Therefore, responses to temperature change will not always be the same; or if a response is in the same direction, it may not be of the same magnitude.

Skin blood flow has an important role both in nutrition and in the maintenance of constant core body temperature of 37°C (98.6°F), and is primarily under the control of sympathetic adrenergic nerves.[18,19] Vasodilation of resistance vessels of the skin will occur as a means of losing heat through local or reflex mechanisms. The skin is unique in that it has specialized vessels, arteriovenous (AV) anastomoses, which have an important role in heat loss.[19] These shunt vessels go from arterioles to venules to venous plexuses, thus bypassing the capillary bed. The blood flow through these anastomoses is under neural control. Activation occurs in response to reflex activation of temperature receptors or stimulation of heat-loss mechanisms triggered in part by the circulation of warmed blood through the preoptic region of the anterior hypothalamus. These AV shunt vessels are found in the hands (palms and fingertips), feet (toes and soles), and face (ears, nose, and lips).

Blood flow changes in the skin, as mentioned previously, can be caused by local[1,10,18,20] or reflex[17] mechanisms. Vasodilation of the heat-exposed skin can be proposed to occur owing to three factors: (1) an axon reflex; (2) release of chemical mediators secondary to temperature elevation; and (3) local spinal cord reflexes. Heat applied to the skin stimulates cutaneous thermoreceptors. These sensory afferents carry impulses to the spinal cord. Some of these afferent impulses are carried through branches antidromically toward skin blood vessels, and a vasoactive mediator is released. This results in vasodilation through an axon reflex (Fig. 5–1).

Heat produces a mild inflammatory reaction. Chemical mediators of inflammation, including histamine and prostaglandins, are released in the area and act on resistance vessels to cause vasodilation. In addition, temperature elevation causes sweat se-

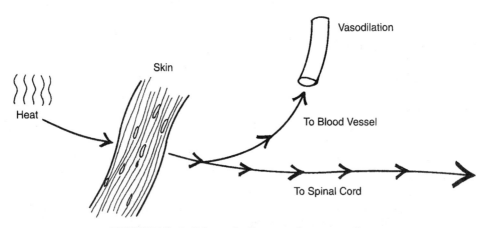

FIGURE 5–1. Schematic diagram of an axon reflex.

cretion and the enzyme kallikren is released from sweat glands. This enzyme acts on a globulin, kininogen, to release bradykinin.[21] Vasodilation of resistance vessels and an increase in capillary and postcapillary venule permeability occur because of the action of these chemical mediators on smooth-muscle tone and endothelial-cell contractility, respectively. Because of an increase in capillary hydrostatic pressure and permeability, outward fluid filtration from vascular to extravascular space is favored. Therefore, heat within the therapeutic range can potentially increase interstitial fluid and cause mild inflammation.

A local spinal cord reflex is elicited through heat-activated cutaneous afferent stimulation. This reflex results in a decrease in postganglionic sympathetic adrenergic nerve activity to the smooth muscles of blood vessels.[22] A schematic of the reflex is diagrammed in Figure 5–2.

Vasodilatory effects of this reflex response are not only limited to the area heated, but there will be a consensual (reflex) response in areas remote from the site of application. When one area of the body (e.g., the low back) is heated, increases in skin blood flow occur in distal extremities in areas of the body that are not directly heated.[23-25] This principle of reflex vasodilation is felt to be safe to use with patients with peripheral vascular disease.[23] For example, cutaneous blood flow to the feet could be increased by the application of heat to the low back.

Skeletal muscle blood flow is primarily under metabolic regulation and demonstrates the greatest response to increases or decreases in levels of exercise. When superficial heating agents are given, minimal to no change in skeletal muscle blood flow is expected. This notion is supported by two reports on heat lamp (infrared) application. Crockford and Hellon[9] measured venous oxygen content following 20- to 30-minute exposures of the forearm. Superficial venous oxygen content increased, but there was no change in muscle blood flow. Wyper and McNiven[26] reported no change in muscle blood flow following heat (infrared) treatment.

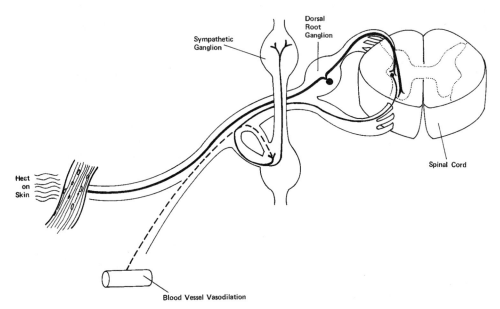

FIGURE 5–2. Heat applied to the skin leads to vasodilation. The change in activity of postganglionic sympathetic adrenergic fibers secondary to local heating is diagrammed.

Cobbold and Lewis[27] measured blood flow to the knee joint of the dog following exposure to superficial (radiant) heat. However, the magnitude of temperature change was not as great as when ice packs were applied to the animals. Their work does not support the earlier suggestion of Horvath and Hollander[28] that heat will cause a reflex decrease in joint temperature and blood flow, and cold will cause the opposite response.

Heat is often used before exercise. Both heat and exercise can increase blood flow. Greenberg[12] compared hot packs alone, exercise alone, and hot packs plus exercise. Heat was applied for 20 minutes; exercise consisted of squeezing a rubber ball once per second for 1 minute. The increase in blood flow from exercise was greater than with heat; however, the effects of hot packs plus exercise in combination were additive and greater than either modality used alone. Johnson and Park[29] found that the onset of vigorous exercise will lead to cutaneous vasoconstriction, the body's method of shunting blood to the muscles. This means that during vigorous exercise, the patient's skin may appear cool to the touch because the blood is being shunted to the muscles.

Neuromuscular Effects

Heat is used therapeutically to provide analgesia[17,18,30,31] and assist in the resolution of pain and muscle-guarding spasms.[1,32] Although the mechanisms of action are not totally understood, the underlying basis for use may relate to the ability of heat to elevate pain threshold,[17,33] alter nerve conduction velocity,[34-36] and change muscle spindle firing rates.[37] (An interesting depiction of the mechanisms of pain relief brought about by heat is illustrated in Fig. 5–3.) In addition, temperature elevation of skeletal muscle can temporarily change the ability to build tension and sustain prolonged activity.[38,39]

Raising subcutaneous tissue temperature using a variety of heating agents has been demonstrated to alter sensory nerve conduction velocity.[35,36] The most pronounced changes appear to occur during the first 1.5°C to 2.0°C (34.7°F to 35.6°F) temperature increase.[35] The relevance of these findings to therapeutic use, however, is not readily apparent.

Heating over the area of a peripheral nerve can elevate the pain threshold. Fifteen minutes of high-intensity heat lamp (infrared radiation) was administered over the medial aspect of the elbow—that is, over the ulnar nerve. Pain threshold measurements distal to the site of application, over the tip of the little finger, revealed analgesia.[33] Direct heating over the area where pain was measured also produced analgesia. Therefore, heat can be a useful adjunct to reduce pain before stretching exercises, joint mobilization techniques, or active exercise.[1-3,5,7,18,40-42]

Muscle spasms can result from the overuse of a muscle during exercise or from activation of a protective mechanism to guard against movement of painful joints. Pain can be the event triggering a reflex, tonic muscle contraction, thus beginning the pain-spasm-pain cycle.[1,5,43] The muscle spindle afferents that alter their rate of firing primarily in response to tonic or static stretch are the type II afferents. Elevation of muscle temperature to about 42°C (107.6°F) will decrease the firing rate of the II afferents and increase the firing of the type Ib fibers from Golgi tendon organs (GTOs).[1,37] Therefore, with decreased firing of the II afferents and increased GTO activity, we could predict a decreased firing of the alpha motoneuron, thus reducing tonic extrafusal fiber activity.

Superficial heating agents most likely will not elevate muscle temperature to the

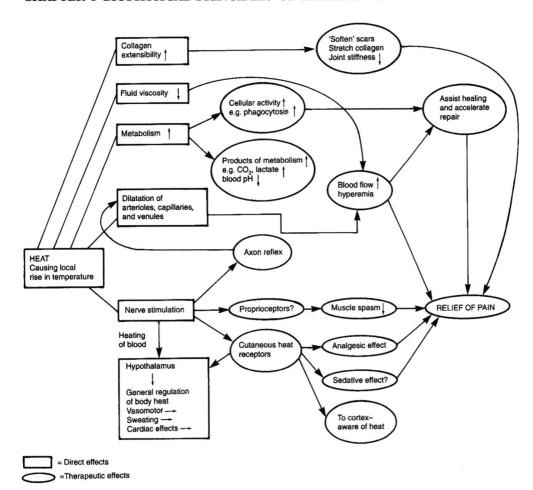

FIGURE 5–3. Mechanisms of pain relief due to heat. (From Wells, PW, Frampton, V, and Bowher, D: Pain Management in Physical Therapy. Oxford, Butterworth-Heinemann, 1988, p 130, with permission.)

degree necessary to alter II or Ib activity. Therefore, another mechanism must be postulated to account for the reduction in muscle spasm when the skin overlying the muscle is heated. Heating the skin has been demonstrated to produce a decrease in gamma (γ) efferent activity.[11] With a decrease in gamma activity, the stretch on the muscle spindle would be less, thus reducing afferent firing from the spindle. This indirect method ultimately results in decreased alpha motoneuron firing, and thus less muscle spasm.

Elevating muscle temperature can also alter strength and endurance. In a study of normal volunteers, Chastain[38] used a deep-heating agent (continuous shortwave diathermy) over the quadriceps. During the first 30 minutes following the termination of the heat, isometric strength was decreased, followed by an increase for the next 2 hours of measurement. Strength and endurance decreases following heating have also been reported in other studies on humans.[39,44] Immediately after immersion in whirlpools ranging from 40°C to 43°C (104°F to 109.4°F), quadriceps strength and endurance were reduced.[44] Edwards and associates[39] found similar results following immersion of the lower extremity in a water bath of 44°C (111.2°F) for 45 minutes. The muscle temperature following the 45-minute immersion had reached a value of 38.6°C (101.3°F) from a normal mean of 35.1°C (95.2°F).

The physical therapist should be aware of the changes in muscle performance following heat application, particularly when planning strengthening programs or performing valid assessments of performance.

Connective Tissue Effects

Temperature elevation in combination with a stretch can alter the viscoelastic properties of connective tissues.[11,45–47] The viscous properties of connective tissue permit a residual elongation of connective tissue after stretch is applied, then released. This is referred to as "plastic" deformation, or elongation.[48] An elastic structure will stretch under tension, but will return to its original length when the load is removed. The elastic properties of connective tissue result in recoverable deformation.[48,49]

Connective tissue will progressively shorten, and joint contractures will develop following injury, if full range-of-motion exercises are not performed.[50] Adhesions, or the loss of ability for tissue layers to glide past one another, also will develop. Lacerations and crush and burn injuries will result in scar tissue, further limiting mobility.

Heat and stretch of connective tissue will result in plastic elongation.[48,51,52] Two factors must be considered in determining effective treatment strategies, including: (1) temperature elevation—site, time, and amount; and (2) stretch—duration, amount, and velocity.

Greater residual length changes with less damage will occur when a stretch is applied during the time the tissue temperature is elevated at therapeutic levels (between 40°C and 45°C [104°F and 113°F]).[6] For in vivo experiments on rat-tail tendon, temperature was elevated in a water bath of 45°C (113°F) for 10 minutes, then elongation was performed and maintained until cooling to resting values occurred.[51] This was compared with stretch in water bath of 25°C (77°F). Length increases were greater in the 45°C (113°F) bath, with less evidence of tissue damage.[52]

There are three techniques reported to provide for permanent elongation of collagen tissue: (1) constant load of enough magnitude to overcome tissue elasticity; (2) rapid stretch followed by a period of holding in that position; and (3) constant rate of stretching using a slow, steady stretch.[6,48,53] Lower loads of longer duration result in less tissue damage[7,48,49,52] and greater increases of joint range of motion.[7,48–50,52,54] Lentell and associates[7] demonstrated an increase in long-term improvement in shoulder flexibility when his subjects were treated with hot packs prior to low-load prolonged stretch. Two groups (ice and stretch, and heat and stretch) showed an improvement in shoulder flexibility compared with controls. However, only the heat-and-stretch group showed significant gains in shoulder flexibility when compared with those who received stretching alone.

Joint stiffness is a common complaint among patients with rheumatoid arthritis and osteoarthritis (degenerative joint disease). Joint stiffness has the physical components of elasticity, viscosity, inertia, plasticity, and friction. Joint stiffness in normal subjects and in patients with rheumatoid arthritis is mainly attributable to the elastic properties of joint capsular structures.[55] Following immersion of the hands in a water bath of 43°C (109.4°F) for 10 minutes, in one study, there was a slight decrease in finger joint stiffness.[47] Superficial heating of the hand to 45°C (113°F) with a heat lamp (infrared) resulted in a 20 percent reduction in metacarpophalangeal stiffness, when compared with heating to a temperature of 33°C (91.4°F).[55] A controlled pilot study involving patients with rheumatoid arthritis was conducted to compare and assess the effects of ice versus superficial heat on shoulder pain and limited mobility.[42] The heat-treated group showed a greater increase in shoulder abduction and flexion than the ice-treated group, although this difference was not statistically significant. Clearly, heating can result in decreased joint stiffness and increased tissue extensibility, thus facilitating ease of motion and gains in range of motion.

PHYSICAL PRINCIPLES OF HEAT

Heat flow through matter (tissues) varies with the nature of the material (type of tissue) and is called thermal conductivity.[18] Changes in surface tissue temperature from superficial heating agents depend on the intensity of the heat applied, the time of heat exposure, and the thermal medium (product of thermal conductivity, density, and specific heat) for surface heat.[56] The greatest degree of temperature elevation with superficial heating agents occurs in the skin and the subcutaneous tissues within 0.5 cm from the skin surface. In areas of adequate blood supply, temperature will increase to a maximum within 6 to 8 minutes of exposure.[8,12,33] Muscle temperature at depths of 1 to 2 cm will increase to a lesser degree and will require a longer duration of exposure (15 to 30 minutes) to reach peak values.[8,16,33] At a depth of 3 cm, using clinically tolerable intensities, muscle temperature elevation can be expected to be about 1°C (31.8°F) or less.[8,57]

In joints of the hand and wrist, or foot and ankle, with relatively little soft tissue covering, superficial heating agents can raise intra-articular temperatures.[3,58,59] In fact, a 20-minute exposure of the foot to dry heat at 47.8°C (118°F) was shown to increase joint capsule temperature in the foot.[3] Even though there can be a reflex vasodilatory response on the unheated opposite extremity, no reflex temperature changes would be expected to occur.[59]

After the peak temperature is reached, there is a plateauing effect, or slight decrease in skin temperature, over the remainder of the heat exposure.[8,12,16,33] Typical temperature responses of areas with intact circulation are diagrammed in Table 5–1.

Fat provides an insulation against heat; it has a low thermal conductivity (see Table 4–1). Therefore, tissues under adipose tissue are likely to be minimally affected by superficial heating agents. In order to elevate deep tissues to therapeutically desired levels without burning the skin and subcutaneous tissue, a deep-heating agent such as continuous wave ultrasound or shortwave diathermy would be selected.

Heat Transfer

The primary methods of heat transfer for superficial heating agents are conduction, convection, and radiation.[1] Conduction is a method of heat transfer where the kinetic motion of atoms and molecules of one object is passed on to another object. This kinetic motion, often described as "atoms jostling one another,"[18] is increased when one object is heated more than another, and occurs more effectively if the objects are solids.[18]

Convection is the bulk movement of moving molecules, either in liquid or gaseous form, such that this bulk movement of liquid or gas transfers heat from one place to another.[18] The fluid movement can be pumped, such as the blood within the body being pumped by the heart, and warming all the parts to which it travels; or, it moves because a heated liquid or gas, being less dense, floats upward.[18]

Radiation is the conversion of heat energy into electromagnetic radiation.[18] All objects at temperatures above absolute zero ($-273°C$) both emit and absorb radiant energy. Any heated object or element, such as an infrared heat lamp, gives off radiant heat. If an object or body part is brought close enough to the radiant energy source, heat will be absorbed. Radiant heat application using infrared lamps is rarely, if ever, used today in rehabilitation as a form of superficial heating, and therefore will not be discussed further.

Conductive Heating Agents: Hot Packs and Paraffin Wax

The two most commonly used superficial heating agents are hot packs and paraffin wax. Both transfer heat to the body via conduction because they are in contact with the skin, and both the hot pack and the paraffin are at a much higher temperature than the skin surface to which they are applied. Therefore, thermal energy is lost from the agent and gained by the tissues. The quantity of heat gained and the subsequent physiologic responses to that heat gain are dependent upon several factors, including but not limited to: (1) thermal conductivity of the tissues; (2) body volume exposed; and (3) time of exposure.

HOT PACKS

Hot packs provide a superficial, moist heat. Commercial hot packs consist of canvas or nylon cases, filled with a hydrophilic silicate or some other hydrophilic substance, or sand (Fig. 5–4). Hot packs are stored in a thermostatically controlled cabinet

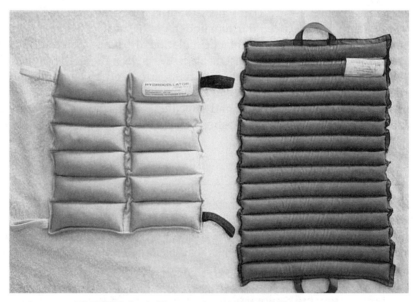

FIGURE 5–4. Two commercially available hot packs.

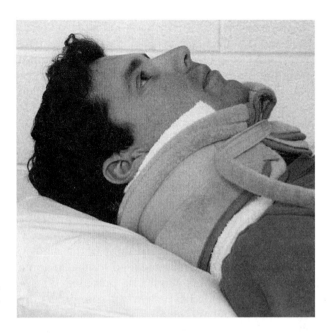

FIGURE 5–5. Hot pack application to the shoulder prior to exercise.

in water at a temperature between 70°C and 75°C (158°F and 167°F).[1,16,18] Hot packs come in a variety of shapes and sizes, and should be chosen on the basis of the size and contour of the body part(s) to be treated.

The packs should totally cover the treatment area and should be secured in place (Figs. 5–5 and 5–6). The pack should not be secured so tightly that the patient cannot remove it if it becomes too hot. The pack should be covered with layers of terry toweling or commercial hot pack covers. While there appears to be no definite number of layers of toweling for wrapping hot packs, the consensus is about six to eight layers, depending on towel thickness. Commercial hot-pack covers often need another layer or two of toweling to ensure adequate insulation from the hot pack.

As with all forms of heating agents, the patient should only feel a mild to moderate sensation of heat during application; the old adage "the hotter the better" could re-

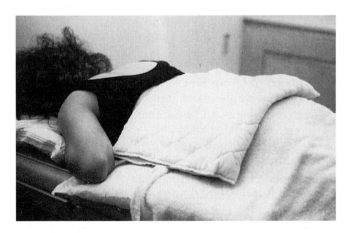

FIGURE 5–6. Hot pack application to the low back before soft tissue mobilization and exercise. Note that the patient is in the prone position. If indicated for patient comfort, a pillow may be added under the abdomen.

sult in skin burns. The therapist should monitor the patient during hot-pack application, and it is advisable to check under the hot pack after about 5 minutes to detect the
skin color and patient's subjective feelings about the amount of heat being perceived.
A significant early change in skin color may suggest overheating. Fair-skinned individuals may turn bright pink/red[16] or blotchy red and white, while darker-skinned individuals may exhibit areas of darker and lighter color. Fyfe[16] suggests frequent monitoring of the patient until about the 9- to 10-minute mark after warmth is first perceived,
when the maximum heating begins to dissipate. If the pack feels too hot to the patient,
or the therapist detects distinct skin color change, more toweling should be added, or
the hot pack should be removed. Patients should be advised not to lie with full body
weight directly on top of hot packs, particularly when the intended treatment area is
on the trunk. Body weight will squeeze water from the pack and may accelerate the
rate of heat transfer. In addition, local circulation could be reduced through compression of vessels, thus reducing circulatory convective cooling (dissipation of the heat).
Both factors could cause overheating of the skin.

If hot packs are recommended for use at home (by caregivers or reliable patients),
adequate instructions should be provided. There are a variety of methods of using
moist heat at home by patients or care givers, including commercial hot packs (hydrophilic silicate) and small water tanks for storage; sand packs, which can be heated
either in water or in a microwave oven; and gel packs, which can also be heated in water or in a microwave oven. A common rubber hot-water bottle covered with moist
toweling will also suffice.

All forms of hot packs should be inspected regularly for leaks and should be discarded if leaking occurs. When hydrophilic silicate hot packs become old and worn,
they leak the pastelike material within them, and they should be discarded, along with
gel packs that leak. Hot packs containing sand can be repaired by re-sewing the seams
of the pack.

Clinically, hot packs appear to be used most often to help reduce pain and muscle
spasm, and to help improve tissue extensibility.[1,2,4-7,17,18,32,42,48] The moist, superficial
heat they provide appears to rate quite highly among patients relative to their comfort,
heating ability, and effectiveness.

When compared with other heating modalities, or other modalities used to treat
pain, hot packs fare well, although not significantly better. Several studies[42,47,55] indicated that while the hot packs decreased pain and muscle spasm and improved range
of motion, they were not significantly better than other modalities. Williams and associates[42] found that hot packs did improve range of motion at the shoulder more than
ice, although not significantly. Interestingly, however, most of the patients in the ice
treatment group asked if they could be treated with heat instead of ice once the study
was completed.

Advantages of Using Hot Packs
1. Ease of preparation and application.
2. Variety of shapes and sizes available.
3. Moist, comfortable heat.
4. Relatively inexpensive to purchase and replace (assuming a tank already owned).

Disadvantages of Using Hot Packs
1. No method of temperature control once applied to patient.
2. Do not readily conform to all body parts.
3. Sometimes awkward to secure in place on a patient.

4. Do not retain heat for longer than about 20 minutes.
5. It is a passive treatment, not requiring active patient participation.
6. Leaking hydrophilic or gel packs must be discarded.

PARAFFIN WAX

Paraffin wax has several physical characteristics that make it an efficient source of superficial heat. First, it has a low melting point, around 54°C (129°F). This can be lowered more by adding more paraffin oil or mineral oil, so that the wax remains molten at temperatures between about 45°C and 54°C (113°F and 129°F). This molten state allows for more even distribution of the wax around the part to be treated (usually distal extremities). Second, paraffin has a low specific heat, which means that it does not feel as hot as water of the same temperature; therefore, there is much less risk of a burn. Third, it conducts heat more slowly than water at the same temperature, thus allowing the tissues to heat up more slowly, also decreasing the risk of a burn. This is particularly important when treating patients with sensitive skin or diminished skin sensation, for example, following burns.[40,60]

The paraffin mixture of a paraffin wax (six or seven parts) to oil (1 part) is commercially available (Fig. 5–7) and is melted and stored for use in thermostatically controlled stainless-steel or plastic containers. These wax baths come in a variety of sizes; the smaller ones are ideal for patient use at home (Fig. 5–8).

Paraffin is most commonly used for the distal extremities, including the fingers, hand, wrist, and perhaps elbow in the upper limb, and the toes, foot, and ankle in the lower limb. There are two principal techniques of application: (1) dip and wrap; and (2) dip and reimmerse. For both methods, the extremity to be treated should be washed and dried, and all jewelry should be removed from the part. When treating the hand and wrist for example the fingers should be slightly spread apart, the wrist relaxed, and the hand and wrist dipped into the wax to a few centimeters above the

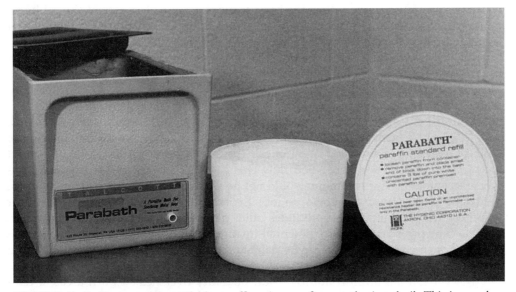

FIGURE 5–7. Commercially available paraffin mixture of wax and mineral oil. This is a replacement pack for a paraffin bath.

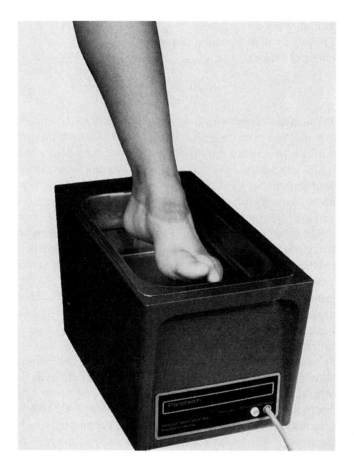

FIGURE 5–8. Application of paraffin to the foot. (Courtesy of Talcott Laboratories, Houston, PA.)

wrist joint. The hand is then removed from the wax and held above the bath until the wax has stopped dripping—then the hand is dipped again. The patient should be reminded not to move the hand and fingers so not to break the seal of the glove being formed. This procedure is repeated about 6 to 10 times until a solid wax glove has formed around the fingers, hand, and wrist. The hand is then placed in a plastic bag and wrapped with a towel to help retain the heat. If there is a potential for edema to increase secondary to the heat, the part should be elevated above level of the heart until the treatment time is over.

With the dip-and-reimmerse technique, after the wax glove has formed, the area covered by the glove is put back into the wax bath and kept there for the duration of the heat treatment (about 10 to 20 minutes). The most vigorous responses with respect to temperature elevation and blood flow changes will occur with the dip-and-reimmerse technique.[61] This technique would not be well suited for most patients who are predisposed to edema, or if they cannot sit comfortably in the position required for treatment. This technique also precludes other patients from using the wax bath during that time period. If there are potential treatment areas that are not amenable to either of these methods, the wax can be painted on using a paint brush, applying up to 10 coats of wax.

When using paraffin to improve skin pliability over healed burn areas, a temperature of 47°C (116.6°F) has been suggested.[40] Paraffin also lubricates and conditions the skin, because of the mineral oil content.[62] This can be particularly useful when treating a scarred skin area. Using wax and stretching, Head and Helms[60] demonstrated a maintainable average increase in range of motion of 7 to 10 degrees in joints of patients with burn scars. If wax is applied over a skin-grafted area, the graft should be stable, nonfragile, and at least 10 days postgraft.[40] Treatment is daily for 2 to 3 weeks.

Paraffin baths are often used as part of a treatment program in patients with rheumatoid arthritis. Wax is used in the nonflare phases to decrease pain and increase tissue extensibility. Dellhag and associates[63] found wax baths to be an effective treatment for this population. Although they found no significant therapeutic effects with wax-bath treatments alone, there was a significant improvement in stiffness, range of motion, and grip function when the wax treatment was followed by active exercise.

Relative to other heat modalities, paraffin wax is not significantly better at decreasing pain or increasing joint range of motion. Hoyrup and Kjorvel[41] compared whirlpool and wax treatments for hand therapy. They measured hand volume, range of motion, and level of pain immediately prior to and following 3 weeks of treatment. While all subjects showed significant improvements in range of motion as well as decreased pain levels, no significant differences were found between the modalities. Hawkes and associates[64] compared wax baths with both ultrasound alone and ultrasound followed by an electrical stimulation hand bath in patients with rheumatoid arthritis of the hands. All treatment groups demonstrated significant improvements in the seven measurements taken (grip strength, joint size, articular index, range of motion, timed task, functional activities, and pain, measured using a VAS), although they found no significant differences among treatment groups.

Paraffin should not be applied over open wounds because of the risk of burning the tissues. Patients with infected skin lesions should not use wax for fear of exacerbating the lesion. When contagious skin conditions or warts are present, prior to immersion in the wax bath, the area is covered with a bandage or some form of plastic skin film, as the wax bath could become contaminated.

Advantages of Paraffin Wax
1. Low specific heat allows for application at a higher temperature than water without the risk of a burn.
2. Low thermal conductivity allows for heating of tissues to occur more slowly, thus reducing the risk of overheating the tissues.
3. Molten state allows for even distribution of heat to areas like fingers and toes.
4. First dip traps air and moisture to create more even heat distribution.
5. Oils used in the wax add moisture to the skin.
6. Wax remains malleable after removal, allowing for use as an exercise tool.
7. Comfortable, moist heat.
8. Relatively inexpensive to replace wax (assuming bath is already owned).

Disadvantages of Paraffin Wax
1. Effective only for distal extremities in terms of ease of application.
2. Most effective method of application is the bath method, which limits accessibility for other body parts to be treated effectively.
3. No method of temperature control once applied.
4. Heating lasts only about 20 minutes.
5. It is a passive treatment; exercise may not be performed simultaneously.

Convective Heating: Fluidotherapy

Fluidotherapy (Henley, Sugar Land, TX) is a dry heat agent that transfers heat energy by forced convection. Borrell and coworkers[3] suggest that for superficial heating, it is irrelevant whether the modality is providing wet or dry heat, provided that the skin temperature is raised to the same temperature by both agents. The Fluidotherapy system uses air-fluidized solids as the heat-transfer medium.[65] Warm air is uniformly circulated through the bottom of a bed of finely divided cellulose particles (finely ground corn cob, dubbed "cellex") in a container.[65] The solid particles become suspended when the stream of air is forced through them, making the fluidized bed behave and demonstrate properties similar to those of liquids.[3,65] The viscosity of the air-fluidized system is low, allowing a patient to submerge body parts into the fluidized bed and suspending these parts similar to being in a fluid, thus permitting exercise with relative ease.[65,66] The heat transfer characteristics within the fluidized bed and to parts submerged in it are similar to those of a mildly agitated liquid.[65] The combination of air flowing around the high surface area of the finely divided particles, and the bulk movement of solids produces high heat fluxes and uniform temperatures throughout, thus providing a strong massaging action, sensory stimulation, and levitation.[65]

Fluidotherapy units come in a variety of sizes (Figs. 5–9 and 5–10). There are

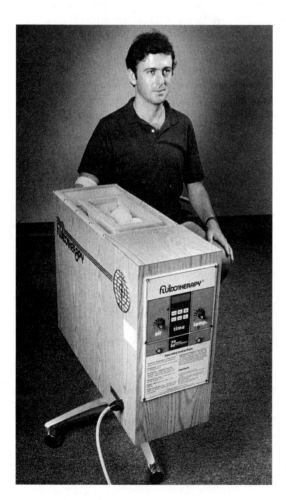

FIGURE 5–9. Fluidotherapy to the hand and wrist.

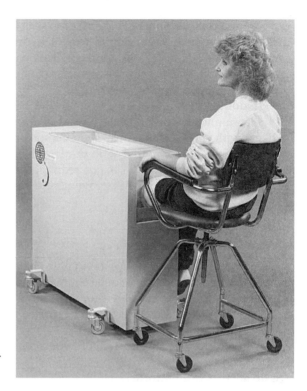

FIGURE 5-10. Fluidotherapy unit designed to immerse the leg and knee. (Photo courtesy of Henley, a division of Maxxim Medical, Sugar Land, TX.)

units for treating the distal extremities and larger joints, and there is a larger model available for the treatment of the back. For joints and distal body parts, the patient places the body part to be treated through the entrance sleeve of the Fluidotherapy unit. The sleeve is then secured to keep the cellulose particles from escaping. As the air stream is blown in, the particles become suspended and the treated body part feels as though it is immersed in a moving liquid bath, such as a whirlpool.

Both temperature and the amount of particle agitation can be varied. Temperature ranges for treatment are typically from 38.8°C to 47.8°C (102°F to 118°F). The lower ranges are recommended for patients who have a greater predisposition for edema formation or who are in beginning programs for desensitization, when they may not be able to tolerate higher temperatures. Agitation can be controlled for patient comfort. In addition, varying degrees of agitation can be used in a program of desensitization for hypersensitive areas.

Patients can carry out exercises while the affected body part(s) are within the cabinet. This is particularly effective for the distal extremities, such as the wrist, hand and fingers, and ankle, foot and toes. If heat and stretch is desired, dynamic splinting can be used during the time of heat treatment to provide a gentle stretch, or stretching techniques can be used immediately following immersion in Fluidotherapy.

If it is desirable to treat a body part that also has an open wound, the wound can be protected by a plastic barrier or bag to prevent any fine cellulose particles from becoming embedded in the wound, and to minimize the risk of cross-contamination.

The effectiveness of Fluidotherapy as a superficial heating agent was compared to paraffin wax and hydrotherapy by in vivo temperature measurements.[3] Joint capsule and muscle temperatures in the hands and feet were measured at various depths, with indication that the Fluidotherapy produced the greatest increase in tissue temperatures in all areas. The authors' conclusion was that the dry whirlpool (Fluidotherapy) delivered more heat than paraffin wax or hydrotherapy because higher temperatures can be tolerated in a dry environment. This conclusion is questioned, particularly in view of the fact that paraffin wax in particular allows tissues to be immersed into a bath with an operating temperature of 45°C to 54°C (113°F to 129°F), compared with the Fluidotherapy range of 39°C to 48°C (102.2°F to 118.4°F).

Alcorn and coworkers[67] used Fluidotherapy and exercise in the management of patients with sickle cell anemia. They demonstrated a marked reduction in the length of hospitalization (compared with the length of hospitalization by the same patients during previous episodes), a major reduction in the dosage of analgesics previously administered, and a marked improvement in spine, trunk and extremity range of motion, and gait.

Advantages of Fluidotherapy
1. Convenient, easy to administer.
2. Temperature of application can be controlled.
3. Agitation of dry particles can be controlled for comfort.
4. Variety of sizes of units allows for most body areas to be treated.
5. Allows for some active exercise to be carried out during treatment.
6. Dry, comfortable heat.
7. Can be used for desensitization of hypersensitive hand/finger(s) or foot/toe(s).

Disadvantages of Fluidotherapy
1. Relatively expensive modality to purchase.
2. Intolerance of some patients to enclosed container (claustrophobic feeling).
3. Intolerance of some patients to dry materials used.

CLINICAL APPLICATION: PRINCIPLES AND INDICATIONS

Superficial heating agents are used in therapeutic programs to assist in reduction of pain and stiffness, to alleviate muscle spasm, to increase range of motion, and to improve tissue healing by increasing blood flow and nutrients to an area. When superficial heat is applied to the trunk, shoulders, hips, or knees, it is usually considered a mild heat. The site of dysfunction is often well below the surface, and the heat will produce desired responses through reflex mechanisms by stimulation of cutaneous afferents. Mild heating usually elevates temperature at the site of pathology to less than 40°C (104°F) and may be thought of as having a soothing, counterirritant effect.[6]

When a higher temperature, for example, between 40°C and 45°C (104°F and 113°F) is desired at the involved structure, then the appropriate agent for the treatment must be chosen. Paraffin, for example, may be a vigorous heater of the finger joints, but only a mild heater of the shoulder. The principles of mild versus vigorous heating are summarized in Table 5–2.

Treatment time with all superficial heating agents usually varies from 15 to 30 minutes. After this time, no further significant increases in blood flow occur.[8] This duration will allow time for maximal tolerable increases in tissue temperature and blood flow.

Despite the widespread clinical use of superficial heating agents, there are very few well-designed clinical studies that address the efficacy of these modalities in a

TABLE 5–2 Comparison of Mild and Vigorous Heating[1]

	Mild	Vigorous
Temperature elevation site of pathology	Low	High
Degree of temperature increase	Comfortable sensation of warmth—up to 40°C	Near tolerance levels up to 45°C
Rate of rise of temperature	Slowly	Rapid
Duration of peak temperature elevation	Relatively short period	Relatively long period
Clinical examples	Hot packs to cervical area for reducing muscle spasm in upper trapezius	Fluidotherapy at 45°C to the hand for increasing tissue extensibility

therapeutic regimen. The remainder of this chapter will discuss some of those studies and will provide treatment suggestions based on purported physiologic rationales and the clinical experience of the authors.

Reduction of Pain and Muscle Spasm

Symptomatic resolution of pain or elevation of pain threshold can be justification for giving a superficial heat agent before exercise, posture training, or gait training. Muscle spasm can perpetuate pain and limited motion. Alleviation of the spasm can be accomplished by using a heat agent.

Heat can be used before stretching exercises to reduce pain. A comparison was made among normal subjects of the effects of heat alone, stretch alone, and heat plus stretch.[68] In one group, an electric heating pad at a temperature of 43°C (109.4°F) was used for 20 minutes over the back and sides of each subject's thigh. Then range-of-motion measurements were taken and compared to pretest values. The second group had exercise only, including contract-relax, followed by passive stretch of the hamstrings. The third group had heat and exercise as described for the first two groups. No changes in range of motion were measured with the heat-only group. The greatest change was measured in hip flexion in the heat-and-stretch group, compared with the stretch-only group. This technique of heat application would not be expected to alter the viscous properties of underlying muscle due to minimal or no temperature elevation of those structures. Therefore, range-of-motion increases could probably be attributed to the analgesic effect of heat, which allowed the person to tolerate the stretch better.

A comparison between hot packs and continuous shortwave diathermy (SWD) was made for trigger-point therapy.[69] Hot packs or SWD were administered for 20 minutes over trigger points in the thoracic, lumbar, or gluteal region. Heat was adjusted to patient tolerance. Pain was measured at the trigger points by tolerable grams of pressure from a pressure algometer. Both hot packs and SWD were effective in reducing pain at the most sensitive trigger points. SWD was more effective in treating less-sensitive trigger points. (An interesting comparison would be between cold versus heat for trigger-point therapy.)

Cervical pain of varying origins (injury, arthritis, or tension) was treated with hot packs, deep massage, and exercise.[70] About one half of all patients were reported to have "good improvement," but the criteria for improvement were not defined by the investigators.

Hot packs reduced muscle spasms in patients with cervical osteoarthritis and neck or hamstring spasms secondary to poliomyelitis.[71] A decrease in spasm was correlated with a decrease in resistance to passive stretch. A static force balance, which measures the force required to initiate movement about a joint, was the measurement tool used. No comparisons were made to the non–heat-treated patients.

Alcorn and associates[67] reported a decreased length of hospitalization for children with pain and loss of motion secondary to sickle cell anemia crises, when Fluidotherapy and exercise were used in combination. The authors also reported decreased dosage of analgesics, increased range of motion, and improved gait. This was compared to the same population of children who were previously hospitalized with sickle cell crises. Fluidotherapy at 45.6°C (114°F), using the unit on which the patient lies, was used two times per day for 30 minutes. This was usually followed by 10 to 30 minutes of exercise. It would be interesting to compare this treatment regimen with one using whirlpools or hot packs.

Williams and associates[42] compared the use of hot packs and exercise versus ice packs and exercise on the shoulder of patients with rheumatoid arthritis of the shoulder. Although both the ice and heat groups demonstrated decreases in pain and increases in shoulder range of motion, there were no significant differences between groups.

Hawkes and associates[64] compared the results of treating the hands of patients with rheumatoid arthritis with wax, ultrasound, and ultrasound followed by an electrical stimulation hand bath. Routine hand exercises were added to each technique. The results showed a significant improvement in pain reduction for all the methods used, although the use of ultrasound alone or ultrasound plus electrical stimulation hand baths had no advantage over the use of paraffin wax.

Hoyrup and Kjorvel[41] compared whirlpool at 43°C (109.4°F) and wax treatments for hand therapy in patients with traumatic hand injuries (excluding burns). Patients were divided into four groups: whirlpool with exercise, whirlpool alone, wax bath with exercise (not in the wax bath), and wax alone. There were significant decreases in pain scores and increases in range of motion for all groups, although there were no significant differences amongst groups. There were no differences in hand volume for any of the groups.

An interesting study compared the effects of active hand exercises and warm wax treatment in 52 patients with rheumatoid arthritis randomized into four groups.[63] The groups were as follows: (1) wax bath and exercise, (2) exercise only, (3) wax bath only, and (4) controls. Treatment was given three times a week for 4 weeks. All groups were measured for pain, digital range of motion, grip function, grip strength, and stiffness before and after the treatment period. The wax bath followed by active hand exercise resulted in significant improvements in range of motion and grip function. Active hand exercise alone reduced stiffness and pain with nonresisted motion and increased range of motion. Wax baths alone had no significant effect. This interesting study demonstrates the absolute need to include exercise as an adjunct to superficial heat in a treatment program where the aim is to decrease pain and spasm, and increase range of motion and function.

When treating a patient with pain, muscle spasm, or both, the patient's position for treatment must be carefully selected and should be the most comfortable position possible, particularly considering that the patient may need to remain in that position for up to 30 minutes. If muscle spasm is present, the muscle(s) should not be in a position of "undue stretch" until some pain relief has occurred. If the patient has joint pain, the joint should be positioned in an open-packed position,[72] with the ligaments and joint capsule in a slackened position. In this position, intra-articular pressure[73] and stress on joint structures will be lessened.

CASE STUDY 1

A 25-year-old female legal secretary is seen in physical therapy 8 weeks following reduction and casting of a right distal radius fracture. The cast was removed yesterday. Her physician indicates that the fracture has healed well, and she can commence physical therapy. She indicates that she is an avid pianist and is concerned about losing the ability to play.

PROBLEMS

1. Pain on active and passive motion of wrist and fingers
2. Mild swelling on dorsum of hand
3. Skin is dry and flaky
4. Functional activities are limited

ASSESSMENT TECHNIQUES

1. Volumetrics of hand and wrist
2. Pain quantity, quality, and location
3. Range-of-motion measurements
4. Strength measurements of wrist, hand, and fingers
5. Functional daily activities assessment

GOALS

1. Reduce and maintain reduction of swelling
2. Reduce pain
3. Increase range of motion of wrist, hand, and fingers
4. Increase muscle strength of wrist, hand, and fingers
5. Increase functional activities

SELECTION OF TREATMENT MODALITY

Superficial Heat—Paraffin Wax Bath

This patient would do well to have her hand and wrist immersed in a paraffin wax bath, initially utilizing the dip-and-wrap method. Following six to eight dips, the hand should be covered with a plastic bag and then wrapped with terry towelling to help retain the heat. After 20 minutes, the wax is removed by the patient, and while it remains soft and malleable, the wax can be used as an exercise tool for the hand and fingers.

This method of treatment could be used for the first few treatments, as it is gentle and takes into consideration the patient's pain with movement. Once the pain has subsided, the method of heating could be changed to either warm whirlpool or Fluidotherapy, where the patient could perform active exercises during the heat treatment.

HOME PROGRAM

This patient should be instructed to carry out active and passive exercises for range of motion for the wrist and fingers, as well as early strengthening exercises such as squeezing a soft rubber or foam ball, as well as rubber band exercises to increase finger abduction/adduction strength. It may be advisable to provide her with a home paraffin unit in order for her to heat the tissue prior to exercise and mobilization. If wax is not feasible, she could soak her hand in warm water in a sink or some form of container. Her home program should be written out in clear and concise terms relative to what she should be doing, how many times, and how often.

RATIONALE FOR CLINICAL DECISION MAKING

Owing to the period of immobilization, one would expect that decreased range of motion is primarily due to capsular shortening and adhesions. Heat followed by exercise can increase tissue extensibility. Paraffin wax application can be expected to increase the temperature of the involved structures. With the wax on, the patient can elevate her forearm and hand during treatment to help prevent further swelling. Passive and active exercises can be performed following removal of the wax. Oils contained in the wax will add moisture to the patient's dry and flaky skin.

CASE STUDY 2

A 49-year-old male taxi driver was involved in a motor vehicle accident 10 days ago, where he was stopped at a red light and struck from behind by another vehicle. He sustained an acceleration-deceleration (whiplash) type of injury, which strained the muscles and soft tissues in his neck. No bony injury or neurologic insult occurred. He has not yet been able to return to driving his taxi, although he is anxious to do so. He is not in need of any assistive devices such as a cervical collar. He has been referred to physical therapy.

PROBLEMS

1. Pain in the neck region, primarily on active movements of rotation and flexion
2. Muscle spasm in the posterior neck muscles, more on the left than the right
3. Decreased active range of motion of all neck movements, primarily rotation, flexion, and side flexion
4. Having difficulty sleeping because of his sore neck

ASSESSMENT TECHNIQUES

1. Pain quality, quantity, and location
2. Range of motion measurements
3. Functional daily activities assessment

GOALS

1. Reduce pain
2. Reduce muscle spasm
3. Increase neck range of motion
4. Increase functional activities

SELECTION OF TREATMENT MODALITY

Superficial Heat—Hot Pack

This patient would benefit from having a cervical hot pack applied to his neck region. He should be in a long sitting position on a treatment bed, with a pillow under his knees and behind his back and shoulders. An alternative position is supine with a pillow under his knees. The hot pack is applied to his neck and left on for about 20 minutes. Following removal of the hot pack, he should be taught active exercises to improve his neck range of motion. He may receive massage to the neck following the heat and preceding the exercises.

HOME PROGRAM

At home, this patient could apply a hot water bottle or electric heating pad to his neck region prior to doing his range-of-motion exercises. He should complete his exercises in front of a mirror, in order to see how well he is performing and improving. His home program should be written out in clear and concise terms relative to what he should be doing, how many times, and how often. He may wish to apply the heating pad or hot water bottle for 15 minutes just before going to bed in the evening in order to help him get a more comfortable sleep.

RATIONALE FOR CLINICAL DECISION MAKING

Muscle spasm and pain can be diminished using superficial heating agents. The sedative effect of the heat will allow this patient to become more mobile in his neck region because of the decrease of pain and spasm. Moist heat is comfortable to most patients, and the increased ability for his muscles to be stretched and exercised after heating will increase his range of motion and thus increase his functional capabilities.

Improving Range of Motion

In addition to heat decreasing the pain associated with stretching, if the temperature of tightened structures is elevated to high but tolerable levels, then tissue is stretched so that range of motion can improve. The stretch should begin after temperature levels have reached their maximum, and a slow, prolonged stretch should be held throughout the period necessary for the tissues to cool back to preheat values. This increased tissue "length" should be maintained over a long duration, that is, up to hours. Devices such as dynamic splints and continuous passive motion machines can be used to facilitate increases in range of motion.[74]

Range of motion during one treatment session could be expected to increase up to 5 to 10 degrees.[6] If increases are more dramatic, one could predict that either tissue was overzealously stretched (thus potentially damaged) or that the cause of the limited range of motion was not alterations in connective tissue.

In addition to those studies described in the previous section that measured changes in range of motion as well as reduction in pain and/or spasm following the use of superficial heating agents, a few others warrant some discussion. Lentell and coworkers[7] described the use of thermal agents to influence the effectiveness of a low-load prolonged stretch (LLPS) to increase shoulder flexibility. Subjects were randomly assigned to one of five groups, which included treatment groups of: (1) low-load prolonged stretch alone, (2) heat applied in the initial phase of an LLPS, (3) cold applied in the final phase of stretch, (4) a combination of heat initially followed by cold, and (5) no intervention. Subjects received three 40-minute treatments over a 5-day period. Results demonstrated that an LLPS associated with the use of heat, ice, or a combination of both facilitated longer improvements in flexibility compared with controls. However, only subjects receiving heat in the initial stages of an LLPS demonstrated significant gains when compared with those who received stretching alone.

Two reports examined the use of superficial heating agents and their effect on burn contractures. Burns and Conin[40] advocated the use of paraffin wax daily for 2 to 3 weeks (on average). The paraffin was applied and left on for 15 to 20 minutes, and the patient's limb was held in a position of maximum stretch, often using a 500-g (1-pound) weight, or some other form of restraint. Their recommendation was to apply the wax to a larger area than necessarily required treatment in order to lubricate the surrounding skin and therefore ease the discomfort of stretching tight skin and scars.

Head and Helms[60] described a similar treatment protocol utilizing paraffin wax and sustained stretch to treat burn contractures. Patients whose joint range of motion had reached a plateau were chosen for this treatment regimen. The temperature of the wax was lowered to 33°C (91.4°F) to accommodate decreases in skin sensitivity and the decreased viability of any newly healed skin. A variety of body parts and joints were treated either by the wax dip method or the wax paint method. The area was covered by a sheet of plastic and several layers of towelling in order to maintain the heat for 20 to 30 minutes. In a review of 20 patients, joint range-of-motion measurements taken immediately upon removal of the wax demonstrated an increase of 2 to 20 degrees, averaging 8 degrees. The skin appeared softer and more pliable, and subjectively more comfortable to the patient. Patients also reported a decrease in joint pain following the wax treatment.

CASE STUDY 3

A 74-year-old retired postal worker underwent arthroscopic surgery 5 days ago to remove a benign cyst from the back of his knee. He has been immobilized in a semirigid knee splint and is allowed to fully weight bear. Currently he is limping slightly and is using a cane for stability. He complains of aching and stiffness in the knee and has some difficulty with sitting, getting up from sitting, and managing stairs. He is in otherwise excellent health, and likes to walk, cycle, and square dance. His sutures are due to be removed in 2 days. He has been referred for physical therapy.

PROBLEMS

1. Stiffness in the knee
2. Aching in the knee
3. Loss of range of motion in the knee
4. Decreased functional activities

ASSESSMENT TECHNIQUES

1. Measure pain quality, quantity, and location
2. Measure knee joint range of motion
3. Measure knee joint stability
4. Measure muscle strength of hip and knee
5. Assess functional activities

GOALS

1. Reduce aching in knee
2. Reduce stiffness in knee
3. Increase knee range of motion
4. Increase muscle strength in hip and knee
5. Increase functional activities

SELECTION OF TREATMENT MODALITY

Superficial Heat—Fluidotherapy

Because this is a soft tissue and joint problem, this patient would benefit from heat as warm as tolerable in order to decrease the aching and stiffness felt in the knee. Fluidotherapy allows the leg to be completely immersed in the fluidized material, and the patient can actively exercise while in the unit (Fig. 5–10). The sutures can be covered by an occlusive dressing so as to not contaminate the wound or cross-contaminate the Fluidotherapy unit.

An alternative to Fluidotherapy would be a whirlpool bath, providing the wound could be properly waterproofed.

HOME PROGRAM

Knee flexion and extension range of motion, hip range of motion, and gait re-education should comprise part of this patient's home program. If pre-exercise heat is required, sitting in a warm bath would work well (where exercises could commence), or perhaps wrapping warm towels, a hot water bottle, or an electric heating pad around the knee would help to decrease the ache and feeling of stiffness prior to exercise. His home program should be written out in clear and concise terms relative to what he should be doing, how many times, and how often.

CONTRAINDICATIONS AND PRECAUTIONS TO SUPERFICIAL HEATING

Before deciding to use heat in a therapeutic regimen, the status of the patient's circulation, and sensitivity to temperature and to pain should be determined by the therapist. The skin overlying the treatment area should be tested for thermal sensation, using hot and cold water in test tubes, or with other hot and cold objects, such as spoons. Pain sensation can be determined by using the pinprick versus blunt test. This information is necessary, because determining the safe level of heat requires that the patient be able to perceive when the pain threshold has been reached. Response of thermal receptors in the skin is illustrated in Figure 5–11.

The following is a list of contraindications to the use of superficial heating agents:

- Application over areas with a lack of intact thermal sensation. (Risk of burn if patient cannot distinguish between hot and cold.)
- Application over areas of vascular insufficiency or vascular disease. (Risk of burn if circulation is inadequate to dissipate heat in tissues.)
- Application over areas of recent hemorrhage or potential hemorrhage. (Heat will increase bleeding.)

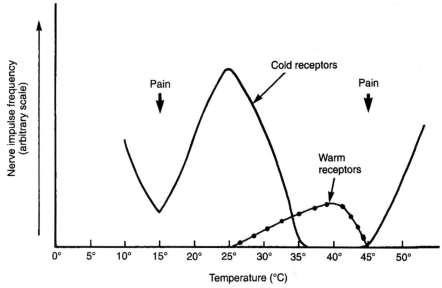

FIGURE 5–11. Responses of thermal receptors in the skin. (From Low, J and Reed, A: Electrotherapy Explained: Principles and Practice. Oxford, Butterworth-Heinemann, 1990, p 177, with permission.)

- Application over areas of known malignancy. (Heat may increase activation and movement of malignant cells.)
- Application over areas of acute inflammation. (Heat will aggravate and potentially increase inflammatory response.)
- Application over infected areas where infection may spread or cross-contamination may occur. (Heat may cause infection to spread to other areas.)
- Application over areas where liniments or heat rubs have recently been applied. (Heat will increase risk of burn because vessels are already dilated because of the presence of liniment; the vessels cannot dilate further to dissipate more heat.)
- Application in any situation deemed unreliable by the physical therapist. (Unreliable situations such as language difficulties put the patient at a risk because they may not understand the therapist's instructions.)

CLINICAL DECISION MAKING

The decision to use a thermal agent as part of a total treatment program should be based on a combination of factors, including the patient's diagnosis and medical status, and the objective findings on physical therapy assessment. It is not until this information is gathered that the treatment goals are established. The plan of treatment to obtain these goals can include a thermal agent, when indicated. It should be noted that, in most situations, it is only appropriate to apply one type of superficial heating agent. To include two, such as paraffin and whirlpool to the hand in one session, would most likely be redundant. Treatment is executed and follow-up done. The procedures for clinical decision making and carrying out the treatment are outlined in Table 5–3.

Heat Versus Cold

There are clinical situations when either heat or cold may be selected to meet treatment objectives, or when one is clearly preferred over the other. Often the choice between heat and cold is empirical, but before the decision is made, certain factors should be considered: (1) stage of injury or disease, (2) area of body treated, (3) medical status, (4) patient preference, which may be determined by cold or heat hypersensitivity, and (5) decision to use thermal agents as part of a home program. Cold is the preferred agent during the acute stages of inflammation—heat at this stage may further aggra-

TABLE 5–3 Procedure for Clinical Decision Making and
Execution of Treatment with a Thermal Agent

1. Assess patient.
2. Establish treatment goals based on results of patient assessment.
3. Select treatment plan including thermal agent when applicable to meet these goals.
4. Choose thermal agent.
5. Select position for treatment.
6. Apply thermal agent (followed by exercise or other appropriate techniques).
7. Reassess and determine if treatment will continue or be modified or discontinued.
8. Establish home program (which can include a thermal agent).

HEAT VS COLD

Heat		Cold	
Advantages: ↓ pain ↑ tissue extensibility ↓ stiffness	*Disadvantages:* May cause ↑ swelling	*Advantages:* May prevent further swelling ↓ pain	*Disadvantages:* ↑ stiffness ↓ tissue extensibility

FIGURE 5–12. Treatment choice: heat versus cold.

vate inflammation. In patients who can tolerate cryotherapy, this may be chosen for reduction of muscle spasm (see discussion, Chapter 4). Cold can also reduce pain around joints before range-of-motion exercises and may be easier for the patient to apply at home. On the other hand, heat may be better psychologically tolerated by persons with pain or muscle spasm, thus increasing patient compliance with treatment programs. Temperature elevation will decrease joint stiffness and increase connective tissue extensibility, so clearly, if either of these is the treatment goal, heat is the agent of choice. In addition, heat to distal extremities seems to be tolerated better than cold. The advantages and disadvantages of using heat or cold are briefly outlined in Figure 5–12.

Superficial Versus Deep Heat

The decision to use superficial versus deep heat primarily depends on the location of the involved structure, the pathophysiology, and the degree of temperature elevation desired (Fig. 5–13). Generally speaking, deep heat is usually selected during the

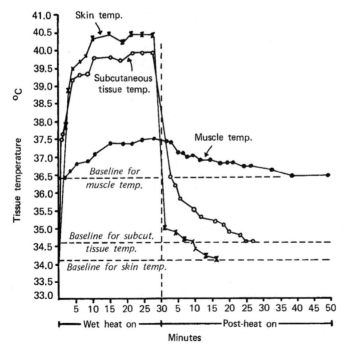

FIGURE 5–13. Curves representing changes in skin, subcutaneous tissue, and muscle temperatures obtained during and after 30 minutes of wet heat topically applied to the forearm. (From Abramson, et al,[8] with permission.)

remodeling phase of an injury or a disease when tissue contractures persist, or heating is required deep into a joint.

Wet Versus Dry Heat

Many patients say that they have heard that moist heat is more penetrating, and thus more effective, than dry heat. Clinical studies that examine the efficacy of one versus the other in obtaining functional treatment goals are not available. It has been determined, however, that dry heat can elevate surface temperatures to a greater degree, but that moist heat can elevate temperature to a slightly deeper level.[75]

Home Application of Superficial Heating Agents

In most cases, it is desirable to provide a patient with a means for pain control and reduction of stiffness before exercise, when they are not within the confines of a supervised clinical situation. Gel packs, sand packs, and bead packs are commercially available that can be heated in either a water container or a microwave oven. Both paraffin wax baths and Fluidotherapy units are available in home use sizes, which are generally for the hands, wrists, and feet. Electric heating pads would also provide superficial heat, and they are available in various sizes. Adequate, clear, and concise instructions should be written down for the home patient, including the treatment time, method, frequency of application, and any special instructions and precautions.

DOCUMENTATION OF TREATMENT

The astute clinician realizes the importance of documenting the specifics of treatment techniques and patient response to therapeutic intervention. Information included in the treatment record should include the thermal agent used, method of application, duration of application, body area treated, patient position for treatment, and any special precautions or application concerns. Without such information, it is often difficult to replicate techniques and to adjust the plan of care as needed. A copy of home instructions should be kept with the patient's file.

SUMMARY

The use of heat in a therapeutic program is predicated on the biophysical effects of temperature elevation, including elevation of pain threshold, decrease in muscle spasm, decrease in joint stiffness, increase in blood flow, and increase in collagen tissue extensibility.

Superficial heating agents used in physical therapy include hot packs, paraffin wax, and Fluidotherapy. Guidelines for their clinical and home use, as well as safety and precautions and contraindications have been presented.

Study Objectives

Having completed this chapter, the reader should now be able to:

1. Explain the methods of heat transfer.
2. Describe the local effects of elevation of tissue temperature.
3. Discuss the effects of heat and pain on muscle spasm.
4. Explain the rationale for elevating tissue temperature before stretching exercises.
5. Discuss the techniques of application of hot packs, Fluidotherapy, and paraffin.
6. Explain why heat should be used with great caution with impaired sensation and decreased circulation.
7. Describe the elements of documentation for treatment with hot packs, Fluidotherapy, and paraffin.
8. Discuss the decisions to be made when choosing among hot packs, Fluidotherapy, and paraffin for heat application.
9. Discuss safety issues regarding the home use of superficial heat agents.

REFERENCES

1. Lehmann, JF and deLateur, BJ: Therapeutic heat. In Lehmann, JF (ed): Therapeutic Heat and Cold, ed 4. Williams & Wilkins, Baltimore, 1990.
2. Baker, RJ and Bell, GW: The effect of therapeutic modalities on blood flow in the human calf. J Orthop Sports Phys Ther 13:23, 1991.
3. Borrell, RM, et al: Comparison of in vivo temperatures produced by hydrotherapy, paraffin wax treatment and Fluidotherapy. Phys Ther 60:1273, 1980.
4. Levi, SJ and Maihafer GC: Traditional approaches to pain (Chap. 3). In Echternach, J (ed): Pain. Churchill Livingstone, New York, 1987.
5. Halvorsen, GA: Therapeutic heat and cold for athletic injuries. Phys Sports Med 18:87, 1990.
6. Warren, CG: The use of heat and cold in the treatment of common musculoskeletal disorders. In Hertling, D and Kessler, RM: Management of Common Musculoskeletal Disorders, ed 2. Harper & Row, Philadelphia, 1989.
7. Lentell, G, et al: The use of thermal agents to influence the effectiveness of a low-load prolonged stretch. J Orthop Sports Phys Ther 16:200, 1992.
8. Abramson, DI, et al: Changes in blood flow, oxygen uptake and tissue temperatures produced by the topical application of wet heat. Arch Phys Med Rehabil 42:305, 1961.
9. Crockford, GW and Hellon, RF: Vascular responses in human skin to infra-red radiation. J Physiol 149:424, 1959.
10. Crockford, GW, Hellon, RF, and Parkhouse, J: Thermal vasomotor response in human skin mediated by local mechanisms. J Physiol 161:10, 1962.
11. Fischer, E and Solomon, S: Physiological responses to heat and cold. In Licht, S (ed): Therapeutic Heat and Cold, ed 2. Waverly Press, Baltimore, 1965.
12. Greenberg, RS: The effects of hot packs and exercise on local blood flow. Phys Ther 52:273, 1972.
13. Krusen, EM, et al: Effects of hot packs on peripheral circulation. Arch Phys Med 31:145, 1950.
14. Randall, BF, Imig, CJ, and Hines, HM: Effects of some physical therapies on blood flow. Arch Phys Med 33:73, 1952.
15. Hardy, JD and Bard, P: Body temperature regulation. In Mountcastle, VB (ed): Medical Physiology, Vol 2, ed 14. CV Mosby, St Louis, 1979.
16. Fyfe, M: Skin temperature, colour, and warmth felt, in hydrocollator pack applications to the lumbar region. Aust J Physiol 28:12, 1982.
17. Wadsworth, H and Chanmugam, APP: Electrophysical Agents in Physiotherapy, ed 2. Science Press, Marrickville, NSW, 1988.
18. Low, J and Reed, A: Electrotherapy Explained: Principles and Practice. Butterworth-Heinemann, Oxford, 1990.
19. Berne, R and Levy, MN: Cardiovascular Physiology, ed 3. CV Mosby, St. Louis, 1993.
20. Fox, HH and Hilton, SM: Bradykinin formation in human skin as a factor in heat vasodilation. J Physiol 142:219, 1958.
21. Milnor, WR: Autonomic and peripheral control mechanisms. In Mountcastle, VB (ed): Medical Physiology, Vol 2, ed 14. CV Mosby, St, Louis, 1979.

22. Guyton AC: Textbook of Medical Physiology, ed 8. WB Saunders, Philadelphia, 1991.
23. Abramson, DI, et al: Changes in blood flow. O_2 uptake and tissue temperatures produced by therapeutic physical agents. III. Effect of indirect or reflex vasodilation. Am J Phys Med 404:5, 1961.
24. Abramson, DI, et al: Indirect vasodilation in thermotherapy. Arch Phys Med Rehabil 46:412, 1965.
25. Wessman, MS, and Kottke, FJ: The effect of indirect heating on peripheral blood flow, pulse rate, blood pressure and temperature. Arch Phys Med Rehabil 48:567, 1967.
26. Wyper, DJ and McNiven DR: Effects of some physiotherapeutic agents on skeletal muscle blood flow. Physiotherapy 62:83, 1976.
27. Cobbold, AF and Lewis, OJ: Blood flow to the knee joint of the dog: Effect of heating, cooling and adrenaline. J Physiol 132:379, 1956.
28. Horvath, SM and Hollander, JL: Intra-articular temperature as a measure of joint reaction. J Clin Invest 28:469, 1949.
29. Johnson, JM and Park, MK: Effect of heat stress on cutaneous vascular responses to the initiation of exercise. J Appl Physiol 53:744, 1982.
30. Kanui, TI: Thermal inhibition of nociceptor-driven spinal cord nerves in rats. Pain 21:231, 1985.
31. Barbour, LA, McGuire, DB, and Kirchott, KT: Non-analgesic methods of pain control used by cancer outpatients. Oncol Nursing Forum 13:56, 1986.
32. Forster, N and Palastanga, A: Clayton's Electrotherapy: Theory and Practice, ed 9. Balliere-Tindall, London, 1985.
33. Lehmann, JD, Brunner, GD, and Stow, RW: Pain threshold measurements after therapeutic application of ultrasound, microwaves and infrared. Arch Phys Med Rehabil 39:560, 1958.
34. Abramson, DL, et al: Effect of tissue temperatures and blood flow on motor nerve conduction velocity. JAMA 198:1082, 1966.
35. Currier, DP, and Kramer, JF: Sensory nerve conduction: Heating effects of ultrasound and infrared. Physiother Canada 34:241, 1982.
36. Halle, JS, Scoville, CR, and Greathouse, DG: Ultrasound's effect on the conduction latency of the superficial radial nerve in man. Phys Ther 61:345, 1981.
37. Mense, S: Effects of temperature on the discharges of muscle spindles and tendon organs. Pflugers Arch 374:159, 1978.
38. Chastain, PB: The effect of deep heat on isometric strength. Phys Ther 58:543, 1978.
39. Edwards, HT, et al: Effect of temperature on muscle energy metabolism and endurance during successive isometric contractions, sustained to fatigue, of the quadriceps muscle in man. J Physiol 220:335, 1972.
40. Burns, S and Conin T: The use of paraffin wax in the treatment of burns. Physiother Canada 39:258, 1987.
41. Hoyrup, G and Kjorvel, L: Comparison of whirlpool and wax treatments for hand therapy. Physiother Canada 38:79, 1986.
42. Williams, J, Harvey, J, and Tannenbaum, H: Use of superficial heat versus ice for the rheumatoid arthritic shoulder: A pilot study. Physiother Canada 38:8, 1986.
43. DeVries, H: Quantitative electromyographic investigation of the spasms theory of muscle pain. Am J Phys Med 45:119, 1966.
44. Wickstrom, R and Polk, C: Effect of whirlpool on the strength endurance of the quadriceps muscle in trained male adolescents. Am J Phys Med 40:91, 1961.
45. LeBan, MM: Collagen tissue: Implications of its response to stress in vitro. Arch Phys Med Rehabil 43:461, 1962.
46. Wright, V and Johns, RJ: Quantitative and qualitative analysis of joint stiffness in normal subjects and in patients with connective tissue diseases. Ann Rheum Dis 20:36, 1961.
47. Backlund, L and Tiselius, P: Objective measurements of joint stiffness in rheumatoid arthritis. Acta Rheum Scand 13:275, 1967.
48. Reid, DC: Sports Injury Assessment and Rehabilitation. Churchill Livingstone, New York, 1992.
49. Sapega, AA, et al: Biophysical factors in range-of-motion exercise. Phys Sports Med 9:57, 1981.
50. Kottke, FJ, Pauley, DL, and Ptak, RA: The rationale for prolonged stretching for correction of shortening of connective tissue. Arch Phys Med Rehabil 47:345, 1966.
51. Lehmann, JF: Effect of therapeutic temperatures on tendon extensibility. Arch Phys Med Rehabil 51:481, 1970.
52. Warren, GC, Lehmann, JF, and Koblanski, JN: Heat and stretch procedures: An evaluation using rat tail tendon. Arch Phys Med Rehabil 57:122, 1976.
53. Akai, M, et al: Electrical stimulation of ligament healing: An experimental study of patellar ligament of rabbits. Clin Orthop 235:298, 1988.
54. Light, KE, et al: Low-load prolonged stretch vs. high-load brief stretch in treating knee contractures. Phys Ther 64:330, 1984.
55. Wright, V and Johns, RJ: Physical factors concerned with the stiffness of normal and diseased joints. Bull Johns Hopkins Hosp 106:215, 1960.
56. Hendler, E, Crosbie, R, and Hardy, JD: Measurement of heating of the skin during exposure to infrared radiation. J Appl Physiol 12:177, 1958.
57. Whyte, HM and Reader, SR: Effectiveness of different forms of heating. Ann Rheum Dis 10:449, 1951.
58. Mainardi, CL, et al: Rheumatoid arthritis: Failure of daily heat therapy to affect its progression. Arch Phys Med Rehabil 60:390, 1979.

59. Wakim, KG, Porter, AN, and Krusen, KH: Influence of physical agents and of certain drugs on intra-articular temperature. Arch Phys Med Rehabil 32:714, 1951.
60. Head, MD and Helms, PA: Paraffin and sustained stretching in the treatment of burn contractures. Burns 4:136, 1977.
61. Abramson, DI, et al: Effect of paraffin bath and hot fomentation on local tissue temperature. Arch Phys Med Rehabil 45:87, 1965.
62. Stimson, CW, Rose, GB, and Nelson, PA: Paraffin bath as thermotherapy: An evaluation. Arch Phys Med Rehabil 39:219, 1958.
63. Dellhag, B, Wollersjö, I, and Bjelle, A: Effect of hand exercise and wax bath treatment in rheumatoid arthritis patients. Arthritis Care Res 5:87, 1992.
64. Hawkes, J, et al: A comparison of three different physiotherapy treatments for rheumatoid arthritis of the hands. Physiother Pract 2:155, 1986.
65. Henley, EJ: Fluidotherapy. CRC Crit Rev Phys Med Rehabil 3:151, 1991.
66. Borrell, RM, et al: Fluidotherapy: Evaluation of a new heat modality. Arch Phys Med Rehabil 58:69, 1977.
67. Alcorn, R, et al: Fluidotherapy and exercise in the management of sickle cell anemia. Phys Ther 64:1520, 1984.
68. Harrison, AS, et al: The effect of heat and stretching on the range of hip motion. J Orthop Sports Phys Ther 6:110, 1984.
69. McGray, RE, and Patton, NJ: Pain relief at trigger points: A comparison of moist heat and shortwave diathermy. J Orthop Sports Phys Ther 5:175, 1984.
70. Cordray, YM, and Krusen, EM: Use of hydrocollator packs in the treatment of neck and shoulder pains. Arch Phys Med Rehabil 39:105, 1959.
71. Fountain, FP, Gersten, JW, and Senger, O: Decrease in muscle spasm produced by ultrasound, hot packs, and IR. Arch Phys Med Rehabil 41:293, 1960.
72. Hertling, D and Kessler RM: Management of Common Musculoskeletal Disorders, ed 2. Harper & Row, Philadelphia, 1989.
73. Eyring, EJ and Murray, WR: The effect of joint position on the pressure of intra-articular effusion. J Bone Joint Surg 46-A(6):1235, 1964.
74. Flowers, K, and Michlovitz, SL: Assessment and management of loss of motion in orthopaedic dysfunction. Postgraduate Advances in Physical Therapy, APTA, 1988.
75. Abramson, DI: Comparison of wet and dry heat in raising temperature of tissue. Arch Phys Med Rehabil 48:654, 1967.

CHAPTER 6

Hydrotherapy: The Use of Water as a Therapeutic Agent

Mark T. Walsh, PT, MS, CHT

Hydrotherapy is one of the oldest therapeutic methods for managing physical dysfunctions.[1] It has been advocated for the treatment of joint stiffness, painful scars, adhesions, and arthritis, and as a warm-up to assist with exercise.[2] Water therapy is used for the effects on body tissues of heating,[3] cooling, debridement,[4,5] pain relief, and relaxation of muscles. When treatment is not well planned or well executed, it can have adverse side effects, primarily on the cardiovascular system.

Hydrotherapy achieves its desired effects through the physical properties of water, temperature, and agitation. A basic understanding of these physical principles, normal physiology, and pathology involved serves as a foundation for the decision to use hydrotherapy in the treatment of a specific dysfunction. The objectives of this chapter are to (1) provide the reader with a knowledge of the physical principles underlying hydrotherapy, (2) discuss the biophysical effects of water immersion, (3) describe equipment preparation and maintenance, (4) discuss specific clinical techniques and pathologies, and (5) discuss safety in hydrotherapy.

PHYSICAL PRINCIPLES

Forces Existing in Water

Water has the inherent forces of buoyancy, pressure, cohesion, and viscosity, which play a role in the effects produced on the body from hydrotherapy. The most important of these is Archimedes' principle of buoyancy. This principle states that a body immersed in a liquid experiences an upward force equal to the weight of the displaced liquid.[6] Thus, the body appears to weigh less in water than it does in air. Buoyancy may be affected by (1) postural alignment; (2) the surface area immersed; (3) the weight of the bones in relationship to muscle and fat; and (4) vital capacity. The buoyancy of water can be used to assist with exercise of the extremities and to minimize stress of joints and muscles. Work can be done in the opposite direction, against the assist of buoyancy, so that resistance to motion can be exerted. In addition, by varying the speed of exercise in water, the difficulty of the exercise can be changed or graded. These concepts will be discussed in more detail.

The principle of relative density is used to provide support of the body and its limbs in water. Specific gravity is the ratio of the weight of a volume of substance to the weight of an equal volume of water. The specific gravity of the body is approximately 0.974. Objects with a specific gravity less than 1.0 will float in water. The specific gravity of the body, therefore, can be advantageous to exercise in water.

Water exerts a perpendicular pressure against the surface of the body. This hydrostatic pressure is the ratio of the magnitude of the force exerted by the fluid per body surface area. This pressure is dependent on the depth of the submerged part and the density of the liquid. Hydrostatic pressure increases as depth and density of the liquid increase. Therefore, motion is performed more easily near the surface of the water than at greater depths.

Water molecules are cohesive; they have a tendency to attract each other. This results in an increase in viscosity of the medium, as compared with that of air, and an increase in resistance to motion. Viscosity is internal friction, the property of liquids that resists relative motion within it. The greater the speed of the liquid, the higher the viscosity. Resistance to motion is also dependent on the shape of the body. The more streamlined the body or object, the less force is required to move it through the water. The larger and more spread out the object moving through the water, the greater the resistance to motion. As will be discussed later, viscosity and pressure will play a role in turbulence created by the whirlpool agitation.

Methods of Heat Transfer

Hydrotherapy is performed in water tanks of varying sizes and shapes. Tanks used for partial body immersion (that is, immersion of one or two extremities) are termed whirlpools. (Often the terms "hydrotherapy" and "whirlpool" are used interchangeably.) Tanks used for full-body immersion are referred to as Hubbard tanks, walking tanks, or hydrotherapeutic exercise tanks or pools. When the body is immersed, thermal energy is exchanged by water in the tank by two methods: conduction and convection.

CONDUCTION

Conduction is an exchange of thermal energy in which there is physical contact between two surfaces. If water temperature is higher than skin temperature, heat will be conducted to the skin and temperature will rise. Since fat acts more as an insulator than as a conductor, it has a tendency to hold heat in or to keep it out. This point is important for two reasons: (1) the effect of superficial heating by conduction will be lessened as the body fat composition increases; and (2) higher body fat content compromises the body's ability to dissipate heat, which may cause an increase in body-core temperature to dangerous levels. With the obese person, therefore, superficial heating with the whirlpool may not achieve the intended effects. Caution must be taken when a large body surface area is immersed; the person may not be able to dissipate internal heat and maintain proper core temperature. This may present a dangerous situation, requiring other methods of heat loss, such as evaporation and convection, to work overtime causing dehydration and increased cardiac output. A particular patient's medical condition may not tolerate this situation, such as a patient with a cardiac or peripheral vascular diseases.

CONVECTION

Convection, which occurs when a portion of the fluid moves from one place to another, is a more rapid process of thermal energy exchange than conduction. Energy transfer by convection occurs when the patient is moving in the water or when the water swirls across the skin surface. Convection plays an important role in heating or cooling tissues, as well as in dissipating or retaining body heat.

Convection occurs between the core and the shell of the body. Surface body heat can be carried by the venous blood toward the core, thus potentially increasing core temperature. Conversely, convection will help with heat dissipation by carrying heat away from areas of the body that are being heated. This method of heat transfer is compromised when the patient has cardiovascular or peripheral vascular disease. In this case, heating an entire extremity or full body may create dangerous overheating because the extremity or body is unable to dissipate heat from the treated area to maintain tissue temperature at safe levels.

Thus far, the methods of heat transfer discussed were used to transport heat in either direction in the body. Two other methods of heat transfer, radiation and evaporation, help to dissipate heat from the body during or following a hydrotherapy treatment.

RADIATION

Radiation is the exchange of electromagnetic energy that occurs when there is a difference in temperature between the skin and the surrounding environment. As convection and conduction bring the heat from within the body to the level of the skin, radiation assists in the transfer of this heat from the skin to the air. This ability to eliminate heat through radiation will be lost in the area immersed in the whirlpool and is further compromised as body surface immersion increases.

EVAPORATION

The other heat transfer mechanism used to dissipate heat is evaporation. No temperature gradient is necessary. Evaporation occurs through the loss of fluid from sweating and by the pulmonary system during exhalation. Any disturbance with the autonomic nervous or pulmonary system's functions may interfere with loss of heat by evaporation. Therefore, when administering hydrotherapy, sufficient body surface must be exposed to the air to allow heat loss; otherwise, water temperatures must be kept below a body temperature between 33.3°C and 36.6°C.

Heat loss is affected not only by the medical condition of the patient and his or her ability to cope with heat, but also by the environmental factors of humidity and temperature. If either humidity and/or ambient room temperature is too high, the body will have great difficulty with heat loss. On the other hand, should the ambient temperature be too low and the area dry, heat loss may occur to a greater extent than needed, thereby causing a chill. Therefore, muscle and joint stiffness secondary to the reduction in peripheral circulation could occur. Strong consideration, therefore, should be given to the design and environment of the hydrotherapy area.

BIOPHYSICAL EFFECTS

Thermal Effects

One of the principal reasons for using hydrotherapy is to gain the therapeutic value of heat or cold. The same physiologic effects of heat and cold apply to hydrotherapy as to other thermal agents, except that a larger body surface area usually is immersed in water than that covered by a hot or cold pack. Therefore, exposure of the body to varying temperatures will have not only a local effect (see Chapter 5), but also systemic effects on the cardiovascular and other organ systems. The greater the difference in temperature between the water and skin, the more intense the reaction. Cold application to the whole body decreases heart rate and lengthens diastole. The tone of the cardiac muscle is enhanced, and blood pressure is raised, as a result of peripheral vasoconstriction. The increase in peripheral resistance requires the heart to work harder to maintain adequate blood flow to the periphery. Other effects of cold immersion can be reviewed in Chapter 4.

The application of heat to the entire body will cause an initial increase in blood pressure, followed by a decrease in blood pressure as a result of vasodilation. The initial rise in blood pressure may be quite marked and prolonged if the temperature of the bath is very high, above 40°C. Respiratory rate will increase with the application of heat or cold, although the increase may be less marked with the application of heat. Dawson and associates[7] studied the effects of hydrotherapy on cardiac output, oxygen consumption, heart rate, and blood pressure, with study subjects in the resting state (positioned supine and sitting) and while exercising (the step test). The subjects were immersed in the whirlpool to hip level for 20 minutes in 40°C water. The mean cardiac output and oxygen consumption increased, but not significantly. Pulse rate increased 1.3 to 1.5 times over the sitting or supine resting level, and the mean blood pressure increased 1.1 times over the supine resting values.

In addition, sweating will increase; the amount is dependent on the temperature, the size of body surface exposed, and the length of treatment. Whether the use of hydrotherapy bath increases diuresis remains controversial,[8,9] but diuresis seems to be affected by the hydrostatic pressure, which increases with the depth of immersion. This influence of hydrostatic pressure may have more of an effect on urinary output than does water temperature itself.

Increasing tissue temperature and blood flow are physiologic effects of heat that can have therapeutic value. The depth to which this vasodilation occurs, and its relationship to tissue temperature, are important. If whirlpool does not increase circulation and temperature to sufficient levels to meet therapeutic goals, it may not be the agent of choice. When one arm was immersed in a water bath of 45°C for 20 minutes, there was a 4.17°C rise in subcutaneous-tissue temperature, a 1.4°C rise in muscle temperature of the forearm, and an increase in blood flow.[10,11] There is a direct relationship between the increase in superficial blood flow and temperature with the arm immersed in a water bath from 37°C to 42°C. Borrell and coworkers[13] confirmed the penetrating ability of whirlpool in their study in which the thumb-joint capsule temperature rose 4°C in a whirlpool bath at 38.9°C when given for a 20-minute period.

Mechanical Effects

WHIRLPOOL AGITATION

Whenever the effects of both cold or superficial heat and water are indicated for a rehabilitation program, the use of whirlpool has been advocated. Physiologically, the whirlpool acts as an analgesic agent, relaxes muscle spasm, relieves joint pain and stiffness, improves mechanical debridement,[14] and facilitates exercise.[15] Based on these facts, its use has been suggested for debriding necrotic tissue and dirt[3,5,8,14,15] before exercising,[3] and for various musculoskeletal problems.[2] The agitation created by the whirlpool serves as a source of mechanical stimulation to skin receptors, which may explain its sedative and analgesic effects. The agitation may act as a counterirritant, or it may act as a stimulus to large sensory afferent nerve fibers, thus blocking pain input.

Cohen and associates[16] studied the effects of agitation on blood flow by comparing agitation and nonagitation on diseased and normal extremities. There was no significant effect on blood flow in limbs immersed in whirlpool baths of 38.6°C without agitation and 37.7°C with agitation.[16]

Determining what effects agitation has on body tissues requires some understanding of the pressure and turbulence created in the whirlpool. This has been studied in several types of whirlpools. In general, pressure was significantly increased when greater amounts of air were entered into the agitation, and there was more turbulence toward the surface than deeper in the water.[17] The importance of these concepts will be clarified further on in this chapter, especially regarding exercise and open-wound care.

GENERAL DESCRIPTION AND UNIT OPERATION

Whirlpool Types

There are basically two types of whirlpools, portable and fixed. In most cases, with the exception of full-body therapeutic tubs, such as the Hubbard tank or walk tank, any size or style of whirlpool can be either fixed or portable. There are three styles of whirlpool baths. They are depicted in Figure 6–1, along with their usual dimensions.[18] The "extremity" tank is used for the treatment of arms and legs. The "lowboy" and "highboy" (hip or leg tank) can be used for lower extremity or trunk immersion. Each of these tank styles has specific applications that will be discussed later.[18]

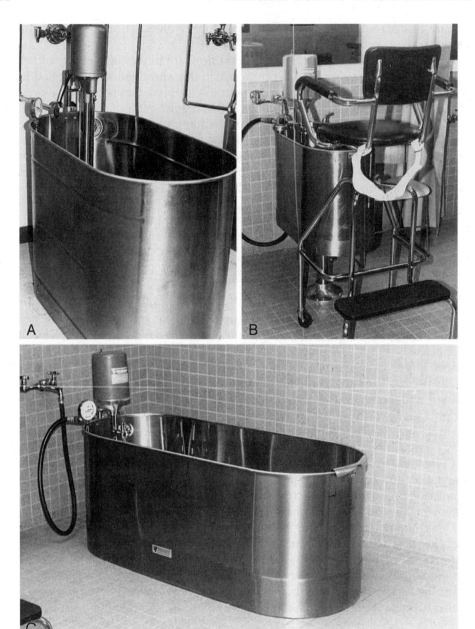

FIGURE 6–1. Styles of whirlpool baths. (*A*) extremity tank width 15 inches, length 28 to 32 inches, depth 18 to 25 inches; (*B*) leg or hip tank (high boy) width 20 to 24 inches, length 36 to 48 inches, depth 28 inches; (*C*) lowboy width 24 inches, length 52 to 66 inches, depth 18 inches.

All tanks require an ample supply of hot and cold water and some means of blending them for the desired temperature. The water may be mixed by a thermostatic control valve or manually using the agitator. The faucet used for filling the whirlpool should include a vacuum breaker to prevent the suctioning of water from the whirlpool into the water system. These tanks are routinely drained and cleaned between patient treatments. The larger walk tanks or therapeutic tanks are used for exercising and conditioning. These are not routinely drained between patients and must be equipped with filtration and chemical additive systems.

Hydrotherapy Area

The room temperature in the hydrotherapy area should be higher than in other treatment areas in the physical therapy department. The area should be adequately ventilated (1) to prevent the condensation of moisture on the walls, floors, and equipment and (2) to remove aerosols of water and additives induced into the air by water turbulence in the whirlpool.[5] The hydrotherapy area is best designed and used when it is kept separate from other treatment areas. There should be adequate storage for bandages and other supplies. A sink for hand and equipment washing and an area for dressing wounds should be available. The room should be of adequate size to allow for maneuvering of wheelchairs and stretchers.

Turbine

The movement of water and air is regulated by the water pump, or turbine. The whirlpool operates by mixing water and air to control turbulence. Turbulence is created and controlled by combining aeration (the amount of air mixed with the water) and agitation (the movement of the water). In general, the more aeration, the greater the turbulence, pressure, and viscosity. Agitation patterns are not uniform from one piece of equipment to another. In any piece of equipment the turbulence is greater toward the surface of the water.[17]

The turbine is mounted on a tubular column, which is often a spring-loaded circular vice attached to the whirlpool. The circular vice functions to help with raising and lowering the turbine, as well as rotating it horizontally. The turbine assembly consists of an electrical motor pump located above the water to which two tubular shafts are connected. The first tube is the drive shaft, which contains an impeller, housed in a casing at the bottom of the tube. A control valve located near the whirlpool motor regulates the opening at the end of the tube, to control the amount of water introduced into the whirlpool system. At the top of the second tube, which is called the breather tube, is a variable-pressure control valve to control the amount of aeration; a water jet is attached at the bottom of this tube. Therefore, by regulating the water and air intake with these valves, the agitation (turbulence and pressure) can be controlled. The various parts of the whirlpool are shown in Figure 6–2.

The agitation pattern may be controlled by rotating the turbine assembly to direct the air and water jet stream to the right or left, creating a circular pattern, or to direct it at various points toward the center of the tube, which decreases the circular motion but increases central turbulence. The agitation can be further controlled by raising or lowering the assembly to increase or decrease the turbulence at various depths.

WHIRLPOOL CARE AND SAFETY PRECAUTIONS

Care of the whirlpool entails cleansing the tank and turbines after each use. The external surface of the tank can be polished with a commercial stainless steel polish. Cleans-

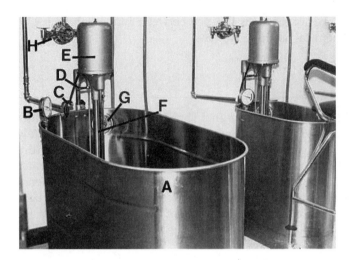

FIGURE 6–2. Whirlpool parts. (*A*) Stainless steel tank; (*B*) thermometer; (*C*) inlet spout; (*D*) water control valve; (*E*) turbine motor; (*F*) impellor and breather tubes; (*G*) overflow drain; (*H*) mixing valve.

ing the inside can be a problem, especially when patients with contagious or infected open lesions are treated in the tank. Proper cleansing can be performed in two steps depending on the whirlpool additive and disinfectant system chosen. After emptying, the inside of the tank should be scrubbed with a commercial disinfectant that will not cause corrosion, rinsed thoroughly with clean water, and dried. Scrubbing alone, however, is not effective in eradicating possible contaminants[19] on the bottom, edges, drains, overflow pipe, thermometers, and agitators, the most frequently contaminated sites. Disinfecting these hard-to-reach places can be achieved through several methods. Chlorine at 200 parts per million (ppm) has been found to be effective in eradicating the common forms of bacteria—*Clostridium* and *Pseudomonas*. However, only glutaraldehyde, formalin alcohol, ethylene oxide, and beta propiolactone have been found to be effective against spore-forming bacteria.[20] A hydrotherapy sterilizing system is probably the most practical system.[21] The exact disinfecting protocol is available from the various manufacturers. The use of povidone-iodine surgical scrub (0.75 percent available iodine) has also been found to be effective in significantly reducing colony counts.[22] Finally, the use of a commercial additive, chloramine-T (Chlorazene), in concentrations of 100 to 200 ppm has proved to be effective at reducing gram-negative organisms and *Pseudomonas*.[23] This product is used at the same time as a whirlpool additive for disinfecting the wound, thus diminishing the amount of time required for sterilization, and it is noncorrosive.[23] If you have any questions about a germicidal product, you may contact either your local or state health department or the Antimicrobial Program Branch, Registration Division, of the Environmental Protection Agency (EPA). Routine culturing of the tanks should be performed. Guidelines for culturing can be obtained through an appropriate clinical laboratory or hospital infection-control department.

Blood-Borne Pathogens

Concern over the transmission of blood-borne pathogens, human immunodeficiency virus (HIV) or hepatitis B virus (HBV) deserves special attention for protection of the health-care worker and other patients. The Centers for Disease Control (CDC) recommends "blood and body fluid precautions be consistently used for all patients regardless of the blood-borne infection status."[24,25] (Note: For the most current update on blood-borne pathogens precautions, contact the Centers for Disease Control, Atlanta, GA.) This would include blood, body fluids containing visible blood, tissues, cerebrospinal fluid, synovial fluid, pleural fluid, peritoneal fluid, pericardial fluid, and amniotic fluid. When treating open wounds with hydrotherapy, protective barriers such as gloves, masks, gowns, and goggles should be used, particularly when dealing with large wounds or an infectious patient, or when there is the possibility of splashing. While cleansing the tank, general-purpose utility gloves and goggles should be used at all times, whether or not an open wound was treated in the tank. A solution of sodium hypochlorite, in concentrations ranging from 500 ppm (1:100 dilution) to 5000 ppm (1:10 dilution), is effective, depending on the amount of organic material (blood, mucus) present on the surface to be cleaned.[26] Sterilization of the tank and its components can be performed in the same manner as previously discussed.

Electrical Safety

Electrical safety is an important matter to consider when using hydrotherapy equipment. The turbines must be grounded. A ground-fault circuit interrupter (GFCI) should be installed either at the receptacle or at the circuit breaker for the receptacle. A GFCI eliminates the hazard of ground-fault circuits (see Chapter 3). Also included in the GFCI circuit would be any electrical motors that may be used to help with patient transfers, such as with the Hubbard, walk, or therapeutic tanks. The tank, motor, and agitation assembly should be checked for any current leakage yearly or, preferably, every 6 months by a biomedical engineering technician.

Finally, if the motor support, which is springloaded and controlled by the vice grip, is released without the counterbalance of the weight of the whirlpool turbine, the assembly spring may catapult the support, creating a hazardous situation.[27] If the support becomes stuck, there should be no attempt to correct the situation while water or a patient is in the tank.

CLINICAL INDICATIONS FOR HYDROTHERAPY

Wound Care

The whirlpool is commonly used in the care of open wounds. The whirlpool provides an effective method of mechanically debriding a wound to remove surface necrotic material and cleansing through the addition of a bactericidal agent. In addition, the mechanical effects of the whirlpool stimulate formation of granulation tissue and, in conjunction with the appropriate water temperature, soften tissues and stimulate circulation of the affected area. The increase in local circulation raises the levels of oxygen, antibodies, leukocytes, and nutrition supplied to the tissues, and enhances the removal of metabolites. The amount of systemic medications, such as antibiotics, available to the wound area may also be increased by the improved circulation, which helps to diminish or to prevent infection. The whirlpool also creates sedation and analgesia, which may aid in reducing pain caused by the open wound or surrounding tissues.

WHIRLPOOL ADDITIVES

The first consideration in the treatment of wounds with whirlpool is deciding which whirlpool additive to use. An antibacterial agent added to the whirlpool water helps prevent or reduce infection. Common additives are a povidone-iodine solution (4 ppm),[22] especially prepared for whirlpools; sodium hypochlorite, 5.25 percent; household bleach; and chloramine-T.[21] Sodium hypochlorite has been found to be effective at reducing colony counts in dilution up to 1:160.[28] The CDC recommends sodium hypochlorite in concentrations of 70 percent/100 gal, which produces 15 mg of pure chlorine per liter.[25,26,29] The 1:60 dilution is sometimes painful, however, and may cause irritation to the surrounding tissues. The aerosols formed from the turbulence also may cause irritation to the eyes with prolonged exposure. Zigenfus and associates[30] found that concentrations of povidone-iodine solution in a minimum concentration of 3 ppm, rounded by 1.2 mL/gal water, to be effective in reducing wound and water colony counts after 18 minutes of exposure. McGuckin and associates[31] studied the cross-contamination of 10 Hubbard-tank wound patients with *Pseudomonas aeruginosa*. The outbreak began after discontinuing sodium hypochlorite additive. The outbreak ceased after reinstituting the sodium hypochlorite additive and disinfecting the tank between treatments for 30 minutes with 12-ppm iodine and 1000-ppm sodium hypochlorite.

The use of chloramine-T (Chlorazene) in concentrations of 100 ppm virtually eliminated positive cultures of all microorganisms on the equipment. Concentrations of 150 to 200 ppm also reduce colonization of a gram-negative organism of the patient's wound. Because of its chemical configuration and stability, chloramine-T is effective in releasing free chlorine, throughout a 20-minute treatment, at effective levels and in reducing the irritating qualities of chlorine. This same solution, with continued agitation of 5 minutes after patient removal, is all that is necessary to sterilize the tank. This is followed by scrubbing with an antimicrobial disinfectant and rinsing. The use of this substance can greatly diminish the amount of sterilization time necessary between treatments. The exact amount of povidone-iodine and chloramine-T to be added for each tank type can be obtained from the manufacturers. The proper dilutions of povidone-iodine, chlorine bleach, and chloramine-T for common tanks can be found in Table 6–1.

Therapists should be aware that the addition of an antibacterial agent in the stronger concentrations, or simultaneous use of more than one whirlpool in the hydrotherapy area with the additives, can produce vapors that have the potential to cause lightheadedness, dizziness, and even syncope. Continuous monitoring of the patient during treatment and adequate ventilation of the hydrotherapy area are essential.

WOUND TYPE AND CONDITION

The second consideration in determining the proper use of whirlpool for wound care is the wound itself. The therapist must consider what effects water temperature,

TABLE 6–1 Betadine and Chlorine Bleach Concentrations in
Standard Whirlpools at Therapeutic Levels

Whirlpool Type	Average Capacity	Povidone-Iodine (Oz)	Chlorine Bleach (Oz)	Chloramine-T Type (Chlorazene)
Foot/hand	22–36 gal	4	26	20–36 g
Leg/hip	100–100 gal	13.5	102	88 g
Lowboy	93–137 gal	10	96	50–88 g

agitation, and duration will have on the wound and surrounding tissues. Evaluation and recognition of the various components of a wound are essential. Tables 6–2 and 6–3 will help the reader to organize wound evaluation and to identify wound characteristics and exudates.

Wounds can be classified in two ways: (1) based on a time frame for closure—primary, delayed primary, or healing by secondary intention; or (2) based on their color—red, yellow, black, or a combination.[32] Primary wounds are surgically closed or closed within 5 days. Delayed primary closures are wounds that are surgically closed after 5 days. Secondary-intention wounds are allowed to close by granulation, marginal or budding epithelialization, and wound-margin contracture. To treat the latter two wound classifications, the clinician would most appropriately use the whirlpool for cleansing, debridement, antibacterial action, and circulation enhancement. An example of delayed primary wound would be a dog bite. Primary closure is not advocated because of the risk of infection and abscess formation. Daily whirlpool could be used un-

---

TABLE 6–2 Components of Wound Evaluation

A. History
　1. Injury—etiology, date onset, injury components
　2. Social/occupational—age, dominance, vocational/avocation, alcohol, nicotine, caffeine, family support
　3. Medical—system review, previous injury, medications, allergies
B. Subjective Report
　1. Pain, sensory changes
　2. Functional problems
C. Objective Evaluation
　1. General observation
　　a. Wound, surrounding tissue, extremity
　　b. Location
　2. Wound
　　a. Size, shape, depth measurement
　　b. Classification
　　　(1) Primary/delayed primary
　　　(2) Secondary
　　　　(a) Red
　　　　(b) Yellow
　　　　(c) Black
　　　　(d) Combination
　　c. Exudate characteristics
　　d. Wound bed
　　　(1) Necrotic, granulative, epithelial budding
　　　(2) Vital structure involvement
　　e. Wound margins
　　　(1) Extent
　　　(2) Change
　　f. Grafts/flaps
　　　(1) Adherence
　　　(2) Drainage
　　　(3) Vascularity

TABLE 6–3 Wound Exudate Characteristics and Relationship
to Wound Type

	Serous	Sanguineous	Proteinious	Purulent
Color	Yellow	Yellow red to red	White to white-yellow	Green Brown White
Odor	No	No	No	Yes
Adherency	No	No	Yes	No
Consistency	Thin	Thin-thick	Gel-like	Viscous
(Viscosity)	Transparent to wound base	Transparent	Nontransparent	Nontransparent
Wound type	Primary Secondary	Primary Secondary	Secondary	Secondary

til delayed closure has occurred, or until the wound heals by secondary intention. An example of secondary intention would be a stasis ulcer. The whirlpool could be carried out until the wound closes or is surgically closed with a skin graft or tissue flap.

SKIN GRAFT AND TISSUE FLAP

Skin-graft viability is still delicate 3 to 5 days postgrafting. The graft may not adhere well to the granular bed, or there may not be sufficient capillary infiltration to provide nutritional support to the graft. A graft at this point will not tolerate the high shearing forces and turbulence that can be created in the whirlpool; therefore, whirlpool agitation is adjusted to minimal levels or turned off and the whirlpool is only administered for 5 minutes. This would allow for softening of the tissues and cleansing with the antibacterial agent, in preparation for mechanical debridement. The whirlpool will also aid in the removal of superficial wound exudates. As the graft ages, and stability improves, the duration and aeration may be increased. Case Study 1 is an example of the clinical reasoning that might occur.

Whirlpool also can be used in the care of tissue flaps, whether they are cutaneous, muscular, or myocutaneous (free or pedicle-type). Considerations must be given to the viability and circulation of the flap. Is it a free flap, where arteries have been anastomosed? Or is it a pedicle flap, where the major circulatory supply in the early phase is dependent on the pedicle? If the whirlpool is too cold, or if the patient suffers a chill while in the whirlpool, vasoconstriction of the small infiltrating vessels may occur. The vasoconstriction may result in ischemia of a portion, or all, of the flap, leading to partial or full loss of the skin flap. Therefore, the temperature of the whirlpool and hydrotherapy area, as well as agitation, is an important consideration. In general, the younger the flap (in postoperative days), the less turbulence and shear force it will be able to tolerate. The common characteristics of skin grafts and tissue flaps are highlighted in Table 6–4.

CASE STUDY 1

A 26-year-old iron worker suffered an avulsion injury to the dorsum of his hand with soft tissue loss including skin and subcutaneous tissues with no

TABLE 6–4 Skin Graft and Flap Characteristics

	Tissue Layers	Vascularity/Take	Common Drainage	Donor Site Closure
Split thickness	Epidermis and superficial dermis	3 days	Serous Sanguinous	Secondary Intention
Full thickness	Epidermis and protein dermal layer	5–7 days	Primary Primary	
Pedicle flap Random Axial	Dermis and subcutaneous fat	Approximately 3 weeks	Serosanguineous	Primary or skin graft
Free flap Cutaneous Myocutaneous Myo Osteo Joint	Dermis and subcutaneous fat Dermis subcutaneous fat and muscle Muscle only Bone alone or in combination Joint and bone	Immediate	Serosanguineous	Primary or skin graft

tendon damage. The wound was primarily closed with a split-thickness skin graft, of which only 50 percent took. The remainder of the graft became necrotic. He is now referred 5 days postgrafting for wound care and range of motion.

PROBLEMS

1. 5-day-old skin graft
2. Necrotic wound
3. Limited digital range of motion
4. Edema of hand
5. Surrounding tissue status questionable
6. Pain in hand

ASSESSMENT TECHNIQUES

1. Wound evaluation—color, size, drainage, photograph
2. Skin graft assessment—adherence, vascularity
3. Edema assessment—volume measurement, circumferential measurements
4. Range-of-motion measurements—goniometry
5. Sensation evaluation—vibration, moving/static two-point discrimination, light touch with monofilaments

GOALS

1. Wound cleansing and debridement
2. Promotion of granulation tissue
3. Pain relief
4. Edema reduction
5. Restore digital range of motion

HYDROTHERAPY TECHNIQUES SELECTED

Arm tank upper-extremity technique. 34°C 10 minutes
Mild agitation

RATIONALE

Because of the need for wound debridement and cleansing, whirlpool would be the appropriate choice. Agitation would have to be gentle to protect the recent skin graft. Sodium hypochlorite (chlorazine-T) additive for antiseptic and wound disinfectant is appropriate. Temperatures less than body temperature are utilized to minimize the swelling. The agitation of the water may also diminish the pain by stimulating large-diameter fibers, and the buoyancy of the water may make exercise easier.

PAINFUL OPEN LESIONS

When an open wound is painful, as in the case of an ischemic ulcer or a burn, agitation should be gentle to avoid stimulating the neural tissue, thereby increasing pain. If used properly, with temperatures below 37°C and gentle agitation, the whirlpool may relieve the discomfort created by the wound and provide a gentle method of debridement. Agitation should be kept at a minimal level and should not be directed at the wound. In the case of a pressure sore, a stasis ulcer, or a traumatic open wound, debridement may be the main objective, and the maximal agitation level may be used. A final consideration is prevention of edema, which a whirlpool may create. The edema could cause compromise by compressing the venous and lymphatic systems, possibly delaying healing or preventing systemic medication from reaching the wound, retarding the development of capillary formation, and removing wound-healing by-products.

SURROUNDING TISSUE CONDITION

A third and final consideration for the treatment of open wounds with whirlpool is the condition of the surrounding tissues, or of the extremity being treated. The circulation, both arterial and venous, must be able to tolerate the increased temperature and turbulence created by the whirlpool. The surrounding soft tissue's neurologic status must also be considered. The sensation in the area must not be compromised to a level that would prevent the patient from being able to protect himself or herself from further injury (caused by the agitation or rise in tissue temperature). Traumatized tissues may not tolerate treatment with a whirlpool because of underlying fractures, joint injuries, or soft-tissue damage.

In summary, the same indications and contraindications discussed for superficial heating must be considered with use of a whirlpool, in addition to (1) the objectives of the whirlpool treatment; (2) the desired physiologic effect; (3) the condition and type of wound; and (4) the condition of the surrounding tissues or extremities.[1]

Exercise Assistance

Pool therapy combines the physical forces of water (buoyancy, pressure, and viscosity) with therapeutic exercise.[11] Buoyancy can help with exercises, as a means of resistance to improve strength, or to reduce undue stress on joints by providing support (to increase range of motion).[33] The general aims of pool therapy are to promote patient relaxation, improve circulation, restore mobility, strengthen muscles, provide gait training with less stress on the weight-bearing joints, and improve psychologic and emotional outlook leading to improved function. Patients are often able to move or ambulate in water in ways they could not achieve without the aid of buoyancy.[34,35]

PRINCIPLES OF EXERCISE IN WATER

Hydrostatic pressure decreases the tendency for blood to pool in the lower portion of the body. Viscosity, the property of friction in fluids, is low in water creating little friction with body movement at low speeds. As speed increases, friction increases, making the movement more difficult, requiring greater muscle strength to perform the exercise. In addition, as speed increases so does turbulence (positive pressure), in the direction of the movement and drag (negative pressure), behind the moving part both creating resistance to movement. One way of varying resistance, therefore, is by regulating the speed at which the body part moves; the greater the speed, the greater the resistance.

The principle of relative density provides support of the body in water. Therefore the stresses placed on weight-bearing joints are decreased, as is the muscle strength necessary to create joint motion.

The final principle, buoyancy, will assist with any exercise when the movement is performed in a direction toward the water surface, such as when abducting the shoulder in the standing position. Buoyancy also produces resistance when the motion occurs in a direction away from the surface of the water, such as when adducting the shoulder in the standing position. The effect of buoyancy can also be varied by (1) changing the length of the lever arm, (2) by adding flotation devices to the extremity, or (3) by performing all extremity exercises in the horizontal position (when the patient is floating on his or her back). In this position, resistance can be adjusted by altering the speed of the movement.

In summary, hydrostatic pressure helps circulation, depending on the depth of immersion. Specific gravity provides support of the body and limbs. Viscosity and the turbulence and drag created by body-parts movement can be used to vary the resistance. The faster the motion, the greater the resistance. Buoyancy can be used to support the body or the limb and provide assistive or resistive exercises. Case study 2 describes using a whirlpool according to the principles of exercise in water for a person with acute arthritis.

CASE STUDY 2

A 55-year-old woman has an acute exacerbation of rheumatoid arthritis in both lower extremities. One ankle, both knees, and both hips demonstrate an antalgic limitation of motion with mild muscle guarding and mild joint effusion. Activities of daily living (ADLs) are reportedly limited by pain, with difficulty transferring supine to sit, sit to stand, and negotiating stairs. She has a history of cardiovascular disease and compromised total vital capacity secondary to reduced motion of her thoracic cavity.

PROBLEMS

1. Pain in both hips and knees
2. Reduced range of motion of both hips and knees
3. Joint inflammation of both hips and knees
4. Muscle guarding and fatigue of lower-extremity muscles
5. Compromised cardiac and pulmonary function
6. Decreased functional activities

ASSESSMENT TECHNIQUES

1. Measure pain—quality, quantity, location
2. Measure range of motion of hips and knees

3. Assess joint inflammation—rate tenderness, note edema, warmth, color
4. Assess sensation of lower extremities
5. Obtain baseline vital signs
6. Assess level of transfer ability
7. Assess overall muscle strength

GOALS

1. Decrease pain
2. Decrease inflammation
3. Increase range of motion
4. Increase transfer ability and ambulation endurance

HYDROTHERAPY TECHNIQUE SELECTED

Lowboy Whirlpool 38°C 20 Minutes

Because of the patient's limited motion and difficulty with transfers, the low-boy whirlpool would be most accessible for this patient. The whirlpool would provide the beneficial effects of heat, muscle relaxation, pain relief via the mechanical effects, and utilization of the properties of water to assist with range-of-motion exercises. Due to the patient's compromised medical status, this technique would also limit the amount of body surface immersion, while gaining the positive effects of whirlpool. The patient's vital signs should be monitored before, during, and following treatment.

PATIENT SELECTION FOR POOL THERAPY

Proper patient selection for the use of pool therapy is very important. The patient should not be incontinent (feces or urine), unless catheterized. No patient for whom exposure to warm water or exercising is contraindicated (including those with open or discharging wounds, upper respiratory infection, uncontrolled blood pressure, febrile conditions, severe mental disorders, uncontrolled epilepsy, or cardiac or pulmonary conditions [especially with vital capacity less than 1500 mL]),[37] and no patient who fears water, should be allowed to participate in pool therapy. When pool therapy is chosen for cardiac- or pulmonary-compromised patients, the intensity of the exercise should be at low levels. There is an increase in oxygen consumption as the exercise level intensifies in young, healthy subjects.[38] Debilitated patients not usually suited to this treatment may be considered when the treatment, based on sound clinical reasoning, is desirable and given for short periods of time. Pool therapy has been recommended for treatment of patients with rheumatoid arthritis,[34] patients with joint injuries or replacements,[35] patients with neurologic disorders (such as paraplegia), or those with poliomyelitis, polyneuritis, multiple sclerosis, and (in certain cases) cerebral palsy.[39]

TREATMENT CONSIDERATIONS: EQUIPMENT AND ENVIRONMENT

Treatment should last from 10 to 20 minutes, with the therapist monitoring vital signs, and neither the therapist nor the patient should remain in the pool for extended periods. In general, the more debilitated or medically compromised the patient, the shorter the duration should be initially. High temperatures of 36°C to 37°C are most suitable for patients with arthritis. Lower temperatures of 30°C to 34.5°C are recommended for patients with spasticity and for any patient whose immersion may last for 20 to 45 minutes. The lower temperatures are chosen to reduce fatigue.[35]

The pool should be at least 12 ft by 6 ft in area, with a built-in filtration and chlorination system; and 3 to 4 ft in depth, with easy accessibility to either a ramp, ladder, or stairs, and a mechanical overhead lift. Adequate room ventilation, which does not allow condensation to accumulate on the walls or windows, is important. There should be a regular maintenance schedule for cleaning at least weekly and tests for water chlorine and pH levels should be performed twice a day.[35,40] Floats (such as rings for the trunk and extremities), paddle boards, slippers, parallel bars or hand rails, as well as weighted stools and chairs, are necessary equipment. There also must be established safety rules and regulations, and procedures for emergencies, including at least one member of the staff present at all times being certified in cardiopulmonary resuscitation (CPR).

The environment should be established as previously discussed for the full-body immersion systems. There should be shower facilities for cleansing before therapy (36°C) and for cooling down after therapy (30°C to 32°C).[41] In addition, adequate space for patients to rest after therapy for 20 minutes and fluid replenishment should be available. Adequate staffing in the pool depends on the condition of the patient population being treated, and there should be one person present to help the patient outside the pool. Case Study 3 is an example of how full-body or pool therapy might be utilized.

CASE STUDY 3

A 54-year-old woman suffered a fracture/dislocation with a rotator cuff tear of her right shoulder after a fall at home. She is otherwise in good health, with no medical problems. She was originally immobilized for 1 month and then underwent rotator cuff repair for a massive tear of her supraspinatus and infraspinatus. Postoperative immobilization included an abduction pillow for 4 weeks. After 8 weeks of therapy she has regained passive functional motion (120 degrees of forward flexion) but is unable to actively forward flex beyond 45 degrees secondary to pain and weakness of her deltoid and rotator cuff strength grade 1/5. As a result of this weakness, she is having significant problems with dressing and hygiene. Her physician is requesting suggestions to improve her recovery.

PROBLEMS

1. Weakness of rotator cuff and deltoid muscles
2. Shoulder pain with active range of motion against gravity
3. Decreased independent ADL abilities

ASSESSMENT TECHNIQUE

1. Measure active and passive range of motion of shoulder
2. Manual muscle test shoulder girdle

3. Assess relationship of pain to motion
4. Assess patient's functional capabilities
5. Assess patient's neurologic status (sensation, peripheral nerve function)

GOALS

1. Increase active range of motion to functional levels
2. Decrease shoulder pain with active motion
3. Increase muscle function and strength
4. Improve proprioception
5. Achieve ADL independence

HYDROTHERAPY TECHNIQUE SELECTED

Therapeutic pool

RATIONALE

The patient has regained sufficient passive motion, but active motion remains limited secondary to pain and weakness. Full-body immersion would allow the patient to utilize the properties of water (buoyancy pressure viscosity) to perform active exercise with the assistance of these properties. This would assist in stimulating proprioception and muscle activation to regain strength through the full available range. As strength improves, the properties of water could be used for resistive exercise, minimizing the compression effects on the joint.

GENERAL GUIDELINES FOR CLINICAL ADMINISTRATION OF HYDROTHERAPY

Preparatory Considerations

Before initiating a whirlpool treatment, objectives of treatment should be determined and may include: (1) stimulation of circulation for wound care; (2) promotion of muscle relaxation and pain relief; (3) mechanical debridement of wound surface exudates and necrotic tissue; and (4) facilitation exercise, either as assistance or resistance.

Next, the proper temperature should be selected, based on the patient's medical condition and treatment objectives. Commonly used temperatures and their corresponding generic names are located in Table 6–5. In general, temperatures from 36.5°C to 40.5°C are reasonable temperatures when using heat,[2] except in the presence of peripheral vascular disease, sensory loss, or full-body immersion. With peripheral vascular disease, the skin temperature of the extremity to be immersed can be a guideline to help determine water temperature and should not be greater than 1°C above skin temperature. In the presence of cardiovascular or pulmonary disease, the temperature should not exceed 38°C.

The part to be treated should be inspected for its temperature, presence of edema,

TABLE 6–5 Whirlpool Water
Temperatures and Frequent
Descriptive Terminology

Descriptive Terminology	°F	°C
Very cold	35–55	1–13
Cold	55–65	13–18
Cool	65–80	18–27
Tepid	80–92	17–33.5
Neutral	92–96	33.5–35.5
Warm	96–98	35.5–36.5
Hot	98–104	36.5–40
Very hot	104–115	40–60

open lesions, color, muscle spasm, sensation, and conditions previously noted. The treatment procedure and unit operation should be explained to the patient to reduce anxiety and promote safety. The patient should be positioned comfortably. The whirlpool may then be activated and the agitation force adjusted initially at a minimal level and increased as desired. Be sure not to direct the agitation specifically toward any body area that could suffer further damage or not withstand the force of the agitation. The patient should not be left unattended during the treatment session. Whenever immersed in a lift chair or stretcher, the patient should be strapped in place. The patient should be strapped into the elevated chair, if used, when employing the extremity tank for treatment of the lower extremities. Table 6–6 summarizes the clinical decision process based on the phases of wound healing.

Whirlpool Duration

The decision on the length of time for treatment in a whirlpool must be based on sound physiologic judgment and on the treatment objectives the therapist is attempting to achieve through the use of the whirlpool. The duration of treatment will change, depending on the specific pathologies involved. When used strictly as a heating modality and the patient's medical condition permits, the usual duration is 20 minutes. Borrell and colleagues[13] demonstrated that 20 minutes was a long enough time to increase skin muscle and joint capsule temperature in the hand and foot. Abramson and associates[11] demonstrated that a 20-minute application of moist heat increased blood flow, and that further exposure of up to 2 hours had no real effect on increasing the peak response obtained at the 20-minute mark. When using the whirlpool for debridement, the duration is 5 to 20 minutes, depending on the amount of necrotic tissue; for exercising, a duration of 10 to 20 minutes is recommended, depending on the patient's medical status. When the treatment is concluded, the agitator should be turned off and the patient should be helped out of the tub. At no time should the patient operate the agitator controls. Occasionally, when full-body immersion has been performed, the patient may experience some lightheadedness. This may be avoided by having the patient sit for 5 to 10 minutes before standing.

TABLE 6–6 Clinical Decision Making for Various Forms of Heating/Cooling Modalities

Healing Phase	Characteristics	Desired Effects	Mild Heating	Vigorous Heating	Cooling	Whirlpool
Active/exudative phase (0–5 days)	Inflammation Vasoactive (histamine) Pain at rest Pain before limitation of motion	Vasoconstriction Dec vasoactive agents Pain relief Dec edema Dec muscle guarding	Contraindicated	Contraindicated	Whirlpool 13–18°C Mild–moderate agitation (extremity) Cold packs	For debridement only 34.4°C (open wounds)
Subacute/fibroblastic phase (5–21 days)	Inflammation Fibroblastic proliferative Stiffness, pain	Vasodilation Dec edema Dec muscle guarding Dec pain	Paraffin Moist heat	Fluidotherapy Circumferential moist heat (latter portion of phase)	Whirlpool 13–18°C Conductive Cooling methods (posttreatment)	Extremity Debridement Only 34.4°C 36.7–38.8°C with caution (open wounds)
Chronic/maturation phase (21 days)	Collagen remodeling Stiffness Pain Pain beyond motion restriction	Vasodilation Tissue Extensibility Sedation analgesia for exercise	Paraffin Moist heat (inc superficial) temperature	Fluidotherapy Circumferential Moist heat (greater penetration depth)	Whirlpool 13–18°C Conductive cooling methods (posttreatment)	Extremity Debridement 34.4°C Heating extremity 36.7–38.8°C w/caution

159

Lower-Extremity Techniques

Lower-extremity immersion, or immersion to the midthoracic level, can be achieved with two of the basic whirlpool types. The highboy tank requires the patient to be able to flex the hip and knee. The length of this tub does not allow for full extension of the average adult lower extremity and limits the amount of range-of-motion exercise of activity a person can perform while in the whirlpool. However, its depth allows a greater body-surface area to be submerged safely and comfortably, to as high as the midthoracic region.

The lowboy tank is not as deep, but has greater length than the highboy, and it affords the patient the ability to fully extend the lower extremities and perform full-motion exercises for the knees. When only the distal portion of the lower extremity has to be immersed, the extremity tank, with the use of the whirlpool chair, is the appropriate choice.

In summary, the highboy and lowboy afford greater body-surface immersion than the extremity tank does, while the lowboy may allow for greater low-extremity extension than the highboy does. In the event that the patient is unable to negotiate transfer into any of the tubs, the highboy and lowboy each can be fitted with a hydraulic chair lift or "hoyer lift," to assist the patient in and out of the tub.

Upper-Extremity Techniques

When treating the upper extremity, the patient should be seated comfortably next to the extremity tank, with a towel or other form of padding on the tank edge to avoid constriction of the circulatory and lymphatic system of the upper extremity (Fig. 6–3). The use of the whirlpool for the upper extremity deserves special consideration, because edema can form. It is well accepted that edema of the hand is one of the adverse effects of whirlpool, and the reduction of edema is the primary concern of the treating therapist.[42] Magness and coworkers[43] studied the effect of whirlpool on volume in the upper extremity. They measured upper-extremity volume in 20 normal male and female volunteers before and after the immersion of this same extremity in a whirlpool bath at temperatures ranging from 33.5°C to 44.4°C for 20 minutes. In addition, 20 patients with various upper-extremity disorders were also treated by whirlpool in the same manner, at temperatures from 37.8°C to 40°C for 20 minutes. The results revealed a significant increase in volume for the normal subjects, which was directly related to the increase in water temperature. There was also a significant increase in volume of the patient's extremity, and the rise in volume was greater than in the normal subjects at the specific temperatures treated.

Several attempts have been made to determine the causes of this edema and how it can be controlled. Schultz[44] used 20 normal subjects and 20 upper-extremity–injured patients to determine the effect of active exercise on edema formation during whirlpool treatment, at 37°C. When comparing active exercise during whirlpool treatment with no exercise during whirlpool treatment for both normal subjects and upper-extremity–injured patients, she found no significant difference in edema formation. Walsh[45] studied the effect of elevation versus nonelevation of the upper extremity during whirlpool on 30 healthy volunteers, at temperatures of 37.6°C and 40°C. He also found a significant increase in extremity volume in the 40°C whirlpool group. Al-

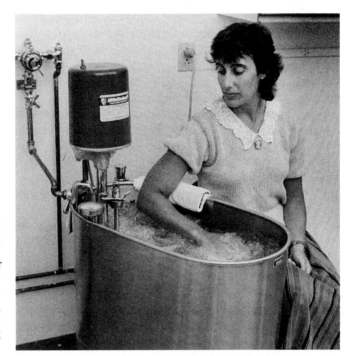

FIGURE 6-3. Whirlpool treatment to the hand and forearm. Caution should be used to avoid a totally dependent position of the hand. If possible, active range-of-motion exercises should be performed during the treatment, to encourage venous and lymphatic return, thus minimizing edema formation.

though not statistically significant, the data supported the theory of nondependency toward the reduction of edema. Recently, Hoyrup and Kjorvel[46] studied the effect of whirlpool and paraffin dips on hand volume, range of motion, and pain of traumatic–hand-injured patients. The patients received whirlpool at 43°C and paraffin dips at 50°C. One half of each group performed exercises; the other half did not. A significant reduction in pain and increase in motion were found. There was no significant change in hand volume during a 3-week period. Daily increases in volume, however, were significant, and the changes were significantly greater in the whirlpool group. Therefore, these studies suggest exercising discrimination when choosing whirlpool for the treatment of upper extremity disorders in patients for whom edema is a primary concern.

Contrast Bath

One special technique in the treatment of distal extremities for which the whirlpool can be used is the contrast bath. This requires the use of whirlpool at a temperature from 38°C to 44°C, and an additional basin containing water kept at a temperature from 10°C to 18°C. The basin should be large enough to enable immersion of the extremity to cover at least the level of the injury. The extremity to be treated is placed into the warm whirlpool for 10 minutes, then immersed in the cold water in the basin for 1 minute, and returned to the warm whirlpool for 4 minutes. The cycle continues for 30 minutes, with the last immersion in the warm whirlpool. Although these specific times do not have to be followed, a hot/cold ratio of 3:1 or 4:1 is typically used. Although not well researched, the theory involves the vasodilation (hot water) and vasoconstriction (cold weather) caused by the contrast bath. The net result is hypothesized to stimulate local circulation in the treated extremity and, to a lesser extent, to increase circulation in the contralateral untreated extremity. If the increase in circulation is caused by an increase in temperature, a recent study by Myrer, Draper, and Durrant[47] would dispute this. They studied 28 normal volunteers in two groups, with the control group receiving whirlpool to the lower extremity at 40.6 °C for 20 minutes and the experimental group receiving contrast treatment in whirlpool at 40.6 °C (hot) and 15.6 °C (cold) at a 4 minutes to 1 minute ratio for four cycles. When measuring tissue temperature in the gastrocnemius at 1 cm depth, there was a significant increase in tissue temperature in the control group (2.83 °C $\pm$ 1.14 °C) as compared with the experimental group's nonsignificant increase (0.39 °C $\pm$ 0.46 °C).

Contraindications for the use of the contrast bath would be small-vessel disease secondary to diabetes, arteriosclerotic endarteritis, and Buerger's disease. Caution should be exercised in patients with any peripheral vascular disease if the water temperature is higher than 40°C. Contrast baths have been advocated for arthritis of peripheral joints, joint sprains, musculotendinous strains, some peripheral vascular diseases (in selected cases), and to toughen amputation stumps. However, no well-controlled studies discussing the efficacy of contrast baths are available in the literature.

Full-Body Immersion

One tank available for full-body immersion is the Hubbard tank, as shown in Figure 6–4. The tank is usually used in conjunction with an overhead lift or stretcher to place the patient into the water. Examples of uses for the Hubbard tank can include treatment of (1) a patient with arthritis who is at present in an exacerbation phase and is unable to negotiate transfer into the smaller tank, but who requires the use of heat and water to help with exercising, maintaining range of motion, and providing pain relief; (2) a patient with neurologically involved paralysis who is actively able to move his or her extremities in the buoyancy of water, but unable to do so in air; (3) a burn patient; or (4) an elderly or debilitated patient with an open wound. The major advantage of the Hubbard tank is that its design allows for motion of all the extremities and accessibility of the patient by the therapist.

The Hubbard tank is shaped with 15-in insets, which permit the therapist access to the patient. Its dimensions are a length of 7 ft 2 in; upper width of 6 ft, middle width 35 in, and lower width 4 ft 2 in; and a usual depth of 22 in. It has approximately a 425-gal capacity, unless the tank has a walking trough, which requires approximately 700 gal of water. It is equipped with two whirlpool turbines that can be moved around the perimeter of the tank to direct and control the agitation pattern. Other accessories include an optional walking trough with parallel bars for gait training. For treating open wounds, the Hubbard tank should be drained and cleaned, as previously discussed, and the same preparatory techniques should be observed.

The walking tank, or larger therapeutic exercise units, because of the greater number of gallons it holds, frequently has its own filtration system. One of the many available therapeutic hydrotherapy units is pictured in Figure 6–5. The primary purpose of these tanks is for exercising or conditioning, while using the inherent forces of water. The patient may be placed into the tank either with or without a flotation device to assist him or her. Full-body immersion systems require some special considerations.

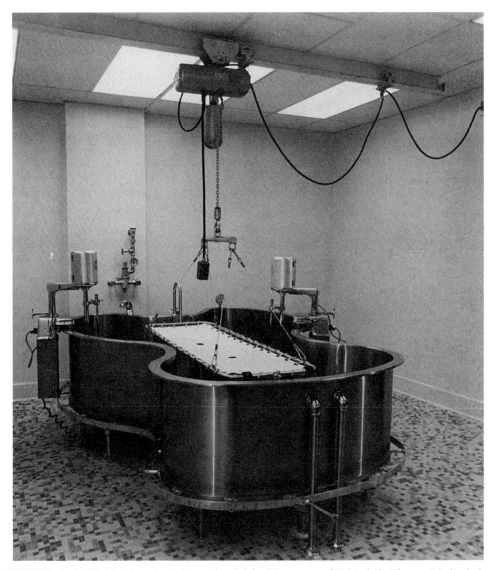

FIGURE 6-4. Hubbard tank with overhead lift. (Courtesy of Whitehall Electro Medical Co., Hackensack, NJ.)

They should be housed in a separate area, with temperature controlled ideally at 25.5°C with 50 percent humidity.[41] An area for showering and cool-down should be available to the patient.

The therapist should be aware of the increased demand placed on the patient's cardiovascular and pulmonary systems. Core temperature can be increased by the water temperature, and muscular contraction places a greater demand on heat dissipation, the respiratory system, and the exposed integument. General considerations should include a maximum immersion time of 20 minutes for noncompromised cardiopulmonary patients, and less time for the elderly, hypertensive, and cardiopul-

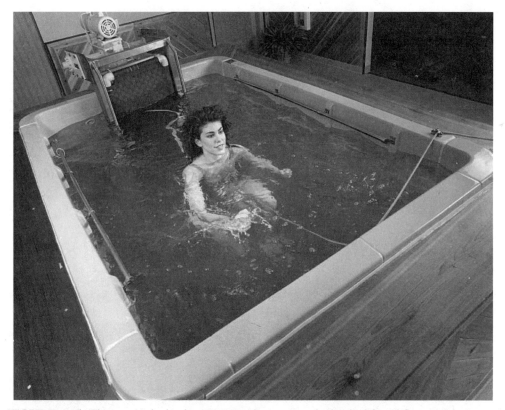

FIGURE 6–5. Therapeutic hydrotherapy unit. Note patient hydraulic lift and flotation device and tethering system. (Courtesy of Aqua Ark Therapeutic Systems, Doylestown, PA.)

monary patients. It may be advisable to initiate treatment for 10 minutes and increase as tolerated. Contraindications are patients who are incontinent of bowel or bladder, presence of skin infection, unstable blood pressure, uncontrolled epilepsy, acute febrile episode, and tuberculosis. Caution should be exhibited with those patients whose vital capacity is less than 1000 ml or in the presence of pulmonary disease.

Hot Tubs and Jacuzzis

With the increase in public awareness for physical fitness, health clubs have been increasing in number and have been including hot tubs or whirlpools as part of their facilities. In addition, Jacuzzis and hot tubs are becoming more popular in the home. One of the rising problems is infection with *Pseudomonas aeruginosa*, causing folliculitis.[48] Organic contaminates reduce the effectiveness of the chlorine as a bactericidal agent. Heavy use of the whirlpool increases the total organic carbon as well as ammonia and organic nitrogen. Because these events are accelerated by high temperatures and turbulence, there is an increased potential for pathogens to be present.

In order to prevent infection, the following steps should be taken. The pool should have a good filtration and chlorination system. Chlorine and pH levels should be monitored as often as hourly during periods of heavy use, and calcium hardness should be checked weekly. Superchlorination should be performed after each cleaning; and the water should be drained, cleaned, and refilled once every 3 months. Finally, the water temperature should not exceed 38.9°C. Maintaining the appropriate temperature is also important because of the physiologic effects of total-body heating and heat dissipation. High temperatures will put a greater demand on the cardiovascular and pulmonary systems. The same precautions and contraindications should be observed for any whirlpool.

DOCUMENTATION OF TREATMENT

After removal from the tank or hydrotherapy pool, the patient should be checked for any evidence of adverse reaction, and the effects of the treatment should be documented. This would include inspection of the patient's skin for marked temperature change, any evidence of skin eruptions, erythema, and blanching time. When treating an open wound, re-evaluation of the wound's appearance and surrounding margins, evidence of exudate and its description, and the amount and type of necrotic tissue present should be noted. If the whirlpool were used for exercising, any change in range of motion, strength, joint appearance, and edema should be noted. Keep in mind that warmer temperatures and full-body immersion may have a tendency to cause transient weakness. If the patient has a medical history of cardiac or pulmonary disease, including hypertension, the patient's respirations, pulse, and blood pressure should be monitored and recorded to determine tolerance to the treatment. Finally, of equal importance are the patient's subjective comments regarding an increase or decrease in pain, joint stiffness, and fatigue. The duration of the treatment, water temperature, techniques, agitation (mild, moderate, full), and additives used should be documented.

SUMMARY

Only with a thorough knowledge and understanding of normal physiology and pathology; the biophysical, thermal, and mechanical effects of whirlpool; the physical properties of water; and methods of heat transfer can the therapist decide on the proper use of whirlpool treatment for the patient. This knowledge plays an important part in the decision-making process and helps with the recognition of contraindications and precautions to be observed in the use of hydrotherapy. Table 6–6 summarizes the clinical decision-making process. Knowledge of the contraindications and precautions (such as those to be considered with patients with medically compromising cardiovascular or pulmonary pathology, peripheral vascular disease—including acute phlebitis—extremely debilitating or disorienting illness, severe infection or febrile process, renal failure, or gangrene), combined with general knowledge, will help the therapist in problem solving in the borderline case. Safe and effective operation of the whirlpool involves a combination of common sense values and an understanding of the whirlpool's operation and components. Another aspect of the decision-making process is recognition of the special consideration that must be taken when using whirlpool for various anatomic parts, such as upper and lower extremities, or full-body immersion.

Wound management, especially, requires that we not only understand the aspects of hydrotherapy, but also have a thorough knowledge of the nature of the wound, its physiology, and the condition of the surrounding tissues.

As we have seen in the example of pool therapy, hydrotherapy does not require agitation to be of value. The inherent properties of water can be combined with therapeutic exercise to effectively treat a portion of the patient population. Finally, we have seen that the use of whirlpool outside the therapist's domain can create potential problems and dangerous situations. Our knowledge, however, can help in properly educating those individuals involved in preventing such situations. The real challenge in hydrotherapy is not necessarily its technical use, but the decision-making process that must occur before its use to achieve the end result of safe, effective treatment for the patient.

Study Objectives

Having completed this chapter, the reader should now be able to:

1. Discuss the significance of buoyancy to hydrotherapy.
2. Discuss the physical principles of turbulence.
3. Explain hydrostatic pressure.
4. Explain the method of heat transfer in relation to hydrotherapy.
5. Discuss the effects of full-body immersion on the cardiopulmonary system.
6. Discuss factors involved in selection of water agitation for hydrotherapy.
7. Discuss the role of hydrotherapy in wound care.
8. Explain the importance of universal precautions during hydrotherapy treatments.
9. Discuss the use of hydrotherapy as a medium for exercise.
10. Explain the contraindications and precautions to hydrotherapy treatment.

REFERENCES

1. Holmes, G: Hydrotherapy as a means of rehabilitation. Br J Phys Med 5:93, 1942.
2. Zislis, J: Hydrotherapy. In Krusen, F (ed): Handbook of Physical Medicine and Rehabilitation, ed 2. WB Saunders, Philadelphia, 1971.
3. Beasley, R and Kester, N: Principles of medical-surgical rehabilitation of the hand. Med Clin North Am 53:645, 1969.
4. Abraham, E: Whirlpool therapy for treatment of soft tissue wounds complicated by extremity fractures. J Trauma 4:222, 1974.
5. Koepke, G: The role of physical medicine in the treatment of burns. Surg Clin North Am 50:1385, 1970.
6. Nave, CR and Nave, BC: Physics for the Health Sciences, ed 2. WB Saunders, Philadelphia, 1980.
7. Dawson, WJ, et al: Evaluation of cardiac output, cardiac work, and metabolic rate during hydrotherapy exercise in normal subjects. Arch Phys Med Rehabil 46:605, 1965.
8. Epstein, M: Water immersions: Modern researchers discover the secrets of an old fold remedy. The Sciences, November: 12, 1979.
9. Boyle, RW, Alisteri, F, and Osborne, F: The value of the Hubbard tank as a diuretic agent. Arch Phys Med Rehabil 45:505, 1964.
10. Abramson, D: Physiologic basis for the use of physical agents in peripheral vascular disorders. Arch Phys Med Rehabil 46:216, 1965.
11. Abramson, D, et al: The effects of altering limb position on blood flow, O_2 uptake and skin temperature. J Appl Physiol 17:191, 1962.
12. Abramson, D, et al: Changes in blood flow, oxygen, uptake and tissue temperatures produced by a topical application of wet heat. Arch Phys Med Rehabil 42:306, 1961.
13. Borrell, R, et al: Comparison of in vivo temperatures produced by hydrotherapy, paraffin wax treatment, and Fluidotherapy. Phys Ther 60:1273, 1980.
14. Nylin, J: The use of water in therapeutics. Arch Phys Med Rehabil 13:261, 1932.
15. Pope, C: Physiologic action and therapeutic value of general and local whirlpool baths. Arch Phys Med Rehabil 10:498, 1929.

16. Cohen, A, Martin, G, and Wakim, K: The effect of whirlpool bath with and without agitation on the circulation in normal and diseased extremities. Arch Phys Med Rehabil 130:212, 1949.
17. Hellerbrand, T, Holutz, S, and Eubank, I: Measurement of whirlpool temperature, pressure and turbulence. Arch Phys Med Rehabil 32:17, 1950.
18. Whitehall Hydrotherapy Equipment, Catalog No. 680, Hackensack, NJ.
19. Turner, AG, Higgins, MM, and Craddock, JG: Disinfection of immersion tanks (Hubbard) in the hospital burn unit. Arch Environ Health 28:101, 1974.
20. Miller, JK, et al: Surveillance and control of Hubbard tank bacterial contaminants. Phys Ther 50:1482, 1970.
21. Ascenzi, J: The need for decontamination and disinfection of hydrotherapy equipment, Vol 1. Asepsis Monograph, Surgikos, Inc., 1989.
22. Simonetti, A, Miller, R, and Gristin, J: Efficacy of povidone-iodine in the disinfection of whirlpool baths and Hubbard tanks. Phys Ther 52:450, 1972.
23. Steve, L, Goodhart, P, and Alexander, J: Hydrotherapy burn treatment: Use of chloramine-T against resistant microorganisms. Arch Phys Med Rehabil 60:301, 1979.
24. Universal precautions for prevention of transmission of HIV, HBV, and other bloodbourne infections. CDC, Document 370150, Nov. 19, 1992.
25. Hospital Infectious Program—Sterilization and disinfection of patient-care equipment—HIV related. CDC, Document 37151, Nov. 19, 1992.
26. Office of Health and Safety Biosafety Branch: Use of bleach in prevention of transmission of HIV in health care settings. CDC, Document 101010, Oct. 13, 1993.
27. Gieck, J: Precautions for hydrotherapeutic devices. Clinical Management 3:44, 1983.
28. Abston, S: Burns in children. Ciba Clin Symp 28;14, 1976.
29. Microbiologic Control Branch Bacterial Disease Discussion, Bureau of Epidemiology. CBC, Sept. 1977.
30. Ziegenfus, RW: Povidone iodine as bactericide in hydrotherapy equipment. Phys Ther 49:582, 1969.
31. McGuckin, M, Thorpe, R, and Abrutyn, E: Hydrotherapy: An outbreak of *Pseudomonas aeruginosa* wound infections related to Hubbard tank treatments. Arch Phys Med Rehabil 62:283, 1981.
32. Cazzell, JS: Wound care forum, the new RYB color code. Am J Nurs 1342, 1988.
33. Daggett, R and Gillespie, A: Pool therapy in the treatment of rheumatoid arthritis. In Lamont-Havers, RW and Hilsop, HJ (eds): Arthritis and Related Disorders. American Physical Therapy Associations, 1965.
34. Golland, A: Basic hydrotherapy: Physiother 67:258, 1981.
35. Robers, P: Hydrotherapy: Its history, theory and practice. Occupational Health 235:5, 1981.
36. Haralson, K: Therapeutic pool programs. Clin Manage 5:10.
37. Harrison, RA: Tolerance of pool therapy by ankylosing spondylitis patients with low vital capacity. Physiotherapy 67:296, 1981.
38. Kirby, RL, et al: Oxygen consumption during exercise in a heated pool. Arch Phys Med Rehabil 65:21, 1984.
39. Stewart, JB and Basmajian, JF: Exercises in water. In Basmajian, JV (ed): Therapeutic Exercise, ed 3. Williams & Wilkins, Baltimore, 1978.
40. Bickle, RJ: Swimming pool management. Physiotherapy 57:475, 1971.
41. Atkinson, G and Harrison, R: Implications of the health and safety at work act of relationship to hydrotherapy departments. Phys Ther 67:263, 1981.
42. Hunter, JM and Mackin, EJ: Edema: Techniques of Evaluation and Management. In Hunter, JM, et al (eds): Rehabilitation of the Hand: Surgery and Therapy, ed 4. CV Mosby, St. Louis, 1995, pp. 77–85.
43. Magness, J, Garrett, T, and Erickson, D: Swelling of the upper extremity during whirlpool baths. Arch Phys Med Rehabil 51:297, 1970.
44. Schultz, K: The effect of active exercise during whirlpool on the hand. Unpublished thesis. San Jose State University, San Jose, CA, 1982.
45. Walsh, M: Relationship of hand edema to upper extremity position and water temperature during whirlpool treatments in normals. Unpublished thesis. Temple University, Philadelphia, 1983.
46. Hoyrup, G and Kjorvel, L: Comparison of whirlpool and wax treatments for hand therapy. Physiother 38:79, 1986.
47. Myrer, JW, Draper, DO, and Durrant, E: Contrast Therapy and Intramuscular Temperature in the Human Leg. J Athl Train, 29:318–322, 1994.
48. Randt, GA: Hot tub folliculitis. Physician Sports Med 11:75, 1983.

CHAPTER 7

Therapeutic Ultrasound

Theresa McDiarmid, MSc, PT, MCSP,
Marvin C. Ziskin, MD, MS, BmE,
and Susan L. Michlovitz, MS, PT

Heating agents are divided into two major types: superficial and deep. In Chapter 5, superficial heating agents were discussed. These agents produce temperature elevations in skin and underlying subcutaneous tissues to a depth of approximately 1 cm. In the next two chapters, deep-heating agents are discussed. Deep-heating agents are capable of causing temperature elevations in tissues to depths of 3 cm or more. Furthermore, these agents are capable of delivering the necessary energy to the deep structures without causing excessive heating of the overlying superficial tissues.

A deep-heating agent is an appropriate adjunct to treatment of ailments such as those that (1) limit range of motion owing to a decrease in the extensibility of periarticular soft tissue; (2) cause skeletal muscle spasms that are not of an acute origin; or (3) produce pain secondary to chronic soft-tissue dysfunction.

There are two different deep-heating agents: ultrasound and diathermy. Ultrasound is by far the most commonly used. Shortwave diathermy is discussed in Chapter 8. However, it should also be noted that ultrasound is receiving increasingly widespread use for its nonthermal effects as well. These are discussed in detail in this chapter.

Ultrasound has been employed in medicine for over 50 years. Biologic effects in tissues exposed to ultrasound (high-frequency sound waves) were first reported by Wood and Loomis in 1927.[1] They demonstrated lysis of red blood cells and decreased mobility in mice following exposure to high-frequency (300 kHz), high-intensity sound waves. The application of ultrasound for medical treatment was introduced in Germany in the late 1930s[2] and in the United States in the late 1940s.[3]

Ultrasound is used in medicine for diagnosis (imaging of internal structures), physical therapy (functional restoration and healing of soft tissue ailments), and tissue destruction (in surgery and hyperthermia for tumor irradiation). The intensity of ultrasound in each classification is different; the lowest intensity is used for diagnostic procedures and the highest for tissue destruction.

The objectives of this chapter are to (1) present the physical principles and biophysical effects of ultrasound; (2) discuss the clinical conditions for which ultrasound is effective; (3) discuss the clinical procedures for the application of ultrasound; and (4) present guidelines for the safe use of ultrasound, including a discussion of the contraindications and precautions for treatment with this agent.

PHYSICAL PRINCIPLES

The purpose of this section is to provide a basic foundation of the physics of therapeutic ultrasound. For a more complete and in-depth study, the excellent textbook by Wells[4] should be consulted.

Nature of Sound

Solids and liquids consist of molecules held together by elastic forces that behave like rubber bands connecting each molecule to each of its nearest neighbors. Thus, if set into vibration, a molecule will cause its neighbors to vibrate, and in turn their neighbors, and so on until the vibration has propagated throughout the entire material. Each individual molecule vibrates back and forth a small distance about its initial position. However, the passage of vibrational energy travels over millions of molecules in propagating through tissue. The propagation of this vibratory motion is precisely what sound is.

Unlike electromagnetic waves such as light and x-rays, sound cannot travel in a vacuum. Very important for the patient is the fact that sound is nonionizing radiation, and, therefore, its use does not impose the hazards, such as cancer production and chromosome breakage, attributed to ionizing radiation.[5]

FREQUENCY

The number of oscillations a molecule undergoes in 1 second defines the frequency of a sound wave and is expressed in units of hertz (Hz); that is, 1 Hz = 1 cycle/second, 1 kHz = 1000 cycles/second, and 1 MHz = 1 million cycles/second. Theoretically, frequency can vary from 0 Hz to infinity; however, the human ear is sensitive only to sound frequencies between 16 Hz and 20,000 Hz. Sound with a frequency greater than 20,000 Hz is called *ultrasound*.

For a given sound source, the higher the frequency, the less the emerging sound beam diverges. Sound at audible frequencies appears to spread out in all directions, whereas ultrasound beams are well collimated, similar to a light beam leaving a flashlight (Fig. 7–1). Ultrasound beams at frequencies greater than 800 kHz are sufficiently collimated to selectively expose a limited target area for physical therapy treatment.

ATTENUATION

Energy contained within a sound beam is decreased as it travels through tissue. This results from two processes: scattering and absorption. Scattering is the deflection of sound out of the beam that results when it strikes a reflecting surface. Absorption is the transfer of energy from the sound beam to the surrounding tissues.

Absorption of sound, and therefore attenuation, increases as the frequency increases. Absorption occurs in part because of the internal friction in tissue that needs to be overcome in the passage of sound. The higher the frequency, the more rapidly the molecules are forced to move against this friction. As the absorption increases, there is less sound energy available to propagate further through the tissue (Fig. 7–2).

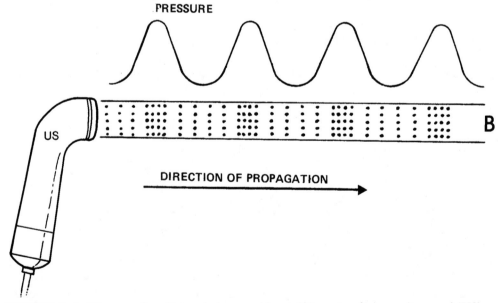

FIGURE 7–1. Diagram of a collimated ultrasound beam (B) coming from an ultrasound (US) applicator. The associated pressure wave is diagrammed; areas of increased molecular concentration (:::) are condensations. Areas of decreased molecular concentrations are rarefactions (:.:).

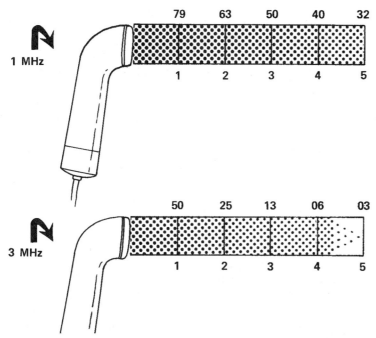

FIGURE 7-2. Attenuation of the sound beam in soft tissue at various frequencies, assuming that uniform attenuation is approximately 1 dB/cm/MHz.

At frequencies greater than 20 MHz, superficial absorption becomes so great that less than 1 percent of the sound penetrates beyond the first centimeter.

For physical therapy applications, 1.0 MHz is the frequency most often used, because it offers a good compromise between sufficiently deep penetration and adequate heating under customary exposure levels. However, as ultrasound is being used more selectively for tissues of varying depth from superficial to deep, ultrasound units offering a 3.0 MHz frequency are widely available.

SOUND VELOCITY

Velocity is the speed at which the vibratory motion is propagated through a material. The more rigid the material, the greater the velocity of sound passing through it. Sound travels through average soft tissue at 1540 m/s and through compact bone at 4000 m/s. The depth of a structure beneath the skin can be determined by measuring the time required for sound to travel to the structure and return. This ability to chart the position of reflecting surfaces forms the basis of the extensive use of ultrasound in medical diagnosis.

WAVELENGTH

A finite period of time elapses before the vibration of a molecule causes its neighbor to vibrate. Because of this delay, the first molecule will reach its point of maximal excursion before its neighbor does, and as long as they continue to vibrate, the second molecule will lag behind the first. These molecules are said to oscillate asynchronously, or be out of phase, and the time delay is called the phase shift. There is an equal phase shift between each of the successive molecules in the path of sound propagation. Because of this overall asynchrony, the concentration of molecules increases in regions called condensations and decreases in alternating regions called rarefactions (Fig. 7–1).

The local pressure is proportional to the molecular concentration and, as shown in Figure 7–1, varies sinusoidally along the direction of propagation with its peak values occurring at regions of condensations. Wavelength is defined as the distance between two successive peaks in the pressure wave.

Wavelength is inversely related to frequency, as indicated in the fundamental equation: Velocity = Frequency × Wavelength. Using the value of 1540 m/s for velocity and 1 MHz for frequency, which are typical values applicable in therapeutic situations, this equation enables one to show that the corresponding wavelength of ultrasound is 1.5 mm.

Types of Waves

Sound waves are classified as longitudinal or transverse, according to the direction of motion of the molecules of the medium through which they travel. A longitudinal wave is one in which the direction of motion of the molecules is parallel to the direction of wave propagation (Fig. 7–3). In a transverse wave, the direction of molecular motion is perpendicular to the direction of wave propagation.

Because gases and liquids are not able to sustain transverse vibrations, transverse

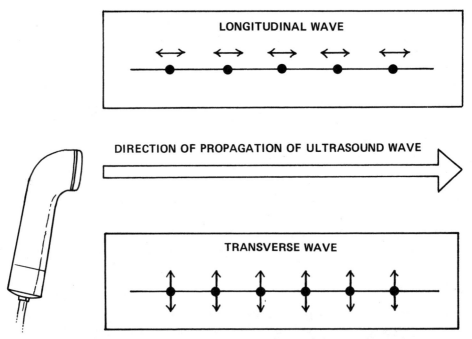

FIGURE 7–3. Schematically depicted types of ultrasound waves.

sound waves do not occur in these substances. In solids, both longitudinal and transverse waves occur. With the exception of compact bone, the tissues of the body behave acoustically as though they were liquids and support only longitudinal waves. Within the body, therefore, transverse waves are found only in bone.

Sound waves can be produced as continuous wave (CW) or pulsed wave. A continuous wave is one in which the sound intensity remains constant (Fig. 7–4), whereas a pulsed wave is intermittently interrupted. Pulsed waves are further characterized by specifying what fraction of time the sound is present over one pulse period. This fraction is called the duty cycle and is calculated using the following equation:

$$\text{Duty cycle} = \frac{\text{duration of pulse (time on)}}{\text{pulse period (time on + time off)}}$$

Typical duty cycles for therapy machines, when in the pulsed mode, range from 0.05 (5%) to 0.5 (50%). The most commonly used duty cycle appears to be 20 percent.

Intensity

The strength of an ultrasound beam is determined by its intensity. Intensity is the rate at which energy is delivered per unit area and is expressed in units of watts per

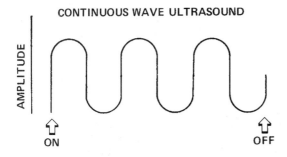

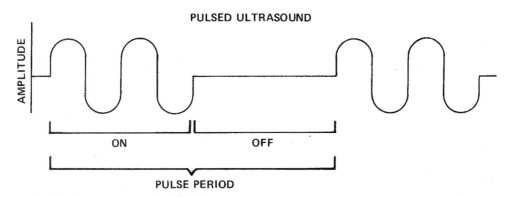

FIGURE 7–4. Continuous-wave and pulsed-wave ultrasound. The duty cycle of the pulsed-wave mode illustrated is $\frac{2\text{ msec}}{4\text{ msec}} = 0.5 = 50\%$.

square centimeter (W/cm^2). Intensities employed in physical therapy range from about 0.25 to 2.0 W/cm^2. With all other factors held constant, the greater the intensity, the greater the resulting temperature elevation.

The measurement of intensity is derived by measuring the total power output (in watts) of the ultrasound applicator and dividing by the area (in cm^2) of the applicator face. Because the ultrasound beam is not uniform, some regions of the beam will be more intense than other regions. The above measurement of intensity gives an average intensity and is referred to as the spatial average intensity. Occasionally, it is desirable to know the greatest intensity anywhere within the beam. This is called the spatial peak intensity (Fig. 7–5).

In the case when the sound beam is pulsed, the intensity will be zero when the sound is off and at its maximum during the pulse (Fig. 7–6). This maximum intensity is called the temporal peak intensity, or the pulse average intensity. The temporal average intensity is obtained by averaging the intensity over both the on and off periods. For example, a pulsed sound beam with a duty cycle of 0.5 (50% and a temporal peak intensity of 2.0 W/cm^2) would have a temporal average intensity of 1.0 W/cm^2 (2.0 W/cm^2 × 0.5 = 1.0 W/cm^2); if the duty cycle had been 0.25 (25%), the temporal average intensity would be 0.5 W/cm^2. In this chapter, unless stated otherwise, all pulsed intensities quoted will be spatial average, temporal peak values along with the duty cycle.

The amount of heating depends on the temporal average intensity rather than the temporal peak. By interrupting (pulsing) a continuous-wave sound beam, the temporal average intensity is decreased proportionately to the amount of time the sound is off. Thus, less heating will occur, even though the temporal peak intensity is unchanged. Pulsing would be of benefit when the desired effect is brought about by a

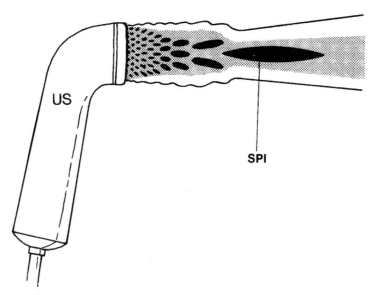

FIGURE 7–5. Schematic diagram of ultrasound (US) beam. The darkest areas indicate more intense regions. The greatest intensity within the beam is the spatial peak intensity (SPI). (Adapted from Stewart, HF, and Stratmeyer, ME [eds]: An Overview of Ultrasound: Theory, Measurement, Medical Applications, and Biological Effects. HHS Publication FDA 82-8-90, 1982.)

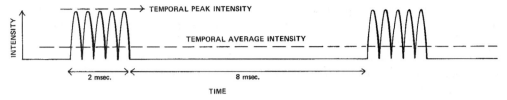

FIGURE 7-6. A typical pulsing pattern. The total pulse period is 10 msec. The pulse duration is 2 msec. The duty cycle is 0.20 (20%).

nonthermal mechanism and when heating is to be minimized, such as in the treatment of stasis ulcers and acute soft tissue injuries.

It should also be noted that the ultrasonic beam is not homogeneous, resulting in high spatial peak intensities within the beam, commonly known as "hot spots." These hot spots may cause damage to the insonated tissues and, therefore, should be avoided. This is best done by always using a moving applicator technique when in direct contact to prevent any build-up of energy in any one spot. The beam nonuniformity ratio (BNR) should also be within the acceptable range. This ratio defines the maximum point intensity on the transducer to the average intensity value across the transducer surface. The BNR should be as low as possible, between 2:1 and 6:1. The lower the BNR, the more even is the distribution of energy from the transducer, and the less risk there is of damage to tissues from areas of concentrated ultrasound energy. In the United States, ultrasound units manufactured since 1979 are required by the Food and Drug Administration (FDA) to have labels indicating the BNR; the therapist should be aware of the BNR of the equipment being used.

When recording the ultrasound exposure administered to a patient, it is important to specify clearly the frequency (in megahertz, MHz), the intensity (in watts per square centimeter, W/cm^2), the duty cycle (in percentage pulsed, p), and the total duration (in minutes, min), for example, 3.0 MHz/0.5 W/cm^2/p 20%/5 min. For continuous-wave exposures, the frequency, the spatial average intensity, the continuous wave (CW), and the duration are reported, for example, 3.0 MHz/0.5 W/cm^2/CW/5 min.

Spatial average intensities ranging from 0.25 to 2.0 W/cm^2 are used in therapeutic applications. The World Health Organization (WHO) limits the spatial average intensity to a maximum of 3.0 $W/1$ cm^2.[5] Intensities above 10.0 W/cm^2 are used to destroy tissue surgically, and intensities (temporal average) below 0.1 W/cm^2 are used for diagnostic purposes.

When considering the intensity applied to the patient, one should also consider that ultrasound vibrations which are propagated through the housing of the applicator into the hand of the physical therapist have been termed "parasitic radiation."[6] This radiation has been reported to possibly result in acute pain in the hand and finger joints of the therapist. The significance or dangers secondary to parasitic radiation are at this point in time speculative at best.

Generation of Ultrasound

Sound within the audible frequency range is normally produced by vibrating membranes, such as the vocal cords or the diaphragm of a loudspeaker. Movement of these membranes sets up corresponding vibrations in the surrounding air molecules, and when this vibration pattern reaches our ears, we perceive it as sound. The frequency of the sound is precisely the frequency of the membrane vibration. Because of their inertia, these membranes cannot vibrate rapidly enough to generate ultrasonic frequencies. However, ultrasound can be generated by replacing these membranes with special crystals that are able to vibrate very rapidly and possess the property of piezoelectricity.

THE PIEZOELECTRIC EFFECT

There are two forms of the piezoelectric effect—direct and reverse (indirect) (Fig. 7–7). The direct piezoelectric effect is the generation of an electric voltage across a crystal when the crystal is compressed. If the crystal is expanded instead of compressed, a voltage of opposite polarity is induced. A sound wave impinging on a piezoelectric crystal will cause the crystal to expand and contract at the same frequency as the sound wave and in turn induce an oscillating voltage across the crystal face. The direct piezoelectric effect is utilized for converting ultrasound into an electrical signal that replicates the sound pattern and can be conveniently and accurately processed and analyzed.

The reverse piezoelectric effect is the contraction or expansion of a crystal in response to a voltage applied across its face. A change in the polarity of the applied voltage causes a contracted crystal to expand, and vice versa. An alternating voltage makes the crystal vibrate at the frequency of the electrical oscillation. In this manner, a piezoelectric crystal can be used to generate ultrasound at any desired frequency.

DIRECT PIEZOELECTRIC

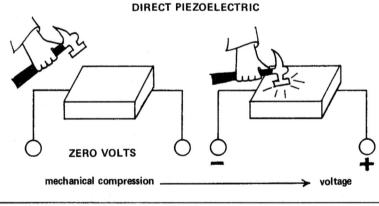

REVERSE PIEZOELECTRIC

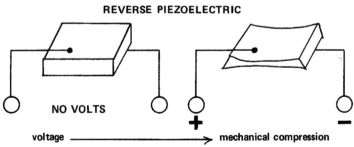

FIGURE 7–7. The direct and indirect (reverse) piezoelectric effects.

THE TRANSDUCER

A transducer is any device that converts one form of energy into another. The piezoelectric crystal is a transducer that converts electrical energy into sound energy, and vice versa.

Many naturally occurring crystals, such as quartz, possess the property of piezoelectricity, but synthetic ceramic crystals, such as barium titanate or lead zirconate titanate (PZT), are almost always used because of their superior mechanical and electrical properties. These crystals are sliced into wafers approximately 2- to 3-mm thick. The diameter may vary from 1 to 3 cm, depending on the intended use. Because of their small size and mechanical fragility, these crystals must be mounted in an applicator to be clinically useful and durable and to facilitate electrical connections. The entire applicator is commonly referred to as the transducer.

BIOPHYSICAL EFFECTS

The biophysical effects resulting from the interaction of ultrasound with tissue can be grouped into two classifications: (1) thermal—those effects produced by the ability of ultrasound to elevate tissue temperature; and (2) nonthermal—those effects that must be attributed to mechanisms other than an increase in tissue temperature. The mechanism of some of the biologic changes produced by ultrasound may be thermal or nonthermal, or a combination of both. For many responses, such as the pain reduction reported following sonation, the underlying physiologic or physical mechanism has not been thoroughly identified and is only speculative at this time.

Thermal Effects

The principal reason for the use of thermal effects of ultrasound is based on the knowledge that ultrasound can elevate tissue temperature to depths of 5 cm or more. The physiologic responses attributed to a thermal mechanism include increased collagen tissue extensibility, alterations in blood flow, changes in nerve conduction velocity, increased pain threshold, increased enzymatic activity, and changes in contractile activity of skeletal muscle. Physiologic changes such as these are reviewed in Chapter 5. Ultrasound intensities at ranges higher than those used for therapeutic application have been demonstrated to retard growth of long bones, damage spinal cord tissue, and destroy various other tissues.

Tissues of high collagen content absorb a large amount of the ultrasound beam and thus are affected to a greater extent by ultrasound energy. The amount of heat produced will depend on the intensity and frequency of the ultrasound, the duration of exposure, and the size and type of tissue sonated. Bone and joint capsular structures have a very high collagen content and are thus the structures that absorb the most ultrasound energy. Ultrasound penetrates through skin and subcutaneous fat with small to moderate attenuation (Table 7–1).

Ultrasound energy absorption and the subsequent tissue temperature elevation are frequency dependent. The higher the frequency, the greater the attenuation of energy in superficial structures. At 3.0 MHz, most of the energy is absorbed within a depth of 1 to 2 cm. At a lower frequency of 1.0 MHz, there is less attenuation in the su-

TABLE 7–1 Attenuation of a 1 MHz
Ultrasound Beam

Tissue	Attenuation (%/cm)
Blood	3
Fat	13
Muscle	24
Blood vessel	32
Skin	39
Tendon	59
Cartilage	68
Bone	96

perficial tissues, allowing more energy to be available for absorption in deeper tissues. This latter frequency is commonly used in the United States in the treatment of musculoskeletal dysfunctions, when an increased depth of penetration and subsequent absorption by a specific structure are desired. However, because many of the conditions commonly treated with therapeutic ultrasound involve superficial tissues, such as ankle sprains, tennis elbow, and stasis ulcers, it is important to use the appropriate frequency in order to treat the injured tissue. In general, a 3.0 MHz frequency should be used in treating tissues up to 1 to 2 cm from the skin surface, and a 1.0 MHz frequency should be used in treating tissues deeper than 1 to 2 cm from the skin surface.

Ultrasound can be used as a deep-heating agent to increase selectively the temperature of periarticular structures[7] and at the bone-muscle interface.[8,9] Intensities required to elevate tissue temperature to a range of 40°C to 45°C vary from 1.0 to 2.0 W/cm² continuous wave for a duration of 5 to 10 minutes. A residual increase in length of amphibian tendons has been demonstrated by elevating tissue temperature with ultrasound and then applying a stretch during the time the temperature remains elevated.[10] In mammalian preparations, similar increases were reported when tissue temperature was elevated by a water bath and a stretch was applied.[11,12] This effect has been attributed to the change in viscous properties of the tissues irradiated, producing a change in the plastic deformation of collagen tissues. This information has been applied clinically to increase the range of motion of contracted joints (see "Clinical Applications section in this chapter).

With an increase of tissue temperature, a mild inflammatory response and an increase in blood flow would be expected. Numerous investigators have measured blood flow in limbs following ultrasound irradiation, some reporting an increase, some a decrease, and some no changes. Intensities, frequencies, duty cycles, and exposure durations of ultrasound application and the methods of measuring changes in blood flow were not consistent among the experimenters. Therefore, drawing clinically useful conclusions is difficult. However, the following statements appear to summarize this information accurately. Following 10 to 20 minutes of ultrasound at intensities greater than 2.0 W/cm², 1.0 MHz frequency, continuous-wave, skeletal-muscle temperature and blood flow increases have been found.[13–15] At lower intensities and for shorter durations, either no change or inconsistent changes in blood flow were noted.[15–17] Considering the length of treatment time required to achieve a clinically useful effect with ultrasound, use of an alternative deep-heating agent, such as continuous shortwave diathermy, should be considered for areas larger than 2 times the transducer size.

Changes in motor and sensory nerve conduction velocity after ultrasound exposure have been reported. Five minutes of ultrasound at 1.0 MHz/1.5 W/cm^2 continuous wave over the lateral cutaneous branch of the radial[18] and superficial cutaneous branch of radial nerves[23] decreased distal latency. No changes were found in the amplitude or duration of the nerve action potential. When sensory nerve latency is decreased, an increase in conduction velocity is implicit. In a similar experimental set-up, latency was decreased in the superficial radial nerve following 1.0 W/cm^2 varying from 5 to 20 minutes.[20] Two groups of investigators compared ultrasound with infrared heating.[19,20] Because latencies were reduced with both agents and temperature increases were similar, the investigators attributed their findings to thermal mechanisms.

Ulnar motor nerve conduction velocity (NCV) increased 3.0 m/s with continuous-wave ultrasound at 1.5 W/cm^2 for 5 minutes and with infrared radiation.[21] Placebo ultrasound and pulsed ultrasound at 1.5 W/cm^2 (1:5 pulse ratio) caused a decrease in NCV. The decrease was proposed to be correlated with the reduction of temperature caused by a cool coupling medium. The thermal effects rather than the nonthermal effects were thought to produce the increased NCV.[21]

Pain threshold was elevated following increases in tissue temperature with 0.8 MHz ultrasound at 1.5 W/cm^2/CW.[22] These findings are consistent with what would be expected when tissue temperature is elevated by a thermal agent.

Nonthermal Effects

Some effects of ultrasound cannot be explained by a thermal mechanism. These nonthermal effects include cavitation and mechanical and chemical alterations. Cavitation is the vibrational effect on gas bubbles by an ultrasound beam. Changes in local pressure produced by ultrasound can cause the expansion and compression of small gas bubbles that may be present in the blood or tissue fluids. During the period of rarefaction, the small bubbles will expand; during condensations, these bubbles will be compressed. If sufficiently intense, the pulsation of the bubbles in the ultrasound field can cause changes in cellular activity and tissue damage. If the bubbles in the field pulse but do not increase much in overall amplitude, stable cavities result. These stable cavities can result in diffusional changes along cell membranes and thus alter cell function.[23] Unstable or transient cavitation refers to the violent collapse of bubbles within the sound field, resulting in tissue destruction. Transient cavitation may be responsible for blood vessel damage.[24] The threshold intensity for unstable cavitation is higher than for stable cavitation. The intensity threshold for stable cavitation may be within the intensity range used in therapy, and although many questions remain, there is some evidence to suggest that cavitation may occur in therapeutic applications. We do not know which, if any, of the beneficial nonthermal effects are caused by stable cavitation.

Acoustical streaming refers to the movement of fluids along the boundaries of cell membranes as a result of the mechanical pressure wave. This streaming has been implicated in the changes in ion fluxes and subsequent changes in cellular activity found with ultrasound application. Increases in cell membrane and vascular wall permeability have been found within the range of therapeutic intensities. Potassium leakage from red blood cells in vitro resulted following sonation at ranges from 0.5 to 3.0 W/cm^2.[25] Increases in fibroblastic activity (e.g., protein synthesis)[26] and increases in calcium fluxes across smooth-muscle membranes of the mouse uterus were found using pulsed ultrasound.[31] These changes may be a result of the mechanical action of ultrasound on cell membranes, rather than of a thermal mechanism.

On the other hand, changes in the diffusion of ions across epithelial cells in isolated frog skin have been attributed to both thermal and mechanical components.[28] Using a stationary applicator, ultrasound at 1.0 MHz/1.5 W/cm^2/CW, applied to the small blood vessels in the hamster cheek pouch resulted in areas of petechiae and demonstrable increases in vascular permeability at the level of the postcapillary venules.[29] The results could have been brought about by thermally induced changes in permeability or by cavitation resulting in damage to vessel endothelial cells. Petechiae in mice were also found after abdominal exposure to ultrasound.[24] Cavitation was implicated as the mechanism producing the observed results.

Other adverse reactions, including stasis of blood flow and endothelial damage, have been demonstrated in chick embryos.[30] Platelet aggregation in blood vessels was shown to occur in guinea pig ears.[31] These responses were attributed to nonthermal mechanisms, because either pulsed ultrasound or very low intensity continuous-wave ultrasound was administered. A stationary transducer was used for all applications. The investigators speculated that such results would not be produced with a moving sound head.

To further elucidate the effects of ultrasound on the microcirculation, Hogan and associates[32,33] have studied the effects of ultrasound on circulation in the rat in an ischemic muscle preparation. When pulsed ultrasound was applied at a frequency of 1.0 MHz at 2.5 W/cm^2 for 5 minutes on alternating days, an increase in capillary density and improved blood flow to medium-size arterioles was found. At higher intensities of pulsed ultrasound, increased vasomotion of small arterioles and decreased flow was found. Although the underlying mechanisms for all the changes seen were not known, they probably were not thermal in origin, because similar findings were not observed when the skeletal muscle was heated in the absence of ultrasound.

In summary, a review of the literature shows that ultrasound can cause many effects. Most of these effects are intensity dependent. With appropriate care to control intensities, ultrasound can be applied to patients in a safe and effective manner.

CLINICAL APPLICATIONS OF ULTRASOUND AT THERAPEUTIC INTENSITIES

Ultrasound is commonly used in rehabilitation as an adjunct in the management of various soft tissue dysfunctions, including joint contracture, scar tissue, tendinitis, bursitis, skeletal muscle spasms, and pain. In addition, ultrasound at therapeutic intensities has been included in treatment regimens for the management of stasis ulcers, pressure sores, and as a noninvasive technique to enhance percutaneous absorption of topical medications (phonophoresis). The basis for the clinical application of ultrasound as a therapeutic agent was developed in the previous section. Although there are now an abundant number of laboratory and clinical reports on the effects and applications of therapeutic ultrasound, much of the material lacks full description of the treatment regimens, and many of the results present contradictory conclusions.[34,35] In this section, the procedures and rationale for the clinical utilization of ultrasound will be discussed.

Joint Contracture and Scar Tissue

Joint contracture is a debilitating consequence of immobilization or trauma. If range of motion is limited owing to periarticular connective tissue changes, stretching exercises are usually employed to increase motion. Elevation of tissue temperature up to 45°C preceding or during a gentle passive or active stretch will be more effective in gaining motion than when either is done in isolation. This concept of "heat and stretch" has been demonstrated in well designed in vitro laboratory studies.[11,12,36] A greater residual increase in tissue length with less potential damage is produced when preheating or simultaneous heating is employed. Length-tension analyses have revealed that tissue extensibility was increased when Gersten[10] applied ultrasound at intensities of 1.0 to 3.0 W/cm², resulting in tissue temperatures ranging from 39°C to 47°C.

Heating has been postulated to alter the viscoelastic (plastic) properties of collagen tissue and collagen molecular bonding, thus facilitating ease of stretch. Deep tissues responsible for decreasing the range of motion at a joint are rich in collagen. Therefore, ultrasound is a logically chosen thermal agent to selectively heat these deep structures.

Lehmann and associates[37] demonstrated that ultrasound was effective in increasing the temperature of the hip joint when applied within therapeutic intensities for at least 5 minutes. A combination of ultrasound and exercise was compared with heat lamp (infrared) and exercise for increasing range of motion of the hips of elderly patients following internal fixation of fractures.[38] Ultrasound was applied to the anterior, lateral, and posterior hip joint at intensities of 1.0 to 2.5 W/cm² for 5 minutes per field. The other group received heat lamp treatment for 30 minutes. Results of treatment were evaluated by range-of-motion measurements. Individuals receiving ultrasound improved in range of motion. Those receiving heat lamp (infrared) showed less or no gain when compared with those receiving ultrasound. Information obtained from these studies can certainly be applied to the treatment of joint contracture in other areas of the body. Joints with a smaller amount of soft-tissue coverage, such as the elbow, wrist, or ankle, are usually treated with ultrasound at intensities averaging 1.0 W/cm² or less.

Ice and ultrasound applications were compared for the treatment of painful "frozen shoulder."[39] Ultrasound therapy was administered to one group at an intensity of 0.5 W/cm² for 5 to 8 minutes, 3 times a week for a total of 15 treatments. Iced towels were applied to the other group for 15 minutes, 3 times a week for a total of 12 treatments. Both groups were placed on a program of passive and active range-of-motion exercises following thermal agent application. All patients reported a decrease in pain and had an increased range of motion that was attributed to their treatment with no apparent differences between the groups. The intensity of ultrasound used for treatment, though, was less than that which has been demonstrated to elevate joint structure temperature at the knee,[7] a joint with approximately as much soft tissue coverage as the shoulder. This observation points out that unless a sufficient intensity is used, one should not expect any greater benefit from the use of ultrasound than with superficial heating or cooling.

Scar tissue is denser than surrounding tissue and can be selectively heated by ultrasound energy prior to friction massage and range of motion exercises. Ultrasound has a definite role in the treatment of joint contractures and scar tissue. However, in order to be used effectively, more work is still needed to determine what intensities and durations should be used to obtain the possible beneficial effects of ultrasound.

CASE STUDY 1

A 28-year-old man sustained partial lacerations to the extensor tendons to the ring and small fingers over the metacarpophalangeal joints when he cut his fingers on a knife in dish water. The tendons were surgically repaired and immobilized for 2 weeks secondary to wound infection. You are now seeing the patient 4 weeks' postoperatively.

PROBLEMS

1. Decreased gliding of the tendon over the metacarpophalangeal joints.
2. Wound infection and slow healing resulted in prolonged immobilization.
3. Limited functional activities.

ASSESSMENT TECHNIQUES

1. Range-of-motion measurements.
2. Wound/scar evaluation.
3. Functional daily activities assessment.

GOALS

1. Increase tendon gliding.
2. Increase range of motion.
3. Increase functional activities.

SELECTION OF TREATMENT MODALITY/RATIONALE

Ultrasound is chosen because of the selective absorption by collagen-rich tendon and joint capsules and because the area to be treated is small. Rehabilitation included ultrasound at 3 MHz/0.5 W/cm^2/CW/4 min. A transducer of approximately 1 cm^2 was used. Active motion into flexion and limited excursion active and full passive motion into extension was used to enhance tendon gliding.

The frequency was chosen because the tissues to be treated are superficial. The intensity was chosen to be moderate because the condition is subacute, but approximately 35 percent of the beam would also be expected to be reflected at the tissue-bone interface, resulting in overall increased intensity. Five minutes was chosen because the area is probably about twice the size of the transducer head (Fig. 7–8). Measure the range of motion before and after each treatment to assess change during treatment and over the course of treatment.

HOME PROGRAM

The patient should be instructed to maintain an increase in mobility by hourly active flexion and passive and active assisted extension.

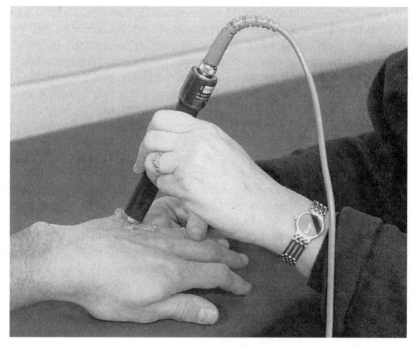

FIGURE 7–8. Ultrasound applied to the dorsum of the hand over the metacarpophalangeal joints of digits 4 and 5. A 1-cm^2 transducer is used with the direct method of coupling.

Reduction of Pain and Muscle Spasm

Following ultrasound application, pain threshold is usually increased. Although the mechanism of pain reduction is not clear, the heat produced by ultrasound could result in counterirritation, heat activation of large-diameter fibers, or an altering of the response to stimulation of the pain receptors (free nerve endings). Pain threshold was elevated following ultrasound application to the arm at 1.5 W/cm^2 for 2 minutes.[22] Because similar changes were found with infrared and microwave diathermy applications (both surface and deep-heating agents), the implicated mechanism of action is through the ability of all three agents to elevate the threshold for activation of the free nerve endings through thermal effects. Williams and coworkers[40] measured a significant decrease in the perception threshold for electrical pain after exposure to ultrasound. This effect developed within 30 to 60 seconds and was increased both with increasing intensity at constant frequency as well as with increasing frequency at constant intensity. When the same amount of ultrasound energy was delivered using a variety of pulsed regimens, exactly the same reduction in pain threshold was obtained. The authors concluded that this indicated a thermal interaction mechanism.

Ultrasound combined with exercise was compared with exercise alone by Munting[41] for patients with shoulder pain. The patients included in the study had no evidence of tendinitis, fracture, or degenerative joint changes. Over a 3-week period, ultrasound was applied for a total of 10 treatments each, at an intensity of 1.5 W/cm² for 3 to 5 minutes, to the anterior, inferior, and posterior aspects of the shoulder. The patients who received ultrasound reported a higher percentage of pain relief (81%) than those who received only exercise (44%). In addition, the gains in active and passive range of motion were greater in the ultrasound-treated groups. At 3-month follow-up, 73% of the patients who had received ultrasound reported no pain, compared with 55% of the "exercise-only" group. Similar results were obtained by Middlemast and Chatterjee,[42] who treated a variety of acute soft-tissue injuries at 1.5 MHz, pulsed wave, for 4 to 10 minutes at intensities varying from 0.5 to 1.0 W/cm² for superficial tissues and 1 to 2 W/cm² for deeply placed structures. They assessed spontaneous pain, tenderness, erythema, restriction of active movement, and swelling and found that after 10 treatments over a 12-day period, those patients treated with ultrasound showed a significantly better overall response when compared with patients treated with infrared radiation, shortwave diathermy, or wax bath. Herrera-Lasso and coworkers found that the use of ultrasound for 10 minutes at 0.5 W/cm² (frequency and duty cycle not stated), in addition to superficial heating and exercises, resulted in improvements in pain and range of motion in painful shoulder syndrome.[43] Similar benefits were found when transcutaneous electrical nerve stimulation (TENS) was applied rather than ultrasound.

Patients with hemiplegia who had painful shoulders were treated using three different regimens: (1) range-of-motion exercises, positioning, and ultrasound at 0.5 to 2.0 W/cm²; (2) range-of-motion exercises, positioning, and sham ultrasound; or (3) range-of-motion exercises and positioning.[44] No statistically significant difference in range of motion was reported among the groups. The authors concluded that in this patient sample, ultrasound was probably not a useful adjunct to treatment with the dosages they administered.

Neuromas in amputation stumps, and as a result of crush injuries, can be sources of pain and can delay the rehabilitation process. Ultrasound has been used in the conservative management of neuromas. When Soren[45] applied ultrasound to patients' painful neuromas, at intensities averaging 1.5 W/cm², five of the six patients studied had decreased pain and improved function.

Ultrasound therapy is often included in the care of patients with low back dysfunction of various etiologies. Considering the extent of use, little had appeared in the literature to support or refute its efficacy in the management of this clinical condition. The technique that is generally employed is paravertebral application with or without sonation along the involved nerve trunk(s). There appear to be only three reports on such application, two from the 1950s and one from the 1980s. Kuitert[46] described six patients with referred pain secondary to osteoarthritis of the spine, damage to vertebral bodies, and/or herniated intervertebral disks. Doses of 0.5 to 1.5 W/cm² were applied paravertebrally on a daily basis for 6 to 12 sessions, averaging 10 minutes per session. Five patients reported decreased pain and muscle spasm, and improved motion. One patient had no change. No other treatments were compared with ultrasound.

Two hundred and nine cases of low back pain secondary to herniated intervertebral disk syndrome were reported by Aldes and Grabin.[47] Symptoms were relieved in 86 percent of the patients when treated with a 12-session course of ultrasound at intensities ranging from 0.3 to 0.8 W/cm². Sonation was administered paravertebrally and along the gluteus maximus, hamstring, and gastrocnemius muscles in patients with radiculitis. Since hot packs and massage were also included in treatment regimens, the relief experienced by the patients may have been produced by these superficial heating agents rather than by the ultrasound. The ultrasound intensities used by the investigators were lower than those customarily used for an area with such a large amount of soft tissue.

Low back pain resulting from herniated intervertebral disks from lumbar four (L-4) to sacral two (S-2) were treated by Nwuga[48] using three different protocols. All patients were seen within 2 weeks after onset of pain. The three groups designated received (1) analgesics and bed rest, (2) sham ultrasound and bed rest, and (3) ultrasound at 1.0 to 2.0 W/cm^2 for 10 minutes and bed rest. Ultrasound and sham ultrasound were given 3 times a week over a 4-week period. Straight-leg raising (Lasègue test) and lumbar spinal flexion, extension, side-flexion, and rotation were measured. Subjective assessments of pain were made. The group treated with ultrasound obtained the best results, with the greatest improvement in flexion, extension, and straight-leg raising and a reduction in pain.

The use of ultrasound combined with high-voltage pulsed current in the treatment of long-standing low back pain (mean = 5 years) was found to be effective in locating and treating "trigger points."[49] The ultrasound transducer was used as the active electrode, and when trigger points in the area insonated were identified by increased pain, they were treated by a stationary technique until the pain decreased (average 5 seconds). All patients reported an analgesic effect, but no attempt was made in this study to differentiate between the specific effects of the two modalities.

Skeletal muscle temperature can be elevated by ultrasound. Temperature measurements of thighs were made, using implanted thermistors.[9] Ultrasound produced temperature elevations at the bone-muscle interface. The ability of ultrasound to elevate tissue temperature may partially explain the basis for the use of this agent in treating skeletal muscle spasm. Ultrasound did seem to reduce muscle spasms in patients with neck dysfunction and with muscle spasms of the lower extremity secondary to poliomyelitis.[50] It also was found to produce a marked reduction in pain, muscle tenderness, and temporomandibular joint clicking when compared to shortwave diathermy (SWD) in the treatment of myofacial joint dysfunction.[51] The authors felt that deeper penetration to muscle tissue by ultrasound accounted for its superiority over SWD.

The mechanism of action for reduction of skeletal muscle spasm with ultrasound is not clear but may be caused by thermal effects that alter the skeletal muscle contractile process directly, reduce muscle spindle activity, or reduce pain, resulting in a break in the pain-spasm-pain cycle.

Ultrasound used alone was not as effective as ultrasound used in conjunction with occlusive splint therapy, acupuncture, and muscle-conditioning exercises in patients with temporomandibular joint (TMJ) dysfunction and associated muscle spasms. When administered for TMJ dysfunction, coupling was achieved through a small water-filled plastic bag. Intensities were kept below 0.6 W/cm^2.[52] Of interest is the suggestion that a higher intensity of ultrasound may have produced even more beneficial results.

The mechanical effect of ultrasound over the affected dermatome in patients with herpes zoster (shingles) is considered responsible for its pain-relieving effects.[53] This mechanical action is thought to increase the activity of the larger nerve fibers, thereby closing the "pain gate" at the substantia gelatinosa and so reintroducing normal inhibition of the smaller unmyelinated fibers. In Payne's study[53] of postherpetic neuralgia, ultrasound was not found to be effective in decreasing pain. However, in studies by Garrett and Garrett[54] and Jones,[55] patients suffering with acute herpes zoster showed good pain relief from treatment. The duration of the condition might help to explain the different results, as well as the use of pulsed ultrasound by Jones, especially if it is the mechanical effects of ultrasound that are thought to be responsible for its benefits.

The effects of ultrasound on peripheral sympathetic nerve fibers as well as increased blood flow are cited as possible explanations for the dramatically beneficial effects produced by the daily use of low-dose ultrasound ($0.5 \ W/cm^2$ for 5 minutes) in the treatment of lower-extremity reflex sympathetic dystrophy.[56]

CASE STUDY 2

The patient, a 45-year-old woman, has had pain in the right cervical and interscapular area for approximately 2 weeks. The onset of pain was caused by repetitive activity during spring cleaning.

PROBLEMS

1. Irritation of right cervical and interscapular pain for about 1 to 2 hours following driving to work.
2. Limited functional activities secondary to limited cervical range of motion and pain.

ASSESSMENT TECHNIQUES

1. Pain quantity, quality, and location.
2. Functional daily activities assessment.
3. Cervical range of motion assessment.

GOALS

1. Reduce pain.
2. Increase functional activities.
3. Improve range of motion.

SELECTION OF TREATMENT MODALITY/RATIONALE

Ultrasound was used because the area to be treated is small and the tissue to be treated (one side of cervical spine) deep. The patient should be lying prone or seated with upper extremities well supported while treatment is administered. Ultrasound was delivered at $1.0 \ MHz/0.5 \ W/cm^2/p$ 20% for 5 minutes on the affected area. The frequency of 1 MHz was chosen because deep tissue was to be treated. The intensity of $0.5 \ W/cm^2$ was chosen because the condition was subacute. Pulsed mode was chosen to enhance the pain relief effect. The 5-minute time was chosen because the area to be treated was approximately 1 to 2 times the size of the 5 cm^2 transducer. Assess change in both duration and intensity of soreness after ultrasound and exercises.

HOME PROGRAM

The patient was instructed to continue exercises 3 to 4 times a day. Instructions in posture awareness were given to be practiced at home and at work.

Bursitis and Tendinitis

Another common use of ultrasound is with patients having bursitis and tendinitis. There is little statistically significant supportive documentation that demonstrates the efficacy of this modality for patients with these problems. However, a study by Binder and associates[57] found that ultrasound applied at 1.0 MHz, 1.0 to 2.0 W/cm^2/p 20%, and a duration of 5 to 10 minutes for 12 treatments over 4 to 6 weeks significantly enhanced recovery in 63% of patients with lateral epicondylitis. In a similar study, using continuous ultrasound at 1.0 W/cm^2 for 10 treatments of 10 minutes, Lundeberg and coworkers[58] found that there was only a significant difference in improvement of "epicondylalgia" between the insonated and rest groups, with no significant difference between the insonated and the mock-insonated groups. The intensity used by Lundeberg was higher than that used by Binder. In addition, the numbers of patients in each study group were fewer.

Decreased pain, increased range of motion, and decreased tenderness have been reported anecdotally in patients receiving ultrasound therapy for subacromial bursitis.[59-61] Similar success was found in patients with bicipital tendinitis.[61] None of these reports, though, compared ultrasound with other forms of therapy.

The combination of sham ultrasound and exercise was compared with actual ultrasound and exercise in patients with subacromial bursitis of greater than 1 month's duration.[62] Ultrasound was administered at an intensity averaging 1.0 to 2.0 W/cm^2 for 6 minutes, 3 times a week for 4 weeks. Intensity levels were determined by increasing power until the patient reported a dull aching or pricking sensation, then reducing the ultrasonic intensity by 10%. Therefore, intensity was determined individually for each case. All medications were held constant during the time of the study. No differences between the groups could be found in pain relief, range of motion of the shoulder, or overall condition. The authors concluded that ultrasound was probably not a useful adjunct in the conservative management of subacromial bursitis.

Falconer and associates[63] reviewed the literature to determine the effects of ultrasound on musculoskeletal conditions. In their review, they suggested that ultrasound appears to be effective in relieving pain and increasing range of motion in acute periarticular inflammatory conditions, but not in chronic periarticular inflammatory conditions. They suggested that the pain relief in these acute conditions might be caused by (1) an increased pain threshold through ultrasound's effect on sensory nerves; (2) a washout of pain mediators by increased blood flow; and (3) ultrasound's effect on cell membrane permeability, resulting in reduced inflammation. However, it is still not certain whether ultrasound produces a pro-inflammatory or an anti-inflammatory effect and what prompters may be responsible for these effects (see "Wound Healing" section in this chapter). Thus, careful clinical monitoring should accompany treatment of acute conditions.

There have also been comparative studies of the therapeutic benefits of ultrasound compared to ice massage, iontophoresis, and phonophoresis in the treatment of shinsplints[64]; ultrasound to phonophoresis, transcutaneous nerve stimulation, and steroid injection in the treatment of lateral epicondylitis of the elbow[65]; ultrasound/ice contrast to ice, phonophoresis, and iontophoresis in the treatment of knee extensor mechanism disorders.[66] All the treatments studied were found to be superior to control groups, but only ice/massage contrast treatments were found to offer any greater improvement over the other treatments. Small numbers of subjects were used in each study. It would be interesting to see if the results were similar with larger sample sizes.

The rationale for the treatment of tendinitis and bursitis with ultrasound appears to lie in its effects of increased blood flow to aid healing, increased tissue temperature to reduce perceived pain, or perhaps a pro-inflammatory effect.

CASE STUDY 3

A 26-year-old male patient has a patellar tendinitis. The insidious onset of pain occurred approximately 3 weeks ago. The patient was told to place ice on the area, rest, and do range of motion exercises.

PROBLEMS

1. Persistent pain in affected area.
2. Limited functional activities.

ASSESSMENT TECHNIQUES

1. Pain quality, quantity, and location.
2. Functional daily activities assessment.

GOALS

1. Reduce pain.
2. Increase functional activities.

SELECTION OF TREATMENT MODALITY/RATIONALE

Ultrasound was chosen for its effect on increasing healing and decreasing pain. Rehabilitation included ultrasound at 3 MHz/0.8 W/cm^2/p 50% for 5 minutes. A frequency of 3 MHz was chosen because tissues are 1 to 2 cm deep from the surface of the body. The intensity was chosen because the condition is subacute. A pulsed mode of 50 percent was chosen because injury is subacute and only a mild heat effect is desired to increase healing. The time is chosen because the area to be treated is 1 to 2 times the size of the transducer. Assess range of motion before and after each treatment and between subsequent visits; assess duration and intensity of pain following treatment.

HOME PROGRAM

Follow progressive exercise program as clinically indicated.

Calcium Deposits

Some clinicians have stated that ultrasound can be a valuable agent in assisting in the reabsorption of calcium deposits in soft tissue. Although case reports[67] have suggested that ultrasound facilitates calcium reabsorption, may increase the perfusion of a calcified bursa, and affect the integrity of the bursal sac,[68] no controlled studies or follow-up studies using radiographic analysis have appeared in the literature. Therefore, statements that ultrasound exposure results in calcium reabsorption may be incorrect. Nevertheless, ultrasound may help relieve the inflammation around a calcium deposit, thus relieving a patient's pain and improving function.

Phonophoresis

Ultrasound energy has been used in an attempt to enhance percutaneous absorption of anti-inflammatory drugs (cortisol, dexamethasone, salicylates) and local analgesics (lidocaine) through the skin to underlying tissue. The technique of delivering medication by ultrasound has been termed phonophoresis. The purported rationale for this technique is that via this technique, the drug will be delivered to the site where the effect is sought. In animal studies, high intensities of ultrasound were used to deliver cortisol to depths of 5 to 6 cm subcutaneously into skeletal muscle and peripheral nerve.[69] More lidocaine was extracted from rabbit tissue following ultrasound than when the lidocaine was applied topically and not followed by ultrasound.[70]

The implicated mechanism that allows the medication to reach underlying tissues could be the changes in tissue permeability following ultrasound. Diffusion rates could possibly be enhanced by acoustic streaming. Thus, theoretically the medication could follow the well-focused pattern of the ultrasound beam.

Griffin and associates[71] studied the effects of ultrasound and a placebo cream versus those of ultrasound and hydrocortisone ointment on patients with osteoarthritis, periarticular arthritis, and rheumatoid arthritis. From the group treated with hydrocortisone and ultrasound (at less than 1.5 W/cm^2 for 5 minutes, once a week), 68% of the patients had improved range of motion and decreased pain. Of those treated with placebo cream and ultrasound at the same dosage, only 25% had marked improvement in the measured characteristics. All patients received other forms of therapy during the experimental period. In the Griffin study, the hydrocortisone[72] may not have transmitted ultrasound energy very well, thus attenuating intensity. Therefore, we speculate that superior results may have occurred because the "phonophoresis" group had ultrasound at a lower intensity than the placebo cream and ultrasound group. Lower intensities of ultrasound may be more appropriate for treating inflammatory conditions. This notion is supported in a study by Ciccone and associates.[73]

TABLE 7–2 Factors to Consider
for Phonophoresis

Transmission of ultrasound through coupling medium and
    drug
Absorption of drug across the stratum corneum
Site for delivery of drug (target tissue)
  • Is the drug delivered in sufficient dosage to the tissue
    intended for treatment?
Clinical efficacy of phonophoresis technique
  • Can ultrasound without drug produce the same result?
  • Can cutaneous application of drug without ultrasound
    produce the same result?

The results of phonophoresis were not shown to be superior to that of ultrasound alone in the treatment of lateral epicondylitis[65] or in the treatment of extensor carpi radialis brevis tendinitis.[74]

Moll[75] treated a series of trigger points comparing three groups treated with (1) a placebo solution and sham ultrasound, (2) a water-based solution and ultrasound, or (3) a decadron-lidocaine solution and ultrasound. The ultrasound dosage was less than 1.5 W/cm^2 for 5 minutes, twice a week for 3 weeks. While the greatest improvement was found in those patients receiving the phonophoresis with decadron-lidocaine solution, the number of subjects in the study was too small to show a statistically significant difference.

More well-controlled studies on the efficacy of phonophoresis are warranted. When studying phonophoresis, many factors should be considered.[76] These are outlined in Table 7–2.

The transmission of the ultrasound energy through the pharmaceutical product should also be considered. Benson and McElnay[77] found that relatively few of the products commonly used for phonophoresis had good transmission characteristics. Considering that such products are usually applied directly onto the skin, it is likely that the effectiveness of the insonation itself will be decreased. Cameron and Monroe[72] also reported that many of the drugs commonly used in phonophoresis transmitted much less than 40%, and often 0% of the ultrasound transmitted by water. They concluded that it was unlikely that the results from phonophoresis with these drugs were caused by the effects of ultrasound if little, if any would have been generated. It would appear, however, that this technique may provide the clinician with a means of administering medication locally in a relatively easy and painless fashion. However, from the studies cited above, as well as from that of Byl and associates,[78] clinicians should be certain that their drug of choice is not only suitable for the lesion to be treated, but also that it transmits ultrasound to at least 80% relative to transmission through water. They should also limit the use of phonophoresis to tissues superficial to the submuscular or subtendinous levels, because diffusion deep to these levels is unlikely. Care should also be taken to monitor any unwanted systemic effects that may result from penetration of the drug through the therapist's own skin. Phonophoresis, however, may continue to be the method of choice for patients who are apprehensive about receiving injections. Certainly this is an area for more study.

CASE STUDY 4

The patient, a 38-year-old man, has a lateral epicondylitis. His symptoms, which first began after prolonged hammering, have continued for approximately 6 weeks. He was instructed to use ice on the affected area and to rest. In addition, anti-inflammatory medication was prescribed.

PROBLEMS

1. Temporary relief only.
2. Aggravation with renewed activity.
3. Limited functional activity.

ASSESSMENT TECHNIQUES

1. Pain quantity, quality, and location.
2. Functional daily activities' assessment.

GOALS

1. Reduce pain.
2. Increase functional use of involved extremity.

SELECTION OF TREATMENT MODALITY/RATIONALE

Phonophoresis was selected in order to introduce dexamethasone to the site of the lesion. Treatment included ultrasound at 3 MHz/1.0 W/cm^2/CW for 3 minutes. The frequency of 3 MHz was chosen because the tissue to be treated is less than 2 cm deep to the skin. The intensity was chosen because this is a subacute to chronic condition. Continuous mode was chosen to enhance the thermal effect, as well has having the maximum effect to increase diffusion of the drug. The time was chosen because the area is approximately equal to, or less than, the size of the transducer in cm^2. Assess ability to perform repetitive movement, resisted activities, and pain-free stretch. Assess periods of decreased or no pain after treatment.

HOME PROGRAM

The patient was instructed to perform stretching of his forearm extensor muscles every 2 hours. A progressive, resisted exercise program should be implemented, as clinically indicated, to increase forearm extensor muscle strength.

Note to the reader: This case study represents an integration of the literature on phonophoresis. How could you determine if the technique suggested is appropriate? (Guidelines for such study are found in Chapter 10.)

Wound Healing

Low-intensity continuous-wave or pulsed-wave modes have been used in the treatment of acute and chronic wounds to enhance the reparative process. During the first 24 to 48 hours following trauma, edema prevention or reduction is an important goal. Persistent edema can prolong the inflammatory process and increase pain, thereby reducing function. Recently, attention has been given to the anti-inflammatory effects of therapeutic ultrasound. El Hag and coworkers[79] reported that ultrasound reduced facial swelling and trismus following removal of lower third molars. The authors could not clarify why the nonthermal effects produced by their use of low-intensity pulsed ultrasound (i.e., increased protein synthesis, increased mast-cell production) should lead to decreased swelling because these changes would be likely to lead to increased vascular permeability. They did feel, however, that the massaging and placebo effects of ultrasound treatment could contribute to its anti-inflammatory effect. The placebo effect was further supported by Hashish and associates[80] when they reported little difference between the anti-inflammatory effects of ultrasound and mock ultrasound as measured by changes in facial swelling, trismus, pain, and serum C–reactive protein levels following removal of impacted lower third molars. The authors reported that although the majority of the anti-inflammatory action appeared to be a placebo effect, increasing the intensity of ultrasound was counterproductive and the most beneficial intensity was 0.1 W/cm². The authors suggest that higher intensities might produce more pro-inflammatory changes, such as increased cell membrane permeability and mast-cell degranulation, which might explain the partial reversal of anti-inflammatory activity seen in their study. They concluded that low-intensity ultrasound might inhibit the release of inflammatory mediators from cells. In a study designed to assess the effect of ultrasound on acute inflammation as measured by temperature differences between inflamed and normal surrounding skin, Snow and Johnson[81] also found little difference between the insonated and mock-insonated groups.

Using an animal model to look particularly at plasma extravasation following soft-tissue damage, Fyfe and Chahl[82] induced edema in abdominal tissue with an intracutaneous injection of silver nitrate. (The release of histamine and prostaglandins, and other chemical mediators of inflammation, can be induced by silver nitrate.) The animals treated with pulsed ultrasound, 0.79 MHz/0.5 W/cm²/p 20% or 50% for 2 to 4 minutes, had less leakage from the capillaries into the interstitial space than did untreated animals.

In a further study,[83] the investigators found that ultrasound treatment increased plasma extravasation during the first 24 hours, but later reduced it significantly compared to controls. The effects of ultrasound on plasma extravasation were found to vary according to both the duration of insonation and the number of insonations. Although early extravasation might result in increased delivery of oxygen and nutrients to enhance tissue repair, the authors questioned whether this early increase represents an advantageous effect in terms of enhancing tissue repair.

In order to further understand the effects of ultrasound on tissue repair, Dyson and Luke[84] considered many variables in an attempt to determine the effect of ultrasound on mast-cell degranulation. Mast-cell degranulation induces inflammation; stimulation of degranulation should be expected to induce the physiologic changes necessary for wound healing. The authors suggest that induction of mast-cell degranulation by low intensities of therapeutic ultrasound in injured tissues may be of significance in the acceleration of tissue repair. It is apparent that the effects of ultrasound on such tissues should be carefully monitored to prevent the possibility of further damage. They conclude that more research into the mechanisms of ultrasound is needed before the effects of ultrasound therapy on human tissues can be "adequately predicted and its safe and efficient use optimized."[84]

Dyson and associates[85] reported that ultrasound facilitated a greater increase in growth of tissue in experimentally wounded rabbit ears, compared with that in untreated control subjects following excision of a small amount of tissue. Ultrasound was initiated 2 weeks after the wound occurred and continued 3 times a week. The dosages found to be most effective were 0.25 and 0.5 $W/cm^2/p$ 20% and 0.1 $W/cm^2/CW$ at 3.5 MHz for 5 minutes. With higher intensities—4.0 to 8.0 $W/cm^2/p$ 25%—swelling resulted. Because tissue temperature increases were only 0.53°C to 1.35°C in the successfully treated wounds, the investigators suggested that acoustic streaming may have been part of the mechanism that facilitated repair. Streaming may in fact alter ion fluxes across membranes.

This work of Dyson and associates[85] on tissue regeneration has served as an impetus for further studies on the use of ultrasound for fresh-wound healing. Roberts[86] applied ultrasound through a "window" in the casts of animals with surgically repaired tendons. The dosage given was 1.1 $MHz/0.8$ W/cm^2 pulsed for 5 minutes, 5 days a week, for 6 weeks. The control animals with tendon repairs were treated only by cast immobilization for 6 weeks. In the casted-only group, the tensile strength of the tendons (as measured by breaking strength) at 6 weeks was within the range of values reported by Lundborg and Rank[87] following tendon repair. In the ultrasound group, none of the tendons showed evidence of healing. The authors conclude that the use of ultrasound in the early period after tendon repair is detrimental to healing. The investigators stated that the intensity of ultrasound chosen for the experiment was similar to that which would be administered to the human hand. Other factors, though, may have clouded their conclusions. The breaking strength of the ultrasound-treated group was less than that of the casted-only group, but the casted-only group had low breaking strengths also. Perhaps the method of immobilization was insufficient, also contributing to difficulty with healing.

A study of the effects of ultrasound following partial rupture of Achilles tendons in rats was carried out.[88] This study reported that the tensile strength of the insonated tendons seemed to be greater and that the insonated tissue appeared to be at a more advanced stage of healing. Treatment in this study was only 3 times a week, for 3 weeks. Stevenson and coworkers[89] also found that ultrasound enhanced the functional return of repaired flexor tendons in the hen. They used ultrasound at 3.0 $MHz/0.75$ W/cm^2 for 5 minutes in 20 daily treatments. Treatment started after 4 weeks of immobilization after surgical repair of the profundus tendon. However, they also reported that ultrasound had no effect on gap formation or tensile strength of the repaired tendons. Enwemeka,[91] however, found that exposure of tenotomized, repaired, and immobilized rabbit tendons to ultrasound at 1 $MHz/1$ W/cm^2 for 5 minutes over 9 consecutive days, resulted in a significant increase in both the tensile and energy absorption capacity of the tendons. The difference between Enwemeka's results and those of Roberts and Stevenson may relate to the number of treatments.

Byl and coworkers[92] used animal models with surgically induced wounds to try to determine what treatment parameters were of most benefit in accelerating early tissue repair. They looked at the effect of low-intensity ultrasound on tensile strength, collagen deposition, and reduction in wound size of full-thickness lesions and mast-cell degranulation. They found that all these factors were significantly greater in insonated wounds when compared to sham-insonated wounds. The dose used was 0.5 W/cm^2 for the first 3 days and then 1.5 W/cm^2 for the next 2 days. The rationale was that low-dose ultrasound used initially would help to decrease edema and increase mast-cell degranulation. The higher dose would then be used to increase collagen deposition and increase circulation. Byl and coworkers[93] then compared the effects of high- or low-dose ultrasound or sham ultrasound, as well as the number of treatment days, on wound breaking strength and collage deposition. They concluded again that insonated wounds were significantly stronger than the controls. They also concluded that thermal effects were most likely the main physical difference between high- and low-dose ultrasound. They, therefore, recommended that low-dose ultrasound should be used to treat acute wounds, whereas high-dose ultrasound should be used in the later stages of healing when wound remodeling takes place.

These preliminary studies on wound healing suggest that the time in the course of healing at which ultrasound therapy is administered is important. The total amount of ultrasound energy delivered into the tissues may also determine the positive or negative effects on healing. When therapy is initiated during the early stages of wound healing, within the first week, repair may be hindered if excessive ultrasound is applied. On the other hand, if therapy at low intensities is initiated after 2 weeks, during the proliferative phase (fibroblastic infiltration and collagen formation) and early into the remodeling phase, ultrasound at low intensities may be beneficial. In contrast to this, it was found that the higher intensity of 1.5 W/cm^2 was highly significant in healing the traumatized soft tissue of experimental animals when compared to the lower intensity of 0.5 W/cm^2.[90] It is clear that further well-designed and well-controlled investigations are needed to determine the efficacy of ultrasound in facilitating tissue healing.

CHRONIC WOUNDS

Ultrasound has been employed in the treatment of chronic skin ulcers, especially when other methods of therapy have failed. Paul and associates[94] used dosages of 0.5 to 1.0 W/cm^2 3 times a week in managing pressure sores in patients with spinal cord injuries. Thirteen of the 23 ulcers treated with ultrasound healed, five improved, and the remainder did not benefit from the treatment. Previous methods of treatment had failed.

McDiarmid and associates[95] found that although no effect of ultrasound was observed on healing rate of "clean" pressure sores, ultrasound therapy appeared to improve the healing rate of "dirty" sores. It was postulated that such an effect might be caused by the stimulation of the production of wound factors by ultrasound.[96]

Dyson and Suckling[97] reported on a series of patients with chronic varicose ulcerations. Sham ultrasound was compared with ultrasound at 3 MHz/1.0 W/cm^2/p 20% for 5 to 10 minutes, 3 times a week. At 28 days after the initiation of treatment, the average size of the ultrasound-treated ulcers was 66% smaller compared with a 10% reduction of size in the sham ultrasound group. Ultrasound treatment to chronic leg ulcers was also given just once a week, at 1.0 MHz/0.5 W/cm^2 for 1 minute per applicator area by Callam and coworkers.[98] A 20% positive difference in ulcer area between the control and treatment group was apparent at 4 weeks and was maintained for the 12-week duration of the study. Although Lundeberg and coworkers[99] and Eriksson and coworkers[100] could not demonstrate significant differences in the proportion of healed ulcers or ulcer area in an insonated group of chronic leg ulcers when compared with placebo groups, both of these studies noted a tendency that ultrasound was indeed more effective than the placebo.

If ultrasound is chosen as an adjunct treatment in ulcer care, coupling can be direct or indirect in water, depending on the location of the ulcer. Another agent, Geliperm, has also been described as a sterile coupling agent particularly suitable in the treatment by ultrasound of broken skin.[101] The ultrasound energy can be applied around the periphery of the ulcer for 5 minutes or increased to 10 minutes in ulcers greater than 2.5 cm^2 in size. It is important to emphasize that other aspects of ulcer care should not be ignored. Prior to ultrasound application, the wound should be cleansed and debrided if necessary. Between ultrasound treatments, the wound should be kept clean and moist, with all pressure kept off the area. All of these measures should aid in preventing further skin breakdown and facilitate healing.

There have also been several reports of the effectiveness of ultrasound therapy at low doses in decreasing pain and increasing the dispersal of bruising following childbirth[102,103] and surgery, including episiotomies,[104] as well as in the pain relief of indurated episiotomy scars of long standing.[105]

CASE STUDY 5

A 40-year-old male factory worker sustained a sprain of the lateral ankle. This occurred when he overturned his foot 1 day ago. Rest, ice compression, and elevation were recommended to the patient by the company nurse.

PROBLEM

1. Swelling and bruising of the ankle.
2. Pain in the ankle.
3. Decreased range of motion in dorsiflexion.
4. Limited functional activities.

ASSESSMENT TECHNIQUES

1. Volumetrics of ankle.
2. Pain quantity, quality, and location.
3. Range of motion measurements.
4. Functional activities assessment, including gait.

GOALS

1. Decrease swelling and maintain the reduction.
2. Reduce pain.
3. Increase range of motion of the foot and ankle.
4. Increase strength of the foot-ankle musculature, when appropriate.
5. Improve gait to normal, as appropriate.
6. Increase functional activities.

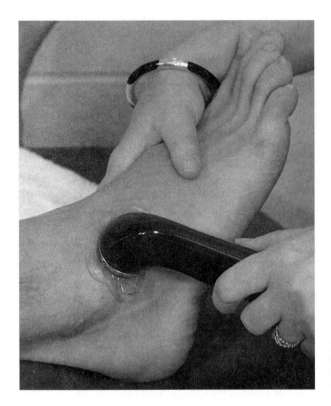

FIGURE 7–9. Ultrasound applied to the lateral ankle using a 5-cm² transducer with a direct coupling technique.

SELECTION OF TREATMENT MODALITY/RATIONALE

Low-dose ultrasound to decrease edema and increase mast-cell degranulation was used. Days 1 to 5, 3 MHz/0.5 W/cm²/p 20% for 5 minutes; days 6 to 14, 3 MHz/1.0 W/cm²/p 20% for 5 minutes. The 3 MHz frequency was chosen because tissues are superficial. Low-dose or high-dose intensity was chosen for a stage of healing as described above. Pulsed mode was chosen to aid healing effects. The time was chosen because the area is 1 to 2 times the size of the 5-cm² transducer (Fig. 7–9). Assess decrease in swelling, bruising, and pain and increase in range of motion, strength, and function over the course of treatment.

HOME PROGRAM

Days 1 to 2: rest, ice, compression, elevation; days 3 to 14: active range of motion, non–weight-bearing strength and knee exercises, increased weight bearing as pain allows; day 14 and onward: increased weight bearing, range of motion, and strengthening exercises.

THERAPEUTIC ULTRASOUND UNITS

The basic components of therapeutic ultrasound units include a power supply, oscillator circuit, transformer, coaxial cable, and ultrasound applicator. The purpose of the therapeutic ultrasound unit is to produce a sound beam at a specific frequency. The frequency is generated by an oscillator circuit carefully tuned by the manufacturer to the preferred frequency for the transducer. Occasional tuning adjustments may be necessary, particularly when a transducer is replaced. These adjustments are best left to the biomedical engineering technician. The intensity is determined by the electrical voltage applied to the transducer. The voltage is controlled by setting the intensity control, which adjusts a variable gain transformer.

A circuit can be added that interrupts the oscillator to produce a pulsed mode. The duty-cycle control selector on the face of the machine can change the on-off times by controlling a pulse timing circuit. The treatment timer limits how long the instrument is energized.

To work properly, the unit is supplied with appropriate voltages obtained through a transformer to which electrical power from the wall receptacle is applied. Appropriate power can also be supplied through a battery.

A coaxial cable connects the ultrasound applicator to the generator (console). The purpose of the coaxial cable is to maximize transmission of the electrical energy and to minimize frequency distortion and interference with the external environment.

All units have a power meter calibrated to read in both watts (acoustic power) and watts per square centimeter (acoustic intensity). For any given applicator, the ratio of the acoustic power to the intensity is a constant, the effective radiating area (ERA). Some machines now also feature self-calibration testing, output power control in response to tissue loading, and automatic shutoff in case of transducer overheating and/or inadequate coupling. A typical ultrasound unit is pictured in Figure 7–10.

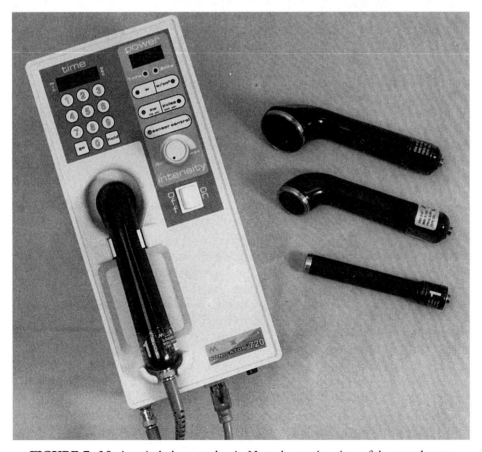

FIGURE 7–10. A typical ultrasound unit. Note the varying sizes of the transducers.

Quality Control

Surveys of ultrasound machines used in physical therapy departments[106,107] revealed that a considerable number of machines were not within acceptable limits, especially with regard to the effective intensity. In light of these reports of machine inadequacies, it would appear that physical therapists should be more vigilant in ensuring that their ultrasound equipment is functioning safely and correctly. A survey of 204 hospital physical therapy departments and 109 private clinics in England and Wales[108] revealed how often the ultrasound machines were calibrated, by whom, and how many physical therapists had access to a radiation balance. In order to ensure that ultrasound machines are performing correctly and safely, factors such as beam shape, power, and pressure should be checked annually, as should all the electrical components. In particular, the transducer assembly is prone to deterioration and so should be frequently checked, especially for watertightness. These factors are generally checked by the manufacturers or a biomedical instrumentation service (see Chapter 3).

GUIDELINES FOR CLINICAL ADMINISTRATION

The therapeutic aim with continuous-wave ultrasound is to elevate the tissue temperature for a given duration at a specific anatomic location. The pulsed-wave mode, or a continuous-wave mode of very low intensity, can be chosen if the goal of treatment is to facilitate soft-tissue healing, and when a significant increase in tissue temperature is not desired (for example, in the case of stasis ulcers). The average intensity for a given power-output machine setting is less with the pulsed-wave mode than with the continuous-wave mode.

To achieve the therapeutic goal that has been delineated, certain procedures should be followed when applying ultrasound. The ultrasound generators for patient care should be properly calibrated and electrically safe (see Chapter 3). Even though the operation of all units is similar, the instructions provided by the manufacturer should be carefully reviewed prior to the use of a machine. The therapist should be present during treatment. Patients should not administer their own ultrasound.

Coupling Techniques

Unlike electromagnetic energy, which can travel well through air, ultrasound energy is markedly attenuated in air and is totally reflected at air-tissue interfaces. Therefore, a coupling medium must be used to transmit ultrasound energy from the transducer to the irradiated surface. When the surface area being treated is larger than the applicator surface and is relatively regular or flat in contour, a direct method of coupling can be employed. With this technique, a thin layer of water-soluble gel is spread over the area to be treated, and the sound head is placed in contact with the gel. The objective of the coupling is to eliminate as much air as possible between the transducer and the skin and thereby to maximize the amount of sound entering the body.

The choice of a coupling agent for the direct contact technique is based on transmission characteristics, viscosity, ease of application, cost, and therapist preference.

Impedance match between the transducer and the coupling medium should also be considered.[109] Substances that may irritate or be driven through the skin should be avoided. The viscosity of the gel should be high enough to prevent any "run-off" during treatment and low enough to permit ease of movement of the transducer across the skin surface. The gel can feel very cold to the patient as it comes directly out of its storage container, and, therefore, some therapists preheat the gel purely for patient comfort. However, overzealous heating of the gel will decrease viscosity and often make the gel "runny." Lehmann and coworkers[110] have suggested that coupling agents such as mineral oil, when applied at a lower temperature (18°C to 20°C), will be more effective in transmitting ultrasound energy to deeper tissues without heating superficial tissues than they will be at a temperature of 24°C. However, the differences produced in deep-tissue temperature elevation were found to be minimal. Therefore, in the interest of patient comfort, it may be best to slightly preheat the gel.

Although a number of agents have been suggested in the past, commercially available gels for ultrasound therapy are usually more practical to use in a busy clinic. The salt found in gels used for electrocardiogram (ECG) or surface electromyogram (EMG) may damage the transducer face, so if these gels are used, after the treatment is complete, they should be carefully wiped from the transducer face and the transducer rinsed with tap water.

If there are bony prominences in the area (e.g., in a small-framed person or over the lateral epicondyle of the humerus) or if the surface is small and irregular in contour (for example, a distal extremity), one of the more recently available small-sized applicators should be used in direct contact. However, if such an applicator is not available, other methods of coupling may be selected.

For treatment of the hand and wrist or foot and ankle areas, a basin can be filled with room-temperature water and the part can be immersed in the bath. Ideally, degassed water is the medium of choice, but its preparation and maintenance render it impractical for clinical use. Forrest and Rosen[111] found that temperature elevations in the extensor tendons of the lateral epicondyles of pigs failed to reach therapeutic levels when treatment was given under water, but did reach such levels when the same treatment parameters (1 MHz, 2.0 W/cm^2) were used in direct contact. Draper and coworkers[112] also found that human muscle tissue temperature at a depth of 3 cm was increased 4.8°C when insonated through topical gel, but only 2.1°C when insonated through tap water (1.5 W/cm^2/CW for 10 minutes). Because these results have not been confirmed by other studies, tap water should be considered a reasonable alternative, especially when an uneven surface would make treatment with direct contact extremely difficult, or when thermal effects are not the aim of treatment.

If treatment is given in a metal basin or whirlpool, some of the ultrasound energy will be reflected off the metal, thus increasing intensity in certain areas near the metal. A plastic or rubber basin will not cause as much reflection. In addition, water in a whirlpool often has a large number of air bubbles, which tend to reduce the transmission of ultrasound. This situation can be particularly troublesome if the turbine has been used before the ultrasound is to be given.

Both mineral oil and glycerin have been tested as couplants for the immersion technique. The use of either can result in greater surface heating and an increase in couplant temperature, compared with a water medium.[112] When coupling is done with the immersion technique, the recommended medium for the bath is water.

When the immersion technique is employed, the transducer should be held 0.5 to 3.0 cm from the body surface area to be treated. Small air bubbles tend to accumulate on the face of the applicator and the skin surface when this method is used. However, the operator can wipe off the accumulated bubbles during exposure, as long as this is done quickly to prevent the therapist's being unduly exposed to the ultrasound energy.

Moving Versus Stationary Applicator

Two treatment methods have been used to deliver ultrasound energy to the tissue to be irradiated: (1) moving applicator and (2) stationary applicator.

Some clinicians have preferred to hold the transducer stationary over the area to be irradiated. This technique has usually been used when the treated area was very small or when the intensity delivered was very low (less than 0.5 W/cm^2). Because of the nonuniformity of the sound beam, the distribution of energy to the tissue is uneven; therefore, some areas within the beam may receive a large amount of energy and other areas effectively none. This situation predisposes the patient to "hot spots" and potential tissue damage. Various effects caused by a stationary sound beam have been noted in laboratory studies using animal models. In particular, stasis of blood flow,[30] venular endothelial damage, and platelet aggregation[31] have occurred at therapeutic intensities. This stationary technique should, therefore, be avoided.

With the moving technique, the transducer is slowly moved over the underlying tissue at approximately 4 cm/s.[21] (Many clinicians have a tendency to move the applicator too rapidly, and thus may decrease the amount of energy absorbed by the tissue.) The purpose of the motion is to distribute the energy as evenly as possible throughout the tissue. Longitudinal stroking or overlapping circular movements can be used. The total area covered is usually 2 to 3 times the size of the irradiating crystal for every 5 minutes of exposure.[113] If a larger area is covered, the effective dosage delivered to any one region is decreased and the tissue temperature rise will be less. With the moving technique, the energy delivered to the target tissue should be evenly distributed, causing no hot spots within the sound field. For this reason, the moving technique is preferred over the stationary technique.

Exposure Factors

Although the dosage delivered to the patient cannot be precisely controlled or calculated, an estimate can be made and duplicated for subsequent treatments if the exposure factors are recorded. These factors include the power output of the ultrasound beam, the effective radiating area (ERA) of the crystal, the ultrasound frequency, and the duration of exposure. The surface area of the body that is irradiated should also be reported.

As mentioned previously in this chapter, the intensity is recorded in watts per square centimeter (W/cm^2, or power per effective radiating area of the crystal). With the continuous-wave mode, the usual method of recording intensity is by the spatial average (the average power across the beam per ERA). With pulsed-wave ultrasound, the duty cycle should also be included.

The intensity selected for ultrasound therapy is based upon the objective of the treatment and the amount of soft tissue being treated. When vigorous heating is desired, Lehmann and de Lateur recommend increasing the ultrasound power until the patient reports a dull, deep ache (indicating elevation of tissue temperature at the periosteum) and then reducing the power by 10%.[114] A mild sensation of warmth may be felt by the patient during the treatment. As crystals with lower BNRs are provided, it may be less likely that a feeling of warmth will be experienced during treatment. This is because there is a more uniform distribution of energy.

When using the continuous-wave mode to elevate tissue temperature over an area such as the hip or low back (where there is a large quantity of soft tissue), intensities as high as 1.5 to 2.0 W/cm^2 are typically used. This intensity should be effective in increasing tissue temperature and should result in the desired physiologic response. However, if large areas are to be heated, the use of other thermal agents should be considered (see Chapter 8).

A lower intensity in the order of 0.5 to 1.0 W/cm^2 and a higher frequency is employed over areas where there is less soft tissue coverage and where bone is closer to the skin surface (for example, over the wrist). At tissue-bone interfaces, about 35 percent of the ultrasound beam is reflected, resulting in increased intensity in the soft tissue overlying the bone, specifically the periosteum.

The higher intensities are usually chosen when the purpose of treatment is to elevate tissue temperature of periarticular structures during or preceding a slow, sustained stretch with limited range of motion. Such raised temperatures should be maintained at least 5 minutes to allow for an increase in extensibility. Treatment, therefore, should last at least 5 minutes after the patient reports the sensation of heat.[115] Draper and coworkers[112] also found that deep tissues (3 cm) did not reach the 40°C therapeutic temperature until after approximately 8 minutes of treatment. When the desired temperature rise is not as high, a lower intensity can be employed for pain reduction and relief of muscle-guarding spasms. The best guideline, though, for determining a maximal, tolerated intensity that will not produce a burn or other tissue damage is patient tolerance, or the patient's report of a feeling of deep warmth underlying the transducer. For that reason, when ultrasound is used for heating, it is important that the patient's pain and temperature sensations are intact. Furthermore, patients should be instructed not to "rough it." Should the patient report deep aching (periosteal pain), either the power can be reduced or a larger area can be covered.

Occasionally, a patient will report an increase in temperature of the transducer, a feeling of surface heating. This sensation can be indicative of inadequate coupling or of loosening of the crystal in its mounting or of "hot spots" caused by a high BNR. If coupling appears to be adequate, then the transducer should be tested by a qualified service technician.

The aforementioned intensities are appropriate for typical-sized transducers and would need to be modified if transducers with smaller or larger effective radiating areas were used. For example, suppose we wish to heat a 10-cm^2 tissue area using a transducer with an effective radiating area of 10 cm^2, and emitting ultrasound at an intensity of 1 W/cm^2. If the transducer is held stationary, the 10-cm^2 area of skin immediately beneath the transducer crystal would receive a total exposure of 10 W (1 W/cm^2 × 10 cm^2). In contrast, a transducer with a smaller effective radiating area—say 5 cm^2—emitting the same ultrasonic intensity would have to be applied with a moving technique in order to cover the 10-cm^2 area of skin. In this latter case, the total exposure would be 5 W (1 W/cm^2 × 5 cm^2). Consequently, heating this area of skin would be reduced by a factor of 2. Thus, in order to produce the same therapeutic effect, the intensity of the smaller transducer would have to be raised to 2 W/cm^2, or exposure time doubled over the same area.

When pulsed-wave ultrasound is applied, the spatial average intensity read from the meter will appear to be the same as in the continuous-wave mode. But the time-averaged intensity will be less, because the energy is delivered in periodic bursts, with the power on for a fixed duration and then off for a fixed duration. The time the power is on is sometimes referred to as the "mark" and the time off as the "space." Thus a mark:space ratio can be reported. Both time on and time off are measured in milliseconds.

A more common way of providing the same information is by reporting the duty cycle. As defined previously, the duty cycle is the percentage of the time the power is on during one pulse period (time on + time off). Some generators are equipped with variable duty cycles. As the duty cycle increases (e.g., from 20% to 50%), the time-averaged intensity will increase. With a low duty cycle, there will be a minimal if any detectable rise in tissue temperature. As duty cycle increases, a rise in tissue temperature can be expected.

Total exposure to ultrasound seems to be an important factor in determining benefits to healing from the ultrasound (see "Wound Healing" section in this chapter). There are still no definitive guidelines available with respect to optimal treatment parameters, and the effects on soft tissue are not readily visible. It would be advised to use ultrasound cautiously during the acute stages of healing, limiting exposure to low intensities. On the other hand, for chronic conditions where thermal effects are being produced, use of ultrasound should be continued as long as the need is still present and benefits are being gained from its use. The thermal effects should be considered transient in nature with no danger of accumulating over time.

If the desired response from the treatment is nonthermal, then a small duty cycle should be chosen. There is increasing evidence that the nonthermal effects of ultrasound may be important in enhancing tissue repair (see under "Wound Healing") and pain relief (see under "Reduction of Pain and Muscle Spasm" section in this chapter). Although there are conflicting recommendations about treatment regimens for specific conditions, in general, one should be advised to use (1) an appropriate frequency for the depth of tissue to be treated, (2) a continuous-wave or pulsed-wave, according to the aims of treatment, and (3) the lowest intensity and duration that achieves the desired result in order to avoid the risk of tissue damage that may or may not be apparent to the treating therapist.

Technique of Phonophoresis

If performing phonophoresis, coupling can be direct or indirect using water. The medication is rubbed directly onto the surface of the skin. Coupling gel is then spread over the medication, and sonation is initiated. With the indirect technique, the ointment is spread over the area to be sonated, then the part is placed in a water bath.

When medication is prepared pharmaceutically, it may have air trapped in it; massaging the ointment into the skin may reduce air bubbles and improve transmissivity. Considering the more recent findings concerning the relative transmission rates of commonly used drugs (see "Phonophoresis" earlier in this chapter), the transmission rate of any agent used with ultrasound should be determined to be greater than 80 percent before it is used.

Patient Positioning and Field Selection

Because ultrasound energy can be well focused at a delineated target, careful patient positioning and determination of areas to be treated is often critically important to produce an effective treatment. The anatomic structures to be treated and the treatment goal should be well delineated by careful evaluation. The site of soft-tissue involvement, whether muscle, joint capsule, tendon, or bursa, should be determined. Depending on the particular pathology, the position of the patient can vary for each joint or body surface area affected.

As a representative example, dysfunction about the shoulder will be discussed. Three different examples of shoulder dysfunction include (1) capsular shortening or contracture, (2) supraspinatus tendinitis, and (3) muscle-guarding spasm and pain secondary to degenerative joint disease. In the first case, the area of the joint capsule around the glenohumeral joint that is likely to shorten or develop tightness is the anterior-inferior aspect. The resulting limitations in motion affect predominantly abduction and external rotation. To facilitate an increase in range of motion, while elevating joint capsular temperature with ultrasound, the therapist can externally rotate and abduct the patient's shoulder and simultaneously apply ultrasound over the anterior and inferior axillary areas (Fig. 7–11).

If the intention is to provide ultrasound at the site of the insertion of the supraspinatus, as in the second example, the position of choice for ultrasound application would be with the arm abducted and internally rotated. This position is chosen in order to expose the supraspinatus tendon from under the acromion process (Fig. 7–12).

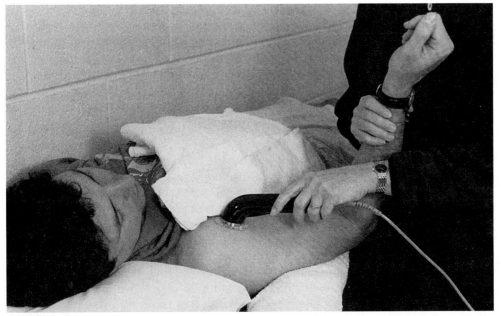

FIGURE 7–11. Ultrasound applied to the anterior aspect of the shoulder for treatment of adhesive capsulitis.

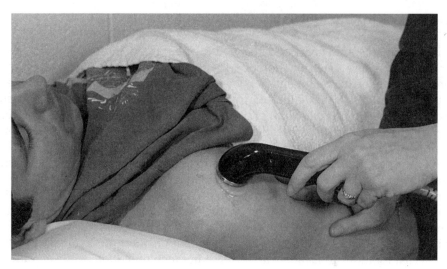

FIGURE 7–12. Ultrasound applied to the insertion of the supraspinatus tendon. Note the position of the arm in internal rotation.

In the third case, the patient with muscle spasm is in pain and is therefore guarding motion. The position of choice would be that in which the patient is comfortable and as relaxed as possible.

In all of these examples, the patients have shoulder dysfunction, but in each case a different anatomic site has been delineated as being problematic. Therefore, ultrasound can be well focused over an area to achieve a particular therapeutic goal if anatomic relationships are appreciated.

TREATMENT PRECAUTIONS

Therapeutic ultrasound should not be applied over the eye. The blood supply to the lens is poor, so that heat applied to that area is not dissipated adequately. Temperature elevations can result in cataract production.[116] Most of the ultrasound energy entering the eye will reach the retina, because the aqueous humor and the vitreous humor minimally attenuate the ultrasound energy. Local destruction of areas of the retina can result.

Irradiation over the heart should be avoided. In preliminary laboratory experimentation, one of this chapter's authors (MZ) found ECG changes (S-T segment elevation) in dogs following direct exposure at 2.5 W/cm^2 to the heart. Cardiac pacemakers should be protected from direct ultrasound exposure because of the possibility of the sound's interference with the electrical circuitry of the pacemaker.

One should not apply therapeutic ultrasound over the pregnant uterus. The fetus should not be exposed to the therapeutic ultrasound beam, because temperature elevation of the fetus has been shown to cause abnormalities such as low birth weight, brain size reduction, and various orthopedic deformities in experimental animals.[119] Unless reassured by the patient that she is not pregnant, it is probably prudent to avoid exposing a woman over the abdominal region or low back during the reproductive years except during the first 10 days following the onset of menses.[118]

Ultrasound should not be applied over the testes. Prolonged temperature elevation in this area can produce temporary sterility.

Except in the special case of treatment for cancer (hyperthermia), ultrasonic irradiation to malignant tissue should be avoided. Research done under in vitro conditions has suggested that this may increase cellular detachment and the possibility of metastasis.[119,120] Recent research in an in vivo model revealed increased tumor growth at therapeutic intensities.[121]

A major safeguard for patients undergoing therapeutic ultrasound at intensities sufficient to heat tissue is their ability to perceive accurately any changes in pain and temperature. For this reason, the therapist must be very cautious when applying ultrasound over areas of impaired pain and/or temperature sensation. This concern is particularly pertinent in areas where sensory nerves may have been severed immediately following surgery (e.g., the extremities or spine).

Caution should be used in applying ultrasound at intensities sufficient to heat tissue over areas with reduced circulation, because of possible excessive temperature elevation. Owing to the reduced circulation, the heat generated cannot be adequately dissipated. Ultrasound should not be administered over areas of thrombophlebitis, because the possibility of clotting or of dislodging a thrombus could be increased.

Epiphyseal areas (growth areas of bone) in children should be exposed to ultrasound only minimally. Literature in the field suggests that intensities used therapeutically would be safe.[114,122] But at intensities above 3.0 W/cm^2 there is some evidence of demineralization of bone, damage to epiphyseal plates, and retardation of bone growth when using a stationary transducer for periods of 3 minutes or greater.[123-125]

There are no reasons to avoid ultrasound application over fracture sites, unless sensation to the area is impaired. In fact, animal studies by Dyson and Brookes[126] have demonstrated that pulsed ultrasound may accelerate fracture healing. Certainly, this subject warrants further investigation.

CLINICAL DECISION MAKING

Ultrasound has become one of the most prevalent treatments in physical therapy clinics. Considering the foregoing material, it should be clear to clinicians that its effects are complex and generally not immediately apparent to the practicing clinician. In order to use this modality efficiently, and to avoid any possibility of increasing tissue damage, one must consider the aims of treatment and then choose the treatment parameters that would be most likely to achieve those aims. The choice of ultrasound as the preferred treatment should also be made with consideration of any other modalities available.

After treatment goals and plans have been established, if a heating agent is desired, the choice of which one to use can depend on a number of factors. These factors include (1) stage of inflammation and repair; (2) site of pathology, including depth and anatomic location; (3) total amount of tissue to be heated; and (4) presence or absence of orthopedic metal implants.

During the subacute stages of healing, a mild heat would be the logical choice. Surface heating agents, such as hot packs, may provide the desired response. If the site of pathology is in deep-seated structures, such as the hip joint, then low-intensity ultrasound at less than 1.0 W/cm^2 may be best. With a chronic condition in which pain and limited range of motion are the key problems, a deep heat, such as that provided by ultrasound at a higher intensity, may be used.

Site of Injury

The site of pathology is also important. If the goal of application is to deliver a deep heat to a well defined area, then ultrasound should be the therapeutic agent of choice. For example, a knee flexion contracture secondary to capsular tightness may respond best to ultrasound followed by a slow, gentle stretch. If a larger area with a large muscle mass is to be heated, then the agent chosen should be continuous short-wave diathermy. For example, limited motion and pain secondary to chronic ham-string strain may be best heat-treated by an agent that can apply heat to the entire muscle belly in the most efficient manner. Of course, ultrasound is capable of elevating hamstring temperature, but only a small area at a time can be heated using ultrasound and therefore would not be effective in heading such a large area (Table 7–3).

Metal Implants

Many patients seen for rehabilitation have surgical metal implants, either for stabilization of fractures or for replacement of damaged joint surfaces. In these cases, ultrasound can be safely employed over the area of the metal implant using the moving technique.[128,129] Shortwave diathermy, however, may not be given over areas of metal implants. Many of the implants used for prosthetic joint replacements have high-density polyethylene components and are fixed in place by methyl-methacrolate cement. If the moving technique is employed, ultrasound can be applied over these joints.[130]

TABLE 7–3 Clinical Decision Making: Ultrasound vs. Diathermy for Deep Heating

Case Problem	Decision	Rationale
70-yr-old women, 2 mo post open reduction and internal fixation of intertrochanteric hip fracture with a nail and plate; now has pain on hip flexion and abduction; muscle-guarding spasms contribute to decreased ROM	Continuous ultrasound	Pain reduction; able to increase temperature of joint structures and overlying muscle; can focus energy to target areas; can apply over metal implant
45-yr-old bricklayer 1 mo postlumbar injury; L–5 to S–1 herniated intervertebral disk with paravertebral muscle-guarding spasms	Shortwave diathermy with induction drum	Capable of increasing temperature of paravertebral musculature; can cover a relatively large area

Note: Case examples are provided with supporting rationale for treatment with the chosen deep heat agent. (Readers should cover the authors' decision and rationale while formulating their own, then uncover and compare with their own decision.)

Ultrasound with Other Agents

Often ultrasound is used in conjunction with other physical agents, such as hot packs, cold packs, and electrical stimulation. Hot packs may provide additional pain relief and encourage relaxation of the patient. Cold packs should not be given prior to ultrasound, because cold alters the patient's perception of pain and temperature, which thereby limits their ability to tell the therapist if the ultrasound intensity is too high.

How Many Treatments with Ultrasound

The authors are not aware of any detrimental, cumulative effects of ultrasound used within therapeutic ranges. The best guideline for continuing treatments with ultrasound comes from assessment of the condition being treated. If improvement in patient status, for example, closure of a wound or reduction in pain, can be attributed in part to ultrasound, then further treatments are warranted. As with many of our techniques, if no positive change occurs, then treatment must be modified or discontinued.

We are not aware of any controlled clinical studies that have shown that multiple treatments with ultrasound are damaging. The adage that only "9 to 12" ultrasound treatments should be given, then discontinued for 2 weeks, to our knowledge, is anecdotal at best. Many times, though, treatment goals may be accomplished before that timeframe of 9 to 12 treatments.

Further Study

It is also clear that ultrasound is likely to have a beneficial effect on the healing of soft tissue. However, as apparent from the literature reviewed, the effects of ultrasound at different stages of healing and with different treatment parameters are not well understood. Therefore, although the use of ultrasound to enhance soft tissue repair generally appears to be recommended, the clinician should be alert for any negative effects and should use the minimum dosage necessary to produce a beneficial effect.

There is also evidence that ultrasound is effective as a pain-relieving modality because of other than its thermal effects.[47,55,56,80,103] As early as 1953, Kuitert[46] suggested that mechanical stimulation of the neural pathways may be the reason for the relief of radicular pain. Investigation of the mechanical effects of ultrasound (i.e., cavitation, microstreaming) on the "pain gate" might yield information that would alter our explanation of its analgesic benefits.

In conclusion, although the effects and mechanics of ultrasound are still not freely understood, its use in physical therapy practice is well established. Therapeutic ultrasound should be used for a specific physiologic effect on a specific part of the body, only for as long as there is evidence of benefit from its application.

Clinical decision-making examples are provided in Table 7–3.

SUMMARY

Ultrasound high-frequency acoustic energy can be employed in a physical rehabilitation program to increase tissue temperature to depths of up to 5 cm. The physiologic effects of ultrasound, including increasing collagen tissue extensibility, decreasing pain and muscle spasm, and facilitating tissue healing, serve as the rationale for its use as a therapeutic agent. In order to maximize effectiveness and appropriateness of treatment with ultrasound, the therapist should be knowledgeable about the physics, biophysical effects, and possibly adverse consequences of ultrasonic energy at therapeutic intensities.

Study Objectives

Having completed this chapter, the reader should now be able to:

1. Explain the physical principles of ultrasound with respect to frequency and intensity as it relates to clinical application.
2. Explain the generation of ultrasound energy from electrical energy, that is, reverse piezoelectrical effect.
3. Explain the thermal effects of ultrasound on human tissue.
4. Describe the nonthermal effects of ultrasound on human tissue.
5. Explain how the nonthermal effects of ultrasound affect physiologic changes in human tissue.
6. Describe the major areas of clinical application where ultrasound has been found to be of benefit.
7. Explain how and why therapeutic ultrasound machines should be maintained in a clinical department.
8. Describe the importance of an effective coupling agent during ultrasound application, including agents used in phonophoresis.
9. List the treatment precautions and contraindications with therapeutic ultrasound.
10. Describe clinical situations where ultrasound would be the treatment of choice in the treatment of soft-tissue injuries.

REFERENCES

1. Wood, RW and Loomis, AL: The physical and biological effects of high frequency waves of great intensity. Philosoph Mag 4:417, 1927.
2. Buchtala, V: The present state of ultrasonic therapy. Br J Phys Med 15:3, 1952.
3. Kuitert, JH and Harr, ET: Introduction to clinical application of ultrasound. Phys Ther Rev 35:19, 1955.
4. Wells, PNT: Biomedical Ultrasonics. Academic Press, London, 1977.
5. Hill, CR and ter Haar, G: Ultrasound and non-ionising radiation protection. In Suess, MJ (ed): WHO Regional Publication, European Series No. 10, World Health Organization, Copenhagen, 1981.
6. Hekkenberg, RT, Oosterbaan, WA, and van Beekum, WT: Evaluation of ultrasound therapy devices. Physiotherapy 72:390, 1986.
7. Lehmann, JF, et al: Heating of joint structures by ultrasound. Arch Phys Med Rehabil 49:28, 1968.
8. Lehmann, JF, et al: Heating produced by ultrasound in bone and soft tissue. Arch Phys Med Rehabil 48:397, 1967.
9. Lehmann, JF, et al: Therapeutic temperature distribution produced by ultrasound as modified by dosage and volume of tissue exposed. Arch Phys Med Rehabil 48:662, 1967.
10. Gersten, JW: Effect of ultrasound on tendon extensibility. Am J Phys Med 34:662, 1955.
11. Lehmann, JF, et al: Effect of therapeutic temperatures on tendon extensibility. Arch Phys Med Rehabil 51:481, 1970.
12. Warren, CG, Lehmann, JF, and Koblanski, JN: Heat and stretch procedures: An evaluation using rat tail tendon. Arch Phys Med Rehabil 57:122, 1976.
13. Paul, ED and Imig, CJ: Temperature and blood flow studies after ultrasonic irradiation. Am J Phys Med 34:370, 1955.

14. Abramson, DI, et al: Changes in blood flow, oxygen uptake and tissue temperatures produced by therapeutic physical agents. I. Effect of ultrasound. Am J Phys Med 39:51, 1960.
15. Bickford, RH and Duff, RS: Influence of ultrasonic irradiation on temperature and blood flow in human skeletal muscle. Circ Res 1:534, 1953.
16. Wyper, DJ, McNiven, DR, and Donnelly, TJ: Therapeutic ultrasound and muscle blood flow. Physiotherapy 64:321, 1978.
17. Paaske, WP, Hovind, H, and Seyerson, P: Influence of therapeutic ultrasonic irradiation on blood flow in human cutaneous, subcutaneous and muscular tissues. Scand J Clin Lab Invest 31:389, 1973.
18. Currier, DP, Greathouse, D, and Swift, T: Sensory nerve conduction: Effect of ultrasound. Arch Phys Med Rehabil 59:181, 1978.
19. Currier, DP and Kramer, JF: Sensory nerve conduction: Heating effects of ultrasound and infrared. Physiother Can 34:241, 1982.
20. Halle, JS, Scoville, CR, and Greathouse, DG: Ultrasound's effect on the conduction latency of superficial radial nerve in man. Phys Ther 61:345, 1981.
21. Kramer, JF: Ultrasound: Evaluation of its mechanical and thermal effects. Arch Phys Med Rehabil 65:223, 1984.
22. Lehmann, JF, Bruner, GD, and Stow, RW: Pain threshold measurements after therapeutic application of ultrasound, microwaves and infrared. Arch Phys Med Rehabil 39:560, 1958.
23. Lehmann, JF and Guy, AW: Ultrasound therapy. In Reid, J and Sikov, MR (eds): Interaction of Ultrasound and Biological Tissues. DHEW Pub (FDA) 73-8008, Session 3:8, 141–152, 1971.
24. Lehmann, JR and Herrick, JF: Biologic reactions to cavitation, a consideration for ultrasonic therapy. Arch Phys Med Rehabil 34:86, 1953.
25. Lota, MJ and Darling, RC: Change in permeability of the red blood cell membrane in a homogeneous ultrasonic field. Arch Phys Med Rehabil 36:282, 1955.
26. Harvey, W, et al: The simulation of protein synthesis in human fibroblasts by therapeutic ultrasound. Rheumatol Rehabil 14:237, 1975.
27. Dyson, M and ter Haar, GR: The response of smooth muscle to ultrasound (abstr). In Proceedings from an International Symposium on Therapeutic Ultrasound, Winnipeg, Manitoba (Canada), September 10–12, 1981.
28. Lehmann, JF and Biegler, R: Changes of potentials and temperature gradients in membranes caused by ultrasound. Arch Phys Med Rehabil 35:287, 1954.
29. Michlovitz, SL, Lynch, PR, and Tuma, RF: Therapeutic ultrasound: Its effects on vascular permeability (abstr). Fed Proc 41:1761, 1982.
30. Dyson, M, et al: The production of blood cell stasis and endothelial damage in the blood vessels of chick embryos treated with ultrasound in a stationary wave field. Ultrasound Med Biol 11:133, 1974.
31. Zarod, AP and Williams, AR: Platelet aggregation in vivo by therapeutic ultrasound. Lancet 1:1266, 1977.
32. Hogan, RD, Burke, KM, and Franklin, TD: The effect of ultrasound on microvascular hemodynamics in skeletal muscle: Effects during ischemic. Microvasc Res 23:370, 1982.
33. Hogan, RD, et al: The effect of ultrasound on microvascular hemodynamics in skeletal muscle: Effect on arterioles. Ultrasound Med Biol 8:45, 1982.
34. Kitchen, SS and Partridge, CJ: A review of therapeutic ultrasound. Physiotherapy 76: 593–600, 1990.
35. McDiarmid, T and Burns, PN: Clinical applications of therapeutic ultrasound. Physiotherapy 73:155, 1987.
36. LaBan, MM: Collagen tissue: Implications of its response to stress in vitro. Arch Phys Med Rehabil 43:461, 1962.
37. Lehmann, JF, et al: Comparative study of the efficiency of shortwave, microwave and ultrasonic diathermy in heating the hip joint. Arch Phys Med Rehabil 40:510, 1959.
38. Lehmann, JF, et al: Clinical evaluation of a new approach in the treatment of contracture associated with hip fracture after internal fixation. Arch Phys Med Rehabil 42:95, 1961.
39. Hamer, J and Kirk, JA: Physiotherapy and the frozen shoulder: A comparative trial of ice and ultrasonic therapy. NZ Med J 83:191, 1972.
40. Williams, AR, et al: Effects of MHz ultrasound on electrical pain threshold perception in humans. Ultrasound Med Biol 13:249, 1987.
41. Munting, E: Ultrasonic therapy for painful shoulders. Physiotherapy 64:180, 1978.
42. Middlemast, S and Chatterjee, DS: Comparison of ultrasound and thermotherapy for soft tissue injuries. Physiotherapy 64:331, 1978.
43. Herrera-Lasso, I, et al: Comparative effectiveness of packages of treatment including ultrasound or transcutaneous electrical nerve stimulation in painful shoulder syndrome. Physiotherapy, 19:251–253, 1993.
44. Inaba, MK and Piorkowski, M: Ultrasound in treatment of painful shoulders in patients with hemiplegia. Phys Ther 52:737, 1972.
45. Soren, A: Nature and biophysical effects of ultrasound. J Occup Med 7:375, 1965.
46. Kuitert, JH: Ultrasonic energy as an adjunct in the management of radiculitis and similar referred pain. Am J Phys Med 33:61, 1954.

47. Aldes, JH and Grabin, S: Ultrasound in the treatment of intervertebral disc syndrome. Am J Phys Med 37:199, 1958.
48. Nwuga, VCB: Ultrasound in treatment of back pain resulting from prolapsed intervertebral disc. Arch Phys Med Rehabil 64:88, 1983.
49. Quirion-de Girardi, C, et al: The analgesic effect of high voltage galvanic stimulation combined with ultrasound in the treatment of low back pain: A one-group pretest/post-test study. Physiother Can 36:327, 1984.
50. Fountain, FP, Gersten, JW, and Sengu, O: Decrease in muscle spasm produced by ultrasound, hot packs and IR. Arch Phys Med Rehabil 41:293, 1960.
51. Talaat, AM, El-Dibany, MM, and El-Garf, A: Physical therapy in the management of myofacial pain dysfunction syndrome. Am Otol Rhinol Laryngol 95:225, 1986.
52. Grieder, A, et al: An evaluation of ultrasonic therapy for temporomandibular joint dysfunction. Oral Surg 31:25, 1971.
53. Payne C: Ultrasound for post-herpetic neuralgia. Physiotherapy 70:96, 1984.
54. Garrett, AS and Garrett, M: Letters: Ultrasound for herpes zoster pain. J Roy Coll Gen Pract, Nov:709, 1982.
55. Jones, RJ: Treatment of acute herpes zoster using ultrasonic therapy. Physiotherapy 70:94, 1984.
56. Portwood, MM, Lieberman, SS, and Taylor, RG: Ultrasound treatment of reflex sympathetic dystrophy. Arch Phys Med Rehabil 68:116, 1987.
57. Binder, A, et al: Is therapeutic ultrasound effective in treating soft tissue lesions? Br Med J 290:512, 1985.
58. Lundeberg T, Abrahamsson, P, and Haker, E: A comparative study of continuous ultrasound, placebo ultrasound and rest in epicondylalgia. Scand J Rehab Med 20:99, 1988.
59. Bearzy, HJ: Clinical applications of ultrasonic energy in the treatment of acute and chronic subacromial bursitis. Arch Phys Med Rehabil 34:228, 1953.
60. Bundt, FB: Ultrasound therapy in supraspinatus bursitis. Phys Ther Rev 38:826, 1958.
61. Echternach, JL: Ultrasound: An adjunct treatment for shoulder disability. Phys Ther 45:865, 1965.
62. Downing, D and Weinstein, A: Ultrasound therapy of subacromial bursitis (abstr). Arthritis Rheum 26 (Suppl):587, 1983.
63. Falconer, J, Hayes, KW, and Chang, RW: Therapeutic ultrasound in the treatment of musculoskeletal conditions. Arthritis Care Res 3(2):85, 1990.
64. Smith, W, Winn, F, and Parette, R: Comparative study using four modalities in shinsplint treatments. J Orthop Sports Phys Ther 8:77, 1986.
65. Halle, JS, Franklin, RJ, and Karalfa, BL: Comparison of four treatment approaches for lateral epicondylitis of the elbow. J Orthop Sports Phys Ther 8:62, 1986.
66. Antich, TJ, et al: Physical therapy treatment of knee extensor mechanism disorders: Comparison of four treatment modalities. J Orthop Sports Phys Ther 8:255, 1986.
67. Cline, PD: Radiographic follow-up of ultrasound therapy in calcific bursitis. Phys Ther 43:16, 1963.
68. Gorkiewicz, R: Ultrasound for subacromial bursitis. Phys Ther 64:46, 1984.
69. Griffin, JE, Touchstone, JC, and Liu, A: Ultrasonic movement of cortisol into pig tissues. II. Peripheral nerve. Am J Phys Med 44:20, 1965.
70. Novak, EJ: Experimental transmission of lidocaine through intact skin by ultrasound. Arch Phys Med Rehabil 45:231, 1964.
71. Griffin, JE, et al: Patients treated with ultrasonic driven cortisone and with ultrasound alone. Phys Ther 47:594, 1967.
72. Cameron, MH and Monroe, LG: Relative transmission of ultrasound by media customarily used by phonophoresis. Phys Ther 72:142, 1992.
73. Ciccone, CD, Leggin, BG, and Callamaro, JJ: The effects of ultrasound on trolamine salicylate phonophoresis on delayed onset muscle soreness. Phys Ther 71:666, 1991.
74. Stratford, PW, et al: The evaluation of phonophoresis and friction massage as treatments for extensor carpi radialis tendinitis: A randomized controlled trial. Physiother Can 41:93, 1989.
75. Moll, MJ: A new approach to pain: Lidocaine and decadron with ultrasound. USAF Med Serv Digest May–June:8, 1977.
76. Byl, NN: The use of ultrasound as an enhancer for transcutaneous drug delivery: Phonophoresis. Phys Ther, 75:539–553, 1995.
77. Bensen, HA and McElnay, JC: Topical non-steroidal anti-inflammatory products as ultrasound couplants: Their potential in phonophoresis. Physiotherapy 80:74, 1994.
78. Byl, NN, et al: The effects of phonophoresis with corticosteroids: A control pilot study. J Orthop Sports Phys Ther 18:590, 1993.
79. El Hag, M, et al: The anti-inflammatory effects of dexamethasone and therapeutic ultrasound in oral surgery. Br J Oral Maxillofac Surg 23:17, 1985.
80. Hashish, I, Harvey, W, and Harris, M: Anti-inflammatory effects of ultrasound therapy: Evidence for a major placebo effect. Br J Rheumatol 25:77, 1986.
81. Snow, CJ and Johnson, KA: Effect of therapeutic ultrasound on acute inflammation. Physiother Can 40:162, 1988.
82. Fyfe, MC and Chahl, LA: The effect of ultrasound on experimental oedema in rats. Ultrasound Med Biol 6:107, 1980.

83. Fyfe, MC and Chahl, LA: The effect of single or repeated applications of "therapeutic" ultrasound on plasma extravasation during silver nitrate induced inflammation of the rat hindpaw ankle joint 'in vivo'. Ultrasound Med Biol 11:273, 1985.

84. Dyson, M and Luke, DA: Induction of mast cell degranulation in skin by ultrasound. IEEE Transactions and Ultrasonics, Ferroelectrics, and Frequency Control UFFC-33:194, 1986.

85. Dyson, M, et al: The stimulation of tissue regeneration by means of ultrasound. Clin Sci 35:273, 1968.

86. Roberts, M, Rutherford, JH, and Harris, D: The effect of ultrasound on flexor tendon repairs in the rabbit. Hand 14:17, 1982.

87. Lundborg, G and Rank, F: Experimental intrinsic healing of flexor tendons based upon synovial fluid nutrition. J Hand Surg 3:21, 1978.

88. Friedar, S, et al: A pilot study: The therapeutic effect of ultrasound following partial rupture of Achilles tendons in male rats. J Orthop Sports Phys Ther 10:39, 1988.

89. Stevenson, JH, et al: Functional, mechanical, and biochemical assessment of ultrasound therapy on tendon healing in the chicken toe. Plastic Reconstruct Surg 77:965, 1986.

90. Stratton, SA, Heckmann, R, and Francis, RS: Therapeutic ultrasound: Its effect on the integrity of a nonpenetrating wound. J Orthop Sports Phys Ther 5:278, 1984.

91. Enwemeka, CS: The effects of therapeutic ultrasound on tendon healing: A biomechanical study. Am J Phys Med Rehabil 68:283–287, 1989.

92. Byl, NN, et al: Low dose ultrasound effects on wound healing: A control study with Yucatan pigs. Arch Phys Med Rehabil 73:656, 1992.

93. Byl, NN, et al: Incisional wound healing: A control study of low and high dose ultrasound. J Orthop Sports Phys Ther 18:619, 1993.

94. Paul, BJ, et al: Use of ultrasound in the treatment of pressure sores in patients with spinal cord injury. Arch Phys Med Rehabil 41:438, 1960.

95. McDiarmid, T, et al: Ultrasound and the treatment of pressure sores. Physiotherapy 71:66, 1985.

96. Dyson, M: Therapeutic applications of ultrasound. In Nyborg, WL and Ziskin, MC (eds): Biological Effects of Ultrasound. Churchill Livingstone, Edinburgh, p. 121, 1985.

97. Dyson, M and Suckling, J: Stimulation of tissue repair by ultrasound: A survey of mechanisms involved. Physiotherapy 64:105, 1978.

98. Callam, MJ, et al: A controlled trial of weekly ultrasound therapy in chronic leg ulceration. Lancet 2(8552):204, 1987.

99. Lundeberg, T, et al: Pulsed ultrasound does not improve healing of venous ulcers. Scand J Rehabil Med 22:195, 1990.

100. Eriksson, SV, Lundeberg, T and Malm, M: A placebo controlled trial of ultrasound in chronic leg ulceration. Scand J Rehabil Med 3:211, 1991.

101. Brueton, RN and Campbell, B: The use of Geliperm as a sterile coupling agent for therapeutic ultrasound. Physiotherapy 73:653, 1987.

102. McLaren, J: Randomised controlled trial of ultrasound therapy for the damaged perineum. Clin Phys Physiol Meas 5:40 (abstr), 1984.

103. Creates, V: A study of ultrasound treatment to the painful perineum after childbirth. Physiotherapy 73:162, 1987.

104. Ferguson, HN: Ultrasound in the treatment of surgical wounds. Physiotherapy 67:12, 1981.

105. Fieldhouse, C: Ultrasound for relief of painful episiotomy scars. Physiotherapy 65:217, 1979.

106. Burns, PN and Pitcher, EM: Calibration of physiotherapy ultrasound generators. Clin Phys Physiol Meas 5:37 (abstr), 1984.

107. Docker, MF: A review of instrumentation available for therapeutic ultrasound. Physiotherapy 73:154, 1987.

108. ter Haar, G, Dyson, M, and Oakley, EM: The use of ultrasound by physiotherapists in Britain, 1985. Ultrasound Med Biol 13:659, 1987.

109. Balmaseda, MT, et al: Ultrasound therapy: A comparative study of different coupling medium. Arch Phys Med Rehabil 67:147, 1986.

110. Lehmann, JF, de Lateur, BJ, and Silverman, DR: Selective heating effects of ultrasound in human beings. Arch Phys Med Rehabil 46:331, 1966.

111. Forrest, G and Rosen, K: Ultrasound: Effectiveness of treatments given under water. Arch Phys Med Rehabil 70:28, 1989.

112. Draper, DO, et al: A comparison of temperature rise in human calf muscles following application of underwater and topical gel ultrasound. J Orthop Phys Ther 17:247, 1993.

113. Reid, DC and Cummings, GE: Factors in selecting the dosage of ultrasound with particular reference to the use of various coupling agents. Physiother Can 63:255, 1973.

114. Lehmann, JF and de Lateur, BJ: Therapeutic heat. In Lehmann, JF (ed): Therapeutic Heat and Cold, ed 4. Williams & Wilkins, Baltimore, 1990.

115. Nussbaum, E: Personal communication, 1994.

116. Sokoliu, A: Destructive effect of ultrasound on ocular tissues. In Reid, JM and Sikov, MR: Interaction of Ultrasound and Biological Tissues. DHEW Pub (FDA) 73-8008, 1972.

117. Edwards, MJ: Congenital defects in guinea pigs: Prenatal retardation of brain growth of guinea pigs following hyperthermia during gestation. Teratology 2:329, 1969.

118. NCRP Report No. 74: Effects of Ultrasound: Mechanisms and Clinical Implications. National Council on Radiation Protection and Measurements, Bethesda, MD, 1983, p 197.
119. Conger, AD, Ziskin, MC, and Wittels, H: Ultrasonic effects on mammalian multicellular tumor spheroids. J Clin Ultrasound 9:167, 1981.
120. Siegel, E, et al: Cellular attachment as a sensitive indicator of the effects of diagnostic ultrasound exposure on cultured human cells. Radiology 133:175, 1979.
121. Sicard-Rosenbaum, L, et al: Effects of continuous therapeutic ultrasound on growth and metastasis of subcutaneous marine tumors. Phys Ther 75:3, 1995.
122. Vaughen, JL and Bender, LF: Effects of ultrasound on growing bone. Arch Phys Med Rehabil 40:158, 1959.
123. Bender, LF, Janes, JM, and Herrick, JR: Histologic studies following exposure of bone to ultrasound. Arch Phys Med Rehabil 35:555, 1954.
124. Cerino, LE, Ackerman, E, and Janes, JM: Effects of ultrasound on experimental bone tumor. Surg Forum 16:466, 1965.
125. DeForest, RE, Herrick, JF, and Janes, JM: Effects of ultrasound on growing bone: An experimental study. Arch Phys Med Rehabil 34:21, 1953.
126. Dyson, M and Brookes, M: Stimulation of bone repair by ultrasound (abstr). Ultrasound Med Biol 8(suppl 50):50, 1982.
127. Gersten, JW: Effect of metallic objects on temperature rises produced in tissues by ultrasound. Am J Phys Med 37:75, 1958.
128. Lehmann, JF, et al: Ultrasound effects as demonstrated in live pigs with surgical metallic implants. Arch Phys Med Rehabil 40:483, 1959.
129. Skoubo-Kristensen, E and Somer, J: Ultrasound influence on internal fixation with a rigid plate in dogs. Arch Phys Med Rehabil 63:371, 1982.
130. Lehmann, JF, et al: Ultrasound: Considerations for use in the presence of prosthetic joints. Arch Phys Med Rehabil 61:502, 1980.

CHAPTER 8

Diathermy and Pulsed Radio Frequency Radiation

Luther C. Kloth, MS, PT
Marvin C. Ziskin, MD, MS, BmE

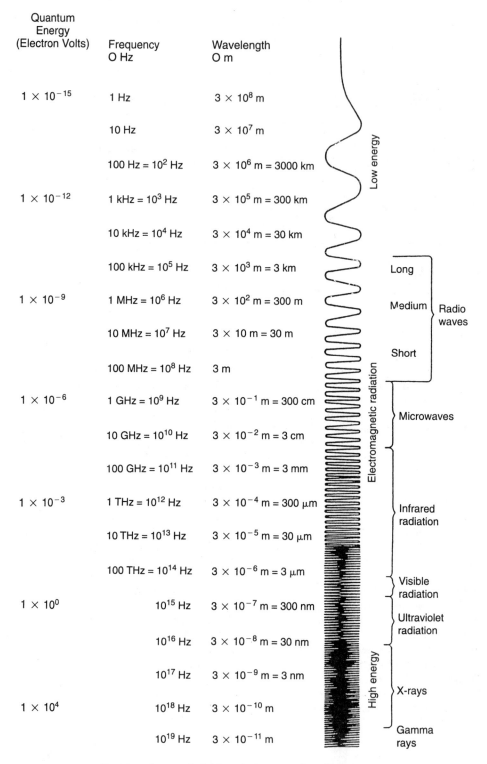

Electric and magnetic fields—electromagnetic radiations

FIGURE 8–1. Electromagnetic radiations—electric and magnetic fields. (Adapted from Low and Reed.)[10]

The application of electromagnetic energy (EM) to the body from the radio frequency (RF) part of the spectrum involves transmission and absorption of nonionizing radiation by the body. RF radiation is the term generally applied to propagating EM waves between 10 kilohertz (kHz) and 300 gigahertz (GHz) (1 kHz is 1×10^3 cycles per second; 1 GHz is 1×10^9 cycles per second [Fig. 8–1]). Therapeutic ultrasound is also nonionizing, but it introduces acoustic, not electromagnetic, energy into the tissue. In the case of continuous shortwave diathermy (CSWD) waves of RF radiation are absorbed by the body and are converted into heat by the resisting tissues.[1,2] When these waves are periodically interrupted at regular intervals, pulses or bursts of RF energy are delivered to the tissues. These pulses of EM energy are referred to as pulsed radio frequency radiation (PRFR). Depending on the average power delivered by these pulses of RF energy, tissue temperature may or may not increase. Thus, PRFR may have either a thermal or nonthermal effect on the tissues. PRFR having low average power produces nonthermal effects (PRFE) on absorbing tissues, whereas PRFR with high average power produces pulsed SWD (PSWD), which has thermal effects.

Therapeutic devices that deliver CSWD and those that deliver PRFR use high-frequency alternating currents that oscillate at specified radio frequencies between 10 and 50 MHz. CSWD and PRFR are most commonly used for physical therapy applications at an RF of 27.12 MHz. MWD, another form of EM radiation, has qualities that allow it to be beamed or directed toward the body and reflected from the skin, owing to its ultra-high frequency (UHF). The frequency most commonly used with therapeutic microwave is 2450 MHz. Clinically MWD is used much less today than either CSWD or PSWD (Table 8–1).

Clinical application of CSWD for its thermal effects was introduced in Germany in the late 1920s. Therapeutic applications of microwave heating began in the United States in the late 1940s. The clinical use of the thermal effects of diathermy and thermal/nonthermal effects of PRFR in the health professions may be divided into three categories: (1) functional restoration and analgesia; (2) facilitation of healing of acutely injured soft tissue and chronic dermal ulcerations; and (3) hyperthermia for tumor eradication. Clinical use of PRFR is less well defined but in general is dependent on the intensity and duration of exposure and the production of thermal or nonthermal physiologic effects in the target tissue.

The objectives of this chapter are to: (1) provide a basic understanding of the physical principles and effects of CSWD and PRFR; (2) discuss the clinical methods for applying CSWD and PRFR; (3) discuss the clinical conditions for which CSWD and PRFR are suggested to be effective; and (4) discuss potential hazards related to the use of these forms of EM energy.

PHYSICAL PRINCIPLES OF ELECTROMAGNETIC RADIATION

The term *diathermy* literally means to heat through. Diathermy is applied to a patient using continuous or pulsed EM waves that produce heat, but are nonionizing. EM waves cover a tremendously wide range of frequencies and corresponding wavelengths (see Figs. 8–1 and 3–1). EM wavelengths range from one billionth of a meter up to miles. All of these wavelengths do not pass through the body with equal ease; in fact, there is no simple relationship between wavelength and the ability of these EM waves to travel through the body almost unimpeded. This explains why you can listen

TABLE 8–1 Radio Frequencies Approved
by the FCC for SWD/MWD and PRFR

Frequency (MHz)	Wavelength	Type of EM Radiation
13.56	22 m	SWD/PRFR
27.12*	11 m	SWD/PRFR
40.68	7.5 m	SWD/PRFR
915.00	33 m	MWD
2450.00	12 cm	MWD

*Most widely used frequency for SWD and PRFR.

to a radio when a person is standing between you and a broadcasting radio. It is this type of EM energy that is used in physical therapy applications of CSWD and PRFR. Wavelengths within the visible light part of the spectrum cannot penetrate more than a few fractions of a millimeter into the skin.

Because of the great demands for the use of various frequencies for communication, the Federal Communications Commission (FCC) has very carefully regulated what frequencies can be used in television and radio transmission, radar, and medical applications. Consequently, all of the medical applications of SWD and PRFR are limited to those frequencies listed in Table 8–1.

Regardless of wavelength, EM waves possess certain properties. First, they transport electrical and magnetic energy through space (hence, they are called electromagnetic waves). Unlike sound waves, they do not require a medium through which to travel. They can travel through a vacuum unimpeded. They do not have mass, and they are composed of pure energy. Although the electromagnetic waves themselves do not contain matter, they do have an effect on the matter through which they travel. This occurs because matter contains electric charges, which are interacted with, and influenced by, EM waves.

Regardless of the type of wave propagation, there is a fundamental relationship between frequency and wavelength, which is given by the equation:

$$\text{Velocity of light} = \text{frequency} \times \text{wavelength}$$

The velocity of light is a constant and equal to 300,000 million meters per second (3×10^8 m/s). If either the wavelength or the frequency is known, the other can be calculated. Because the product of the wavelength and the frequency is constant, a higher frequency will automatically shorten the wavelength, as seen in Table 8–1.

Whenever a therapist applies any form of energy to the body, safety is a concern. (See Chapter 3 for more details pertaining to the biological effects of electrical current flowing through the body.) With one exception, SWD and PRFR are not a source of electrical shock. The one exception is when a patient has direct contact with a metallic portion of the SWD or PRFR device when it is in operation and there happens to be an excess of what is referred to as "leak current" (see Chapter 3) that enters the ungrounded patient's body.

The harmful effect of current depends on the magnitude of the current and the

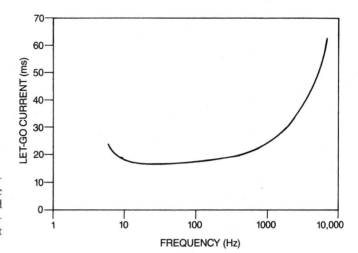

FIGURE 8–2. When electrical currents pass through the body at certain frequencies and amplitudes, muscular contraction is so strong that one is not able to let go.

frequency of the energy. Figure 8–2 illustrates a curve of the amount of current required to produce a "can't let go" effect, as a function of frequency. If current exceeds a certain threshold, muscular contraction is so severe and so persistent that a person is not able to release his or her grip from the source of a dangerous electrical shock. This is most dangerous in the range of approximately 40 to 100 Hz, which is the frequency range in which ordinary household electrical supply lies. In this frequency range, the "can't let go" current is 10.5 mA or more for women and 16.0 mA or more for men. The threshold increases significantly, however, with increases in frequency. Consequently, at sufficiently high frequencies, we do not have to worry about currents causing a persistent muscular contraction.

The RF frequency used for CSWD and PRFR applications (27.120 MHz) is not capable of depolarizing motor nerves or eliciting a contractile response from innervated or denervated skeletal muscle. To excite nerve or muscle tissue currents with minimal amplitude require pulses of about 0.1-ms duration or longer. At 27.12 MHz the pulse duration would only be 36 nanoseconds (36×10^{-9} s); therefore, excitation of these tissues, resulting in depolarization, does not occur because the wavelength (duration) of each cycle of the high-frequency alternating current does not last sufficiently long to cause migration of ions through cellular membranes of nerve or muscle. This is an important reason why such a high frequency is used in CSWD and PRFR applications. Another important reason for using EM radiation in the RF range is that it is nonionizing radiation, which means that there is insufficient energy concentration to dislodge orbiting electrons from atoms. EM energy from the RF part of the spectrum provides energy that may or may not be cutaneously perceived by the human body. Regardless of whether it is perceived by the body or not, RF energy delivers only a fraction of the energy level required to produce ionization in tissue. For example, the energy at a frequency of 100 MHz (in the FM radio frequency band) is approximately 300 million times too weak to produce ionization.[3,4] Therefore, with RF energy, no mutations are induced nor the DNA single-strand uncoupling that results from ionizing x-ray radiation therapy used in cancer treatment.

ELECTROMAGNETIC PHENOMENA

Electrical Charges

The forces created by electromagnetism are responsible for holding protons, neutrons, and subatomic particles together within the nucleus of the atom. These forces not only determine the chemical properties of atoms but also their emission of EM radiation. The emission of EM radiation also depends on how electric charges are affected when they are accelerated. When alternating currents are generated at high frequencies, the rapid acceleration of charges causes a significant emission of EM radiations. The radiations produced by high-frequency (HF) alternating current (sometimes referred to as oscillating current) are known as radio frequency (RF) waves. At frequencies of 100 kHz, 1 MHz, and 10 MHz, the respective wavelengths are 3 km, 300 m, and 30 m. The radiowave frequencies around these three spectral regions, including 27.12 MHz, are respectively categorized as long, medium, and shortwave bands. The term shortwave is used to denote the shorter wavelengths in only the RF spectrum (Fig. 8–1) and does not refer to EM energies having even shorter wavelengths than RF waves, such as microwaves and infrared and ultraviolet radiations.

Electrical charges exist in either a positive or a negative state. The characterization of charges actually stems from Benjamin Franklin, who decided to call one type of charge positive and the other negative. Other than the fact that oppositely charged particles attract, and similarly charged particles repel each other, not much about these charges is known. Nevertheless, a great deal is known about how charges behave. The forces of attraction and acceleration can be precisely quantified. The same is true of quantifying effects of how electrically charged particles behave when EM waves pass in their vicinity.

Within molecules, charges can exist in both free and fixed forms, depending on how tightly they are bound to the atomic nucleus. Free charges are so loosely bound that they can readily leave the molecule when an electrical voltage is applied. Fixed charges, on the other hand, are confined within the boundaries of the molecule and can only move within that molecule.

In order to explain and quantitatively predict the behavior of charges, physicists have found it convenient to define an electrical field, which relates the force that will be exerted on a charged particle when it is brought into a particular region of space. Electrostatics refers to the electric force between electric charges. In this context, the forces between charges and their strength and direction are described by drawing lines called lines of electric force. The area in which this force acts is called an electric field, which is measured in volts (Fig. 8–3). When a charge of the same polarity is brought within this field, the charge will experience a repulsive force. If the particles are oppositely charged, there will be a equal force, but one of attraction. The mechanism by which this force acts over a distance to cause attraction or repulsion is not understood. When an electric field is produced near a conductor carrying an alternating electric current, the changing electric field in turn creates a changing magnetic field that travels through space in phase with, but at right angles to, the electric field and the direction of the alternating current charge motion (Fig. 8–4). Both electric and magnetic fields are represented by lines of force that represent their magnitude and direction. Regardless of frequency, when alternating (electric) current changes direction (e.g., 60 Hz/s), the resulting magnetic field changes in amplitude and direction in the same manner.

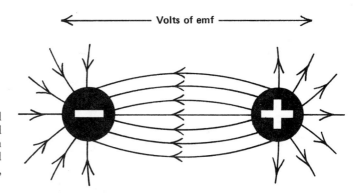

FIGURE 8-3. The electrical field pattern around charged particles. (Adapted from Grob, B: Basic Electronics, ed 4. McGraw-Hill, New York, 1977, p. 289.)

GENERATION OF RADIO FREQUENCY RADIATION (RFR) FOR SWD AND PRFR

Table 8–1 lists the three radio frequencies approved by the FCC for CSWD and PRFR applications. Of the three frequencies, the one that is permitted to drift the most off the assigned frequency (27.12 MHz) without causing radio broadcast interference is the one that is used most often in designing CSWD and PRFR devices. The technology required to control the same amount of drift for the other two frequencies would be more complex and cost prohibitive. Therefore, various commercial enterprises only manufacture and market devices with the 27.12 MHz frequency. In producing the

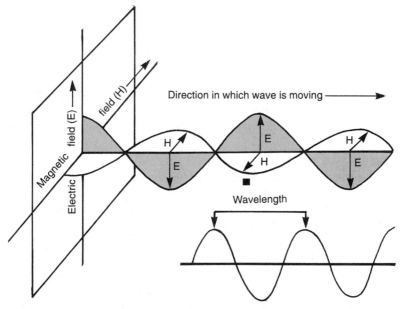

FIGURE 8-4. Electric and magnetic fields at right angles to each other and travelling in the same direction. (From Yost, MG,[4] p. 2, with permission.)

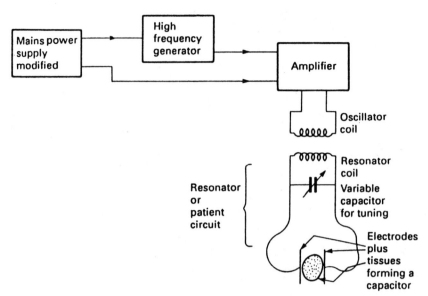

FIGURE 8–5. Components of the high frequency generator and patient circuits of a diathermy device. (From Low and Reed,[10] p. 228, with permission.)

high-frequency current delivered by these devices, two circuits with special electronic components are needed (Fig. 8–5). The first or high-frequency generator circuit is connected to house current power supply of 110 V, 60 Hz AC. This circuit consists of a high-frequency generator that will allow electrons to oscillate at a frequency of 27.12 MHz. Other components of this circuit consist of an amplifier used to increase the power output to a level that is appropriate for therapy and a transformer containing a primary or oscillator coil that is physically in close proximity to the secondary or resonator coil of the second circuit, also known as the resonator or patient circuit. The patient circuit also has a variable capacitor for manual or automatic tuning, and when tuned, both circuits have the same resonant frequency.

TRANSMITTING CSWD OR PRFR TO THE PATIENT

To deliver EM energy to the patient circuit from the high-frequency generator circuit, the tissues of the patient to be treated are first placed in the patient circuit as shown in Figure 8–5. It must be understood that the patient circuit, through the resonator coil, is inductively coupled to the oscillator circuit through the oscillator coil. Thus, when high-frequency continuous RF energy passes through the (primary) oscillator coil, the magnetic field generated by the oscillator circuit induces a current in the (secondary) resonator coil of the patient circuit. When the two circuits are tuned to the same resonant frequency, energy will be most effectively transferred from the high-frequency generator circuit to the patient circuit. Because the frequency of both circuits is proportional to $1/(2 \pi \sqrt{LC})$, the only requirement is that the product of capacity and inductance in one circuit match the product of capacity and inductance in the other. Because the tissues placed in the patient circuit contribute to the capacitance of the resonator circuit, a variable capacitor must be tuned (adjusted manually or automatically) to bring both circuits into resonance. Once both circuits are tuned to the same resonant

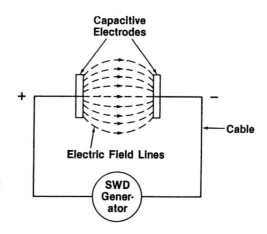

Electric (E) Field

FIGURE 8–6. With capacitive diathermy applicators an electric field occurs between two electrodes of opposite charge. The relative field density is greater near the electrodes where there is less distance between field lines. (From Kloth, L, Morrison, MA, Ferguson, BH: Therapeutic Microwave and Shortwave Diathermy: A Review of Thermal Effectiveness, Safe Use and State of The Art. HHS Publication FDA 85-8237 December 1984, with permission.)

frequency, the amount of thermal energy transmitted to the tissues is controlled by adjusting the output of the diathermy device. Some diathermy devices require manual tuning, while others tune themselves automatically.

Using appropriate treatment applicators or electrodes, there are two ways tissues may be coupled to the EM field generated by the CSWD or PRFR device. The first method involves using an applicator system that requires making the patient's tissues part of the dielectric of a capacitor. This technique, which is called the capacitive or electric field method, primarily influences the tissues by an oscillating electric field (Fig. 8–6). The second method involves using an inductive applicator in which an oscillating magnetic field induces oscillating "eddy" currents in the tissues (Fig. 8–7). This approach is referred to as the inductive or magnetic field method. Because of the high-frequency RF used with CSWD and PRFR, the EM energy can be transmitted

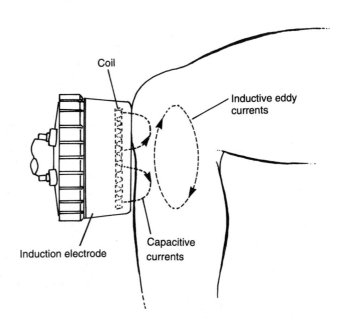

FIGURE 8–7. With magnetic field diathermy applicators eddy currents are induced in the tissues having the highest conductivity. (Courtesy of Delft Instruments, Delft, the Netherlands.)

through "wireless airwaves" to the patient with an airspace or insulating material placed between the applicator and the skin surface. Methods of applying CSWD and PRFR are discussed later in this chapter.

BIOPHYSICAL PRINCIPLES OF TISSUE HEATING WITH RFR

Heating Effects of CSWD

The ability of a CSWD device to induce a heating effect in tissues depends largely on the power output of the device. For CSWD devices, the power output range is 55 to 500 W.[5] This power range is usually more than adequate, because for most CSWD applications, in which the goal is to raise the tissue temperature to within the physiologically effective range of 37.5°C to 44°C, a power output of between 80 and 120 W is required. Although the range of peak (instantaneous) pulse power for most pulsed shortwave devices is 100 to 1000 W, the potential for producing a heating effect with these devices is dependent on the mean power delivered to the tissues with successive bursts of pulse trains. As mentioned previously, the highest mean power that can be delivered with pulsed shortwave devices (80 W) is lower than the usual power output delivered during CSWD treatments.[6]

The effects of CSWD heating on skin bloodflow in humans was studied by Millard,[7] who showed that clearance of radioactive sodium increased nearly 150% after exposure, resulting in an average temperature rise of 5.3°C. In the same study, muscle clearance rates increased by 36%, with a muscle temperature rise of 5.2°C. Using 2450 MHz microwave diathermy, McNiven and Wyper[8] produced a 400% increase in vastus lateralis muscle blood flow in five subjects. This occurred after an 8-minute exposure at a power output adjusted to a "comfortable" level.

The effect of CSWD application on the circulation of knees resulted in a 100% increase, according to Harris[9] in a study of radio-sodium clearance from the knee joint. Similar CSWD treatment of chronic (quiescent) knees in persons with rheumatoid arthritis showed a circulation increase of 60%, whereas with most acute knees with rheumatoid arthritis treated there was a resultant decrease in circulation. This decrease was comparable to decreases found with intra-articular hydrocortisone. Harris[9] suggests that this provides some rationale for using mild local heat therapy in rheumatoid arthritis with acutely inflamed joints.

The physiologic effects obtained with other forms of therapeutic heat are also produced with CSWD. Generally the power of EM fields from CSWD devices allows greater depth of heating than occurs with superficial heating agents. Logically, then, the selection of CSWD is correct when the desired treatment outcome is to increase extensibility of deep collagen tissue, decrease joint stiffness, relieve deep pain and muscle spasm, increase blood flow, and assist in resolution of inflammation.

The primary effect of delivering RF currents at a sufficient power (wattage) level into the body is to cause tissue heating. Recall that heat is energy and that the quantity of heat depends on the amount of random motion of atoms, ions, and molecules in a material. Tissues contain large numbers of ions, and when these charge carriers are exposed to a 27.12 MHz oscillating electric field of CSWD, the ions are accelerated first in one direction, and then in the other. As a result of the increased ionic motion, ions collide with nearby molecules, increasing their random motion, which in turn leads to increased internal kinetic energy and heat generation in the tissues (Fig. 8–8A).[10] Additional significant heating occurs because many tissues, especially muscle and blood, are primarily composed of water. Although water molecules are electrically neutral, they are also polar or have polarity because one end of the molecule is positively charged while the other end is negatively charged. Because it has ends of opposite charge, the water molecule is called a dipole. When exposed to the high-frequency oscillating electric field, the polar water molecules undergo dipole rotation, and in the process of spinning, they collide with other molecules, increasing random motion and heat generation (Fig. 8–8B).[10] Other atoms and molecules that are not electrically charged (nonpolar) may have the paths of their orbiting electrons shifting by the oscillating electric field, which results in a back-and-forth oscillation

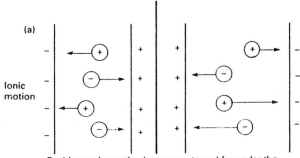

(a)

Ionic motion

Positive and negative ions move to and fro under the influence of an oscillating electric field.

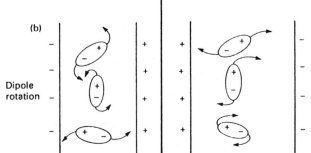

(b)

Dipole rotation

Polar molecules rotate to and fro as the electric field oscillates.

FIGURE 8–8. The effects of oscillating high-frequency electric fields on the molecules and ions of the tissues. (*a*) Ionic motion: positive and negative ions move to and fro under the influence of an oscillating electric field. (*b*) Dipole rotation: polar molecules rotate to and fro as the electric field oscillates. (*c*) Electron cloud motion-molecular distortion: the paths of orbiting electrons are distorted first in one direction then in the other as the electric field oscillates. (From Low and Reed,[10] p. 230, with permission.)

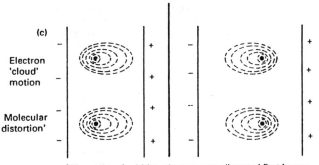

(c)

Electron 'cloud' motion

Molecular distortion'

'The paths of orbiting electrons are distorted first in one direction then in the other as the electric field oscillates.

of their electron cloud. This distortion of the electron cloud allows for only minimal friction and movement between adjacent molecules, which in turn results in minor heating (Fig. 8–8C).[10] According to Ward,[11] the most efficient mechanism involved in the conversion of high-frequency current to heat is the mechanism of increased ionic motion.

Heating Effects Using the Electric Field Method

The primary difference between the electric and magnetic field methods relates to the way EM energy is introduced into the tissues, which leads to different patterns of heating because tissues are not homogeneous. The heating pattern produced by the electric field method is altered by the types and arrangements of the tissues through which the field passes. As described and shown in Figure 8–8, tissue heating from 27.12 MHz alternating current occurs as a result of ion oscillation, dipole rotation, and electron-cloud distortion. Whereas heating by ionic oscillation depends on tissue conductivity, heating by dipole rotation and electron-cloud distortion depends on ease of polarization of polarizable molecules. The amount of this depolarization of polarizable molecules is characterized by a property of insulators known as the dielectric constant. Generally, tissues that have high dielectric constants, such as skin and muscle, are good conductors, while tissues with low dielectric constants, such as fat and bone, have low conductivity (Table 8–2). Electrical conductivity is inversely related to resistance. Therefore, a tissue like fat, which has low electrical conductivity, has high electrical or ohmic resistance. Because different tissues have different conductivities (see Table 8–2), an electric field tends to be refracted when passing through various tissue interfaces near the body surface and between deeper tissue layers. The resulting effect is to spread the field and the area of heating within the tissues.

There is another way to describe how the dielectric constant influences the electric field and its ability to heat the tissues. Tissues with higher dielectric constants, like skin and skeletal muscle, have greater numbers of the polarizable dipole, water. The importance of this is that the greater the number of dipoles, the more charge the tissue can hold for a given imposed voltage across the treatment applicator plates. It is possible, however, to speak instead of the capacity. The dielectric constant is nothing more

TABLE 8–2 Dielectric Constants and
Conductivities of Select Tissues and Materials*

Tissues/Materials	Dielectric Constants (ϵ)	Conductivity (σ)
0.9% saline/blood	80	11.7
Muscle/skin	85–100	0.7–0.9
Bone marrow	7–8	0.02–0.04
Fat tissue	11–13	0.04–0.06
Distilled water	80	2×10^4
Oil	2	10^{11}
Metals	—	10^4–10^7

*Values are given for tissues and materials at 37°C and 50 MHz. The values are temperature and frequency dependent. The unit for conductivity is siemens per meter (S/m).

than the ratio of the capacity of a material (tissue) to that of free space. Capacity is perhaps more easily understood and is simply defined as the amount of charge that a material can hold for a given voltage imposed upon it. In using the electric field or capacitive application technique with applicators known as air-spaced plates to deliver EM energy to the body from a CSWD device, tissues with large capacitance (and dielectric constant) will be most affected and will be the sites at which the greatest heat production will occur.

When using the electric field method of applying CSWD (Fig. 8–6), care must be taken when positioning the treatment applicators to heat tissues that are beneath a thick layer of subcutaneous fat. Schwan[12] has reported that thick subcutaneous fatty tissue may be heated considerably more than muscle when both tissues are exposed to the CSWD electric field. One explanation for this is that the numerous blood vessels that pervade a thick layer of fat tissue carry blood, which has high conductivity and therefore is preferentially heated.[13] In addition, subcutaneous fat is more superficial than muscle.

Heating Effects Using the Magnetic Field Method

As previously mentioned, magnetic field heating is produced mainly by inducing eddy currents in the tissues (Fig. 8–7). The magnetic field passes easily through the tissues and tends to be more intense close to the treatment applicator and less intense as the field spreads out into deeper tissues. However, with this method of applying CSWD there is less heating of subcutaneous fat and more heating of superficial muscle.[14] With this method a strong magnetic field enters the body and induces small, circular-shaped electrical (eddy) currents in the target tissue that alternately change direction with fluctuations of the magnetic field. The amount of heating will occur in those tissues having the lowest impedance and the greatest eddy current density or activity. The magnetic field technique is particularly effective for heating tissues with high conductivities and high electrolyte content, particularly those well perfused with blood, such as muscle. High temperatures are also produced in areas surrounding joints. This method of application does not cause as much heating in fat, bone, or collagen tissues as the electric field technique because these tissues have lower conductivity than muscle. Figure 8–9 shows the relative pattern of heat distribution for the electric

FIGURE 8–9. (*1*) With the electric field (contraplanar) method, for instance, air-spaced applicators, heating occurs in superficial tissues like skin, fat, and some superficial muscle; (*2*) with the magnetic field method, for instance, monode and diplode, more heating occurs in muscle tissue and less heating of fatty tissue. (From Siemens/Physical Medicine: High Frequency Heat Therapy-Basic Information, p. 9, with permission.)

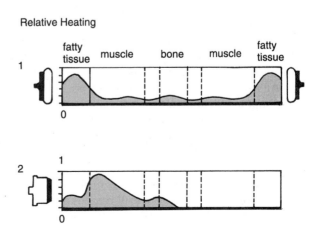

Relative Heating

fatty tissue   muscle   bone   muscle   fatty tissue

and magnetic field heating methods. Thus, the amount of heating (*H*) occurring in a specific tissue is given by Joule's law in the following equation where I^2 indicates current, *R* indicates resistance, and *t* indicates time.

$$H = I^2 Rt$$

When the capacitive applicators are applied to a patient for tissue heating, the plates, plus the intervening air and the patient's tissues placed between the plates, form a capacitor (Fig. 8–10). Thus, with air-spaced plates, the charge of the high-frequency electric field oscillates from one plate to the other 27 million times per second, with the intervening body part of the patient playing an integral part of the system.

With air-spaced plates, a glass or plastic plate guard surrounds each plate to prevent contact between the plate and the patient's skin. A severe electrical burn may occur if either the therapist's or the patient's skin contacts the bare metal plate with the diathermy device in operation. To prevent concentration of the electric field on moisture that may accumulate on the skin from perspiration, a single layer of terry-cloth toweling should be placed between the plate guards and the patient's skin to absorb the moisture. Most plates are manually movable through a distance of about 3 cm within the guard. In some older models, the plate is not movable, but the plate guard can be manually adjusted so the plate-to-skin distance is 1 to 2.5 cm. For optimal heating, the guard should be as close to the towel on the skin as possible, and the plate should be as far away from the skin as the plate guard allows (2.5 cm). This positioning of the plate and guard, with reference to the skin, provides for an increased relative heating depth of the tissues absorbing the energy.[15] In fact, when applied correctly and to patients whose subcutaneous fat layer is less than 1 cm thick, the capacitive-field technique may be capable of delivering energy into tissue depths that correspond to the depths heated with inductive applicators.[16] This is achieved with diathermy devices engineered with deep-field–efficient circuitry that automatically increases wattage (power) output as the plate-skin distance increases, and decreases output as the plate-skin distance decreases. In practice, most CSWD devices maintain constant power output with changes in plate-skin distance. Power or dosage is determined by the patient's subjective perception of heat, and the closer the plates are to the skin, the greater the heat sensation. Air-spaced plates should always be positioned so the distance between any part of the two plates is at least as great as the diameter of the plate. As the plate-to-skin distance increases, heat perception decreases, allowing for power output to be increased so more heating can reach deeper tissues.

Air-spaced plates may be positioned in two different arrangements that produce different tissue heating patterns. In the contraplanar arrangement, the plates are placed in series with the cross section (on opposite sides) of a body part (Fig. 8–9) to treat more deeply located structures. In this arrangement, tissue heating will be proportional to the impedance that each type of tissue offers to the oscillating molecules. Since fat has a higher impedance than muscle or bone, fat will be heated more than muscle or bone.[17] In the coplanar arrangement, the plates are positioned in parallel on the same body surface, rather than placing the body part between the plates. In this arrangement, both superficial and deep tissues are in parallel with respect to the two applicator plates (Fig. 8–10). Tissues that receive more heating in a parallel plate arrangement are those with low impedance (higher conductivity). Thus, muscle tissue will be selectively heated (Fig. 8–10) because current takes the path of least resistance

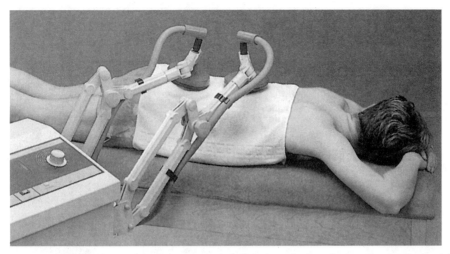

FIGURE 8–10. Capacitive applicators (air-spaced plates) applied to thoraco-lumbar area with single layer of towelling used to absorb moisture. (From Enraf Nonius Catalogue 89/90: Equipment for Physiotherapy and Rehabilitation, p. 12, with permission.)

in more highly conductive tissue. The coplanar method may be more beneficial when treating problems of the lumbar or thoracic paravertebral musculature.

INDUCTIVE OR MAGNETIC FIELD METHOD OF APPLICATION

As mentioned previously, this method involves using an applicator system in which an oscillating magnetic field induces oscillating electric "eddy" currents in the tissue (see Fig. 8–7). Once the magnetic field enters the body part, an electrical current is induced within the tissues having the lowest impedance. The induced electrical eddy currents alternate in direction with changes of the magnetic field. Thus, the greatest density of eddy current activity and therefore the greatest amount of heating occurs in low-impedance tissues containing the highest electrolyte content, such as skeletal muscle and blood (see Fig. 8–9).

Two types of coil applicators are used to deliver the magnetic field energy to the patient from the patient circuit. The applicators most frequently used consist of a cable shaped into a coil that is contained within two types of rigid plastic insulator housings. The treatment surface of the plastic applicator serves the same function as the plate guard of the air-spaced plate applicator to space the inductive coil away from the skin.

The monode (Fig. 8–11) is used to treat a single body surface and requires additional spacing and moisture absorption from the skin with a single layer of terry-cloth toweling. The diplode (Fig. 8–11) is hinged so that one or more body-part surfaces can be treated simultaneously. The diplode consists of a rectangularly arranged induction coil contained within an insulator housing, which also serves to space the coil away from the patient's skin. Because of the coil's closer proximity to the treatment surface within the diplode, approximately 1 cm of terry-cloth toweling is recommended to

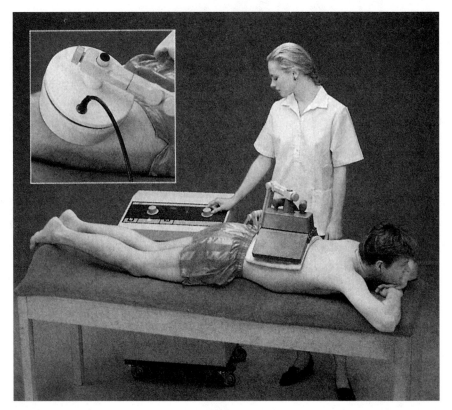

FIGURE 8–11. Two types of magnetic field applicators diplode applied to patient with 2 to 4 layers of towelling used for additional spacing and monode (*inset*). (From Enraf Nonius Catalogue 89/90, p. 10, with permission.)

separate the applicator from the patient's skin to prevent excessive surface heating and to absorb moisture caused by perspiration.

All CSWD and PRFR devices have external cables that connect the applicator to the console and deliver the EM energy from the high-frequency oscillating circuit to the applicator. Cables on older devices may not be adequately shielded and may emit radiation in all directions when the applicators are energized. In this case, care must be taken to prevent the cables from directly contacting the patient or any metal or synthetic materials.

PREPARING THE PATIENT AND DEVICE FOR TREATMENT

Prior to treatment, the therapist should evaluate the patient and carry out the necessary operating and safety checks of the CSWD device as follows:

1. Test and record the patient's thermal sensation of the body part to be treated.
2. For determining adequacy of blood flow to an extremity, check arterial pulses in the distal part of the limb; also check results of other vascular laboratory tests.

3. Inspect the body part to be treated for any metal on or near the patient. Ask the patient, or refer to medical records to determine, whether there is any metal (shrapnel, sutures, prosthetic implants, metal intrauterine device) within his or her body.

4. Remove all metal objects, clothing, or other synthetic materials and electronic devices from the body part to be treated. Watches and hearing aids may be demagnetized if exposed to the EM field if within 1 m of the operating CSWD device.

5. Ask the patient, or refer to medical records to determine, if other electronic devices are present within the patient's body (for example, cardiac pacer, bladder stimulator, spinal cord stimulator, electrodes for a myoelectric prosthesis).

6. Dry any damp skin area that will be exposed to the CSWD applicator. Do not treat over moist wound dressings.

7. Place the patient in a comfortable, relaxing prone, supine, sitting, or side-lying position so she or he does not have to move during treatment; when treating to increase extensibility of contracted soft tissues, position the patient and the body part to encourage a gentle stretch of the tight tissues.

8. Do not place the patient on a metal surface, in a metal wheelchair, or on a mattress containing metal springs when giving a CSWD treatment because the EM field may selectively heat the metal, which could burn the patient.

9. Select an appropriate CSWD treatment applicator (capacitive or inductive field). Apply capacitive applicators using contraplanar or coplanar method.

10. Expose and cover the body part to be treated with one layer of terry cloth if using capacitive applicators (for moisture absorption) or two to four layers if using inductive applicator for additional spacing and moisture absorption.

11. Explain to the patient what the treatment consists of and why it is being done.

12. Position the treatment applicator appropriately with sufficient spacing; if the CSWD device is older and has nonshielded cables connecting the device console to the applicator(s), make sure the cables are no closer than the terminals they plug into on the device.

13. Tell the patient about how much heat sensation to expect. Advise the patient that she or he should only experience "comfortable warmth" and that if it is hotter than comfortable, she or he should either notify the therapist or pull the emergency off switch.

14. To avoid possible shock, instruct the patient not to touch any part of the CSWD device and not to touch any object that may be grounded (such as water pipe, electrical outlet, radiator, metal sink).

15. Switch on the CSWD device; tune and adjust the heat output to comfortable warmth based on patient feedback.

16. If the patient complains of any pain or discomfort during treatment, immediately reduce the output to zero. Determine if the pain was caused by excessive heating or uncomfortable positioning and make the necessary corrections before treatment is re-initiated.

17. Immediately after treatment, assess the patient's skin for normal erythema by observation and palpation.

TREATMENT AND DOSAGE CONSIDERATIONS FOR CSWD

Because it is not clinically possible to measure the amount of EM energy actually transferred from the CSWD device to the tissue, the therapist must use the patient's subjective heat-sensation response as a guide for dosage. Before beginning treatment individuals with a suspected thermal sensory deficit should be tested for pain and temperature sensation to determine if they are capable of reporting reliable changes in cutaneous heat sensation.

However, even if a patient is able to distinguish changes in thermal skin sensation, he or she may not be able to rely on skin sensation to distinguish temperature changes in deeper tissues that are normally warmer than superficial tissues. To more objectively predict deep-tissue temperature changes from diathermy, the National Council on Radiation Protection and Measurements has quantified the amount of EM energy in watts that can be safely absorbed per unit (kg) of tissue mass. This quantity, expressed in watts per kilogram and called the specific absorption rate (SAR), ranges from 50 to 170 W/kg, which to some extent corresponds to the rate of increase of temperature in tissue being treated by CSWD. For example, in well-perfused tissues a low rate of increase in tissue temperature of 0.4°C (0.7°F)/min may occur at a low SAR dosage of 25 W/kg. For the same well-perfused tissue a high rate of increase in tissue temperature of 2.7°C (4.9°F)/min may require a high SAR dosage of 170 W/kg (Table 8–3). Recall that the maximum tissue temperature reached regardless of the heat modality (as expressed by Joule's law) depends not only on the square of the intensity and tissue impedance but also on how long the heat treatment is given. In addition, how much the tissue temperature is elevated is dependent on the adequacy of blood perfusion through the tissues. Poor blood perfusion, such as occurs in arterial insufficiency of the lower extremities, may not adequately allow for heat dissipation when heat from any source is applied directly to the poorly perfused tissues. In this case, tissue burning may occur owing to a high SAR, in which case heat gain may exceed heat loss, which will compromise the ability of the vasculature to remove heat from the local area. When tissues are adequately perfused, the body's thermoregulatory mechanism increases heat removal from the local tissue until a new higher-temperature steady state is reached, thus avoiding tissue damage from excessive heat. Thus, it must be emphasized that the thermal perceptions of the patient are the only safe guide to heating tissue with diathermy.

When using CSWD, therapists should always keep in mind that the extent of biologic reactions elicited depends on the tissue temperature reached at the end of treatment. Since the therapeutic range for increasing tissue temperature is between 37.5°C and 44°C, it is imperative that the therapist know how intensely, how long, and how frequently the treatment should be applied, based on the stage of the condition. According to Thom,[18] a lower dose of CSWD administered over a longer period of time is more effective therapeutically than a more intense dose given over a shorter time. This concept warrants further research.

Heat dosage, or the amount of thermal energy delivered to the tissues per unit time, is very important when specific treatment outcomes are desired. Lehmann's[19] definitions of mild and vigorous heating discussed in Chapter 5 may be used in conjunction with the doses described by Schliephake[20] for CSWD application. The following dosage scheme may also be used for pulsed SWD and for MWD application:

Dose I: Lowest—just below the point of any sensation of heat (acute inflammatory process).

Dose II: Low—mild heat sensation, barely felt (subacute, resolving inflammatory process).

Dose III: Medium—moderate, but pleasant, heat sensation (subacute, resolving inflammatory process).

TABLE 8–3 Dosage Guide for Diathermy Treatments

Condition Being Treated	Treatment			Heat Sensation Reported by Patient	Percentage Output of Energy from the Device	Specific Absorption Rate (SAR) (W/kg)	Rate of Tissue Temperature Rise (°C/min)	Tissue Temperature Increase Goal
	Dosage Level	Duration of Treatment	Frequency of Treatments					
Acute inflammation	1. Lowest	1–3 min	Daily for 1–2 wks	None; dose is just below any sensation of heat	1/4 maximum output	25–50	0.4–0.8	37.5–38.5
Subacute resolving	2. Low	3–5 min	Daily for 1–2 wks	Barely felt	1/2 maximum output	50–75	0.8–1.2	38.5–40.0
Repair phase	3. Medium	5–7 min	Daily for 1–2 wks	Distinct but pleasant heat sensation	3/4 maximum output	75–125	1.2–2	40.0–42.0
Usual chronic conditions	4. High	5–7 min	Daily or 2 times/wk for 1 wk to 1 mo	Definite heat sensation, well within tolerance	Maximum output	125–170	2.0–2.7	42.0–44.0

Dose IV: Heavy—vigorous heating that produces a well-tolerated sensation (chronic conditions). The pain threshold may be reached, but the output is immediately lowered to just below maximal toleration.

It has been suggested that acute conditions like soft-tissue trauma should be treated 2 or 3 times daily, with either dose I or II, for 15 minutes.[21] The acute condition will not require the deep-tissue temperature rise that results from longer, more intense applications (vigorous heating). Chronic conditions (for instance, contracture) call for either dose III or dose IV and longer treatment periods of 15 to 30 minutes. Remember, for moderate to vigorous heating effects, a comfortable feeling of warmth perceived by the patient during the entire treatment is the best guide for adjusting the dosage of CSWD.

TREATMENT INDICATIONS

Indications for CSWD

All of the common indications for thermotherapy are also indications for treatment with CSWD. In fibrous muscular or joint capsular contractures, prior heating of the shortened tissues may enhance collagen extensibility[22] when followed by stretching done manually, with continuous passive-motion devices, with splints or with neuromuscular electrical-stimulation devices. CSWD may be used, because it is capable of heating superficial to deep muscle layers.

Muscle guarding and pain, which occur as a result of injury to tendons and joint structures, degenerative joint disease, bursitis, sacroiliac strains, and ankylosing spondylitis, may be relieved by CSWD applications to the muscles in spasm.[23]

Joint structures may be selectively heated by CSWD when the joint is covered by a thin layer of soft tissue (such as the elbow). Vigorous heating of a synovial joint should only be done in chronic disease conditions, such as contracture or the advanced degenerative (quiescent) stage of rheumatoid arthritis. The purpose of such treatment is to improve joint range of motion by decreasing stiffness and improving resilience of contracted soft tissues. In the subacute stage of traumatic arthritis, CSWD at dose level II may be beneficial in joints with a thin soft-tissue cover to improve blood circulation, thereby aiding in the resolution of edema and hemorrhage. This concept may also apply to acute or subacute epicondylitis, for which mild heating from CSWD may help in reabsorption of inflammatory exudates.

Very mild heating, at dosage level I from CSWD, may be used in recurring inflammatory conditions to improve blood flow and facilitate diffusion of oxygen and metabolite clearance.[23] Lehmann[23,24] advocates the use of CSWD to induce mild heating, which produces a mild physiologic response, in the later stages of traumatic arthritis, chronic pelvic inflammatory disease, epicondylitis, degenerative joint disease, ankylosing spondylitis, and other chronic arthritic conditions.

Continuous shortwave techniques may be used for selective heating of pelvic organs in chronic inflammatory pelvic diseases. According to Lehmann,[23] this treatment produces a significant increase in vascularity and blood flow, with the result that cardiac output is increased in women. As a result of the improved vascularity, antibiotic levels to inflamed tissues may be enhanced.

A reflex or consensual mild heating response of a body part (such as an extremity) is achieved by applying the source of heat proximal to the site of vascular occlusion.[25–27] If this approach is used in treating peripheral arterial insufficiency, it avoids the potential for overheating tissues that are poorly perfused and are, therefore, incapable of adequately dissipating direct applications of heat. It is not known whether improved deep collateral circulation occurs with this method, in addition to the reflex dilation of skin blood vessels that is evoked.[8] Additional research is needed to establish the efficacy of this technique.

Allberry[28] and Barnett[29] have reported positive results with CSWD in enhancing the drying up of blisters from herpes zoster and in alleviating the associated pain. Both reports emphasized the importance of applying mild heating within a few days of the onset of rash, or on the first day if possible. Treatment consists of daily 20-minute applications at the level of the involved dorsal root ganglia until pain is decreased or the scabs fall off.

Precautions and Contraindications for CSWD

The literature cites numerous potential hazards of nonionizing radiation from CSWD. Hazards may result from high levels of unintended exposures to tissues or materials inside the patient's body, adjacent to the patient, or adjacent to the therapist applying the treatment.

Foremost among the potential hazards to be considered with CSWD are internal and externally worn metallic objects and electromedical devices. CSWD should not be applied over surgical metal implants or tissues containing other foreign metallic objects, because focusing of field lines causes excessive current density within the metal and raises its surface temperature, resulting in transfer of excessive heat that may burn adjacent tissues.[11,17,23] Women with metallic intrauterine devices should not receive SWD to the lumbar, pelvic, or abdominal areas.[30,31] Likewise, externally worn metallic items (jewelry and zippers, for instance) should be removed and placed outside the EM field during CSWD treatment.[15] Metal objects within the immediate treatment area (such as metal in the treatment table, chairs, or swivel stools) should be removed.

In addition to biologic hazards, electromagnetic interference (EMI) may cause disturbances in the function of electromedical or other devices. Wrist watches, other RF devices, diagnostic medical equipment (that is, electroencephalographs, electrocardiographs, and electromyographs), unshielded cardiac pacemakers, transcutaneous electrical nerve or muscle stimulators, electrophrenic pacers, and cerebellar and urinary bladder stimulators[23,32,33] may malfunction when CSWD is applied in their immediate vicinity. Unpleasant paresthesias or burning sensations may occur beneath transcutaneous electrodes that connect an electromedical device to the patient, whether or not the device is in operation. Therefore, therapists should avoid directing EM fields over or near externally worn or implanted electronic devices, their lead wires, or their electrodes.

Of prime concern regarding EMI are devices that transmit high-frequency, high-voltage electric and magnetic field energy into, and in the vicinity of, the patient. EMI may cause an unshielded cardiac pacemaker to stop pacing, revert to a prefixed rate, or to pace rapidly and erratically, if the unshielded pacemaker comes within 4.5 m of an operational device.[11] Secondary to the induced malfunction, the patient's cardiac rhythm may revert to asystole or ventricular fibrillation. Improvements in pacemaker engineering and design have reduced their susceptibility to EM fields and have even eliminated this problem in some pacemakers.[33] However, it behooves the therapist to place adequate warning signs outside the area where devices with EM fields are being used and to select another nonelectromagnetic thermal agent to treat the patient who is equipped with an unshielded cardiac pacemaker.

Specific tissues or anatomic structures that may be adversely affected by the thermal effects of CSWD include high fluid volume areas, such as the eyes[16,24,34–39] and fluid-filled joints[40]; testes; space-occupying lesions; ischemic, hemorrhagic, malignant, and acutely inflamed tissues; as well as sensory-impaired skin. Moist wound dressings, moist clothing,[23] or accumulations of excessive perspiration[15] also will focus field lines, because of the higher dielectric constant and conductivity of isolated body fluids in comparison to surrounding tissues. The same focusing effect applies to blood vessels that run through adipose tissue. The potential for overheating of the fluids in each case from charge accumulation at the fluid-tissue interface may result in burning of adjacent tissues. Terry-cloth toweling used with all CSWD applicators absorbs surface perspiration, and wide spacing between skin and air-spaced applicators helps to minimize the risk of excessive heating of surface moisture.

When moisture is present on the skin or in moist wounds or wounds packed with moist dressings, CSWD should not be applied in a way that would allow energy absorption and selective heating of the moisture.

The high fluid volume of the eye makes it susceptible to selective absorption of unintended or accidental doses of energy from CSWD.[34] If CSWD is to be applied to the maxillary sinuses of a person wearing contact lenses, the lenses should be removed before treatment to avoid a concentration of field energy that could cause excessive heating of the ciliary body.[39]

As mentioned previously, the synovial joint that has accumulated excess fluid from effusion may also pose a hazard if the temperature of the fluid is raised a few degrees. The intra-articular temperature of normal synovial joints ranges between 30°C and 31°C.[40] Harris and McCroskery[41,42] have demonstrated in vitro that an increase of 5°C produced a fourfold increase in enzymatic lysis of human cartilage by rheumatoid synovial collagenase. The intra-articular temperature in knees with rheumatoid arthritis is about 36.5°C, and that a significant increase in temperature greater than this may accelerate destruction of cartilage.[43] Based on this knowledge, therapists should use caution when considering whether mild, moderate, or vigorous heating from CSWD is appropriate for the patient who is suspected of having an inflamed joint condition.

The exacerbation of acutely inflamed, fluid-filled joint cavities may occur as a result of selective heating by vigorous treatment (dose IV) using CSWD when the joint is covered by a thin soft-tissue layer.[24] Vigorous heating should be avoided in acute inflammatory processes because of the potential for causing tissue necrosis by imposing an inflammatory reaction on an existing acute inflammatory process.[24] Likewise, vigorous heating of tissue adjacent to a space-occupying lesion, such as a protruded nucleus pulposus, may exacerbate symptoms by increasing swelling and congestion of tissue surrounding the disk lesion.[23,24]

In Chapter 5, it was pointed out that a local application of heat from any source to ischemic tissue is hazardous, because the compromised blood flow may not meet the increased metabolic demand placed on the tissues by the thermal energy buildup.[25] The time rate of change of temperature for vascularized tissues treated with CSWD should range between 0.4°C and 2.7°C per minute, achieving a therapeutic temperature of 37.5°C to 44°C within 10 minutes.[24]

Because an increase in tissue temperature increases blood flow owing to dilation of arterioles, CSWD should not be used to treat individuals who are predisposed to hemorrhage, such as patients with hemophilia, since the increase in blood flow secondary to the induced vasodilation would enhance the tendency to bleed.[25-27]

Patients with pain and temperature-sensory deficits may be unable to appreciate thermal changes applied to their skin. Since dosage depends on the patient's ability to determine when heat sensation is just comfortably warm, only mild to moderate doses (based on the therapist's knowledge of previous output settings) should be applied in these situations. The patient's condition and the equipment should be checked frequently by the therapist.

Animal studies have demonstrated deleterious effects of MWD on gonad structure and function.[44-46] Although both the testicles and the ovaries in humans are generally considered to be sensitive to temperature rise, the testicles (because of their superficial location) are more susceptible to stray radiation than are the ovaries. Unnecessary exposure of the testes to diathermy, therefore, should be avoided.[47]

CSWD should not be applied to the low back, or to the abdominal or pelvic regions of pregnant women, because of the possibility of thermal damage to the fetus.[48] Studies on the effect of CSWD on fetal and embryonic growth and development have demonstrated that anomalies occurred in rat fetuses exposed to a frequency of 27.12 MHz.[49] The observed effects were attributed to hyperthermia. The risk of miscarriage was not significantly increased in pregnant women who operated SWD devices during the 6 months prior to the first trimester or during the first trimester of pregnancy.[50]

Although exposure of pregnant laboratory animals to CSWD[49] does cause fetal abnormalities, it is not known whether the fetus in the human can be reached with significant RF radiation at clinically used intensities. Despite the possibility that amniotic fluid may selectively absorb CSWD energy, there are no clinical reports in the literature to substantiate whether selective heating of the pregnant uterus does or does not occur during exposure to this energy. Based on the finding that temperatures of 39.8°C or more are damaging to the human fetus,[51] CSWD should not be administered with vaginal electrodes to pregnant women.[23]

When diathermy has been applied to the lumbosacral region in menstruating women, clinical reports have indicated that an increase in menstrual flow occurred.[23] The low-back area of a woman may be treated during the menstrual period, but women should be forewarned that their menstrual flow may increase temporarily following treatment.

Regarding the effect of diathermy on bone, it must be emphasized that there is a potential for disturbing bone growth in children when CSWD creates a significant rise in temperature of the epiphyses.[52] Animal studies have demonstrated that CSWD may either enhance[52] or inhibit[54] bone growth. Therapists applying CSWD to children should therefore be aware that bone is not effectively heated when covered by an adequate thickness of soft tissue,[23] and that a disturbance in bone growth will occur only at intensities that produce pain.[23] However, the size of the CSWD applicator relative to the size of the child may prevent application in a way that avoids superficial bone-growth centers.

Concern that the therapist who operates CSWD equipment may receive unintended, hazardous exposure of EM energy is not supported by published reports. Stuchly and colleagues[55] reported that overexposure to the therapist from CSWD is not possible when the distance between the therapist and the applicator is 20 cm or more.

Materials and objects that may be hazardous during application of CSWD include certain synthetic substances such as nylon, foam rubber, and plastics. Objects like pillows, pillow cases, treatment tables, sandbag coverings, and clothing often contain these materials, which are nonconductive. It has been reported, however, that a pillow being used by a patient receiving CSWD treatment was charred at areas of contact with, or directly adjacent to, the unshielded induction power cables of the device.[56] Therapists should avoid such potential fire hazards by correct placement of equipment and by keeping unshielded cables and electrodes well away from synthetic materials.[57]

In summary, the general precautions and contraindications associated with any thermal modality should be observed. Any significant tissue heating should be avoided if acute inflammation is present; if there is a tendency for hemorrhage; if perfusion is restricted by vascular compromise; or if the patient is febrile or has insensate skin that prevents accurate reporting of heat sensation. In addition, SWD treatment should be avoided in the following instances:

1. When metal is on or in the tissues.
2. Over implanted or near externally worn electronic devices.
3. Over organs or tissues containing high fluid volume.
4. Over cancerous tissue.
5. Over accumulated surface or wound moisture.
6. Over lumbar or abdominal area of pregnant women.
7. Over synthetic materials.

CASE STUDY 1

PATIENT

- Retired 38-year-old male former professional football player; now administrator of his own gourmet restaurant.

DIAGNOSIS

- Right knee extension limited to minus 18 degrees.

HISTORY

- Repeated tears of biceps femoris and semitendinosis muscles during previous 12 years.

PREVIOUS TREATMENT

- Ice and immobilization following each acute tear.
- Hamstring and triceps surae stretching after subacute phase following each tear.

PROBLEM

- Difficulty with ambulation and lower-extremity mobility activities because of contracture.

DECISION MAKING/CHOICE OF TREATMENT

- Consider size of area to be treated, that is, extent of contracted tissue.
- Heat with stretch?
- Superficial or deep-heat modality?
- Cold with stretch?
- Cold with contract-relax?
- There is springy end-feel into passive knee extension.

TREATMENT GOAL/DESCRIPTION

- Reduce contracture with heat-and-stretch.
- Treatment daily for 5 days using CWSD.
- Vigorous heating (dose IV) of right hamstrings with inductive drum, patient prone for 30 minutes; maintain this dose just below maximal toleration.
- 10-lb sandbag applied to calcaneus.
- After 30-minute heat-stretch treatment, patient remains prone with 10 lb applied to calcaneus for 20-minute cooldown to facilitate plastic elongation of contracted hamstring muscles.

HOME PROGRAM

- 2 times per day right hamstring stretch sitting with left knee flexed over table edge and right knee extended on the table for 15 minutes.

TREATMENT OUTCOME

- Daily ROM measurements for 5 days results in active right knee extension to minus 10 degrees.
- Recommend another 5 days' daily treatment same protocol.

PULSED RADIO FREQUENCY RADIATION: PULSED SHORTWAVE DIATHERMY AND PULSED RADIO FREQUENCY ENERGY

Pulsed Shortwave Diathermy

Keep in mind that we've been discussing CSWD, which utilizes continuous (uninterrupted) high (radio)-frequency EM radiation (27.12 MHz) for the primary purpose of inducing heat in the tissues. A previously mentioned alternative approach is to interrupt the CSWD waves at regular intervals. Using a timing circuit to electronically

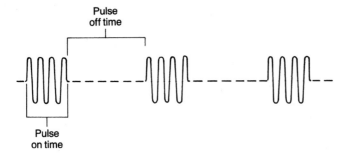

FIGURE 8–12. PRFs are created by interrupting the 27 MHz wave output at regular intervals to deliver pulse trains or bursts of energy during successive "on times" separated by longer lasting "off times."

interrupt the 27.12 MHz waves, bursts of pulse trains containing a series of high-frequency sine wave oscillations are emitted from the PSWD treatment applicator. Each pulse train has a preset duration, or "on time," and is separated from successive pulse trains by an "off time" (Fig. 8–12) that is determined by the pulse repetition rate or frequency. Depending on the PRFR device, the pulse frequency can be varied from 1 to 7000 pulses per second[6] and is selected with a pulse-frequency control on the equipment-operation panel. The desired effect is production of PRFR that, like CSWD, has the ability to raise tissue temperature. This variation of diathermy is called pulsed shortwave diathermy (PSWD). Whether PRFR induces heat in tissues depends on three parameters that in combination give a mean power output that ranges between 38 and 665 W. The three parameters are: (1) peak pulse power, (2) pulse frequency, and (3) pulse duration. The measure of heat production with PSWD devices is the mean power (Fig. 8–13). Gradual increases in tissue heating above 37°C that result in increased vascular perfusion with PSWD, begin to occur at a mean power of 38 W. For most PRFR devices, the peak pulse power (the power in watts delivered during a pulse) ranges between 100 and 1000 W. If the pulse duration is 400 μs (0.4 ms) and the peak power and pulse frequency are known, the mean power may be easily calculated. For example, at a peak pulse power of 800 W, if the pulse frequency is 200 pps, then the pulse period (the pulse on time plus the pulse off time) may be calculated as the

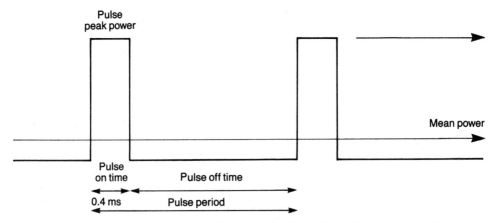

FIGURE 8–13. A subjective measure of heat production with pulsed shortwave is the mean power. The highest mean power produced by pulsed shortwave devices is always lower than the power produced by most continuous shortwave devices. (From van den Bouwhuijsen,[6] p. 20, with permission.)

pulse period (ms) ÷ pulse frequency or in this case 1000 ÷ 200 = 5.0 ms (see Fig. 8–13). In this example, the percentage of time during which the pulsed shortwave output is delivered is 0.4 ÷ 5.0 = 8 percent. Consequently, the mean power is 8 percent of 800 W or 64 W. As shown in Table 8–4, this and other mean wattage values greater than 38 W produce a significant tissue heating effect that elicits expected physiologic responses from accumulated thermal energy. PSWD devices produce heat in tissues the same way heat is produced in tissues by CSWD, that is, by increasing random motion and kinetic energy between atoms, ions, and molecules. Generally, with most PSWD devices the highest mean power output that can be delivered is always lower than the power delivered (80 to 120 W) during most CSWD treatments.

Treatment and Dosage Considerations for PSWD

As stated earlier, the heating effect of a PSWD device is related to the magnitude of the mean power output. For example, low mean power values between 38 and 80 W would be appropriately used to treat acute and subacute inflammatory conditions and would thereby respectively correspond to dosages I and II. Mean power values between 80 and 300 W may be used in late subacute conditions in which the signs and symptoms of inflammation are almost resolved (dose III). Dose IV for PSWD would require higher mean wattages above 300. The dosage level should be adjusted to never exceed a comfortable, well-tolerated heat sensation.

Application Technique for PSWD

PSWD is applied to the body in the same way as CSWD. Most PSWD devices have the drum type of inductive applicator with the tissue heating pattern as described for CSWD. Thus, one would expect less heating of superficial fat and more heating of tissues like superficial muscle, which has a high electrolyte level. The drum applicator, covered with an elastic surgical cap (Fig. 8–14) for hygienic purposes and is placed close to or in contact with one layer of terry-cloth towel over the area to be treated. The strongest heating effect with a PSWD device is achieved by selecting high peak pulse power and high pulse frequency settings. If the PSWD device also allows selection of different pulse durations, then in combination with high peak pulse power and frequency, a longer pulse duration should be chosen. For very mild to almost imperceptible heating, the lowest values for peak pulse power, pulse frequency, and pulse duration that give a mean power in the range of 38 to 80 W should be selected.

Some PSWD devices, like the Curapuls 419 (Delft Instruments, 2600 AV Delft, the Netherlands), not only provide heating effects above 38 W of mean power but also provide athermal effects at mean power values below 38 W (Table 8–4). Thus, when appropriate, these devices can be used in either a thermal or athermal mode. Athermal PRFR is discussed in the next section.

Treatment Indications, Precautions, and Contraindications for PSWD

All of the indications, precautions, and contraindications previously discussed for CSWD apply to PSWD. In addition, all of the steps taken to prepare the patient and

TABLE 8–4 Mean Power Values for the Curapuls 419 PSWD*

Position of Intensity Control	1	2	3	4	5	6	7	8	9	10
Peak Pulse Power	100 W	200 W	300 W	400 W	500 W	600 W	700 W	800 W	900 W	1000 W
Pulse Frequency					Mean power					
15 Hz	0,6	1,2	1,8	2,4	3,0	3,6	4,2	4,8	5,4	6,0
20 Hz	0,8	1,6	2,4	3,2	4,0	4,8	5,6	6,4	7,2	8,0
26 Hz	1,0	2,1	3,1	4,2	5,2	6,3	7,3	8,4	9,4	10,4
35 Hz	1,4	2,8	4,2	5,6	7,0	8,4	9,8	11,2	12,6	14,0
46 Hz	1,8	3,7	5,5	7,4	9,2	11,0	12,9	14,7	16,7	18,4
62 Hz	2,5	5,0	7,4	9,0	12,4	14,9	17,4	19,8	22,3	24,8
82 Hz	3,3	6,6	9,9	13,2	16,4	19,7	23,0	26,3	29,6	32,8
110 Hz	4,4	8,8	13,2	17,6	22,0	26,4	30,8	35,2	39,6	44,0
150 Hz	6,0	12,0	18,0	24,0	30,0	36,0	42,0	48,0	54,0	60,0
200 Hz	8,0	16,0	24,0	32,0	40,0	48,0	56,0	64,0	72,0	80,0

*Device manufactured by Delft Instruments, the Netherlands; has a pulse duration of 400 μs.

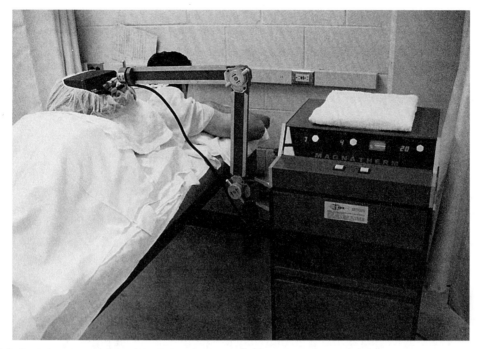

FIGURE 8–14. A PSWD device (Magnatherm) with surgical cap covering a drum treatment applicator.

the PSWD device for treatment as described in the previous section for CSWD are also the same.

CASE STUDY 2

PATIENT

- 54-year-old male Army veteran on disability from multiple war-related injuries.

DIAGNOSIS

- Arterial insufficiency in the right lower extremity (RLE) secondary to vasospastic disease.
- Intermittent claudication, right calf.

HISTORY

- Left below-knee amputee 5 years ago; wears below-knee prosthesis. Right great toe amputed 1 year ago; weak posterior tibial artery and dorsalis pedis pulses.

- Smoked cigarettes for 25 years but quit 18 months ago.
- Trophic changes right leg and foot include thick, brittle nails; scant leg and foot hair; areas of shiny skin.

PREVIOUS TREATMENT

- Heparin to prevent blood clotting.
- Vasodilator medication to preserve perfusion to vessels of RLE.

PROBLEMS

- Right calf pain after walking 50 feet.
- Coldness of right distal LE.
- Tendency for recurring small skin ulcerations right foot/ankle.

DECISION MAKING/CHOICE OF TREATMENT

Consider the following choices:

- Warm whirlpool 100°F, 20 min/day to RLE in dependent position.
- Fluidotherapy at 104°F, 20 min/day to RLE in dependent position.
- CSWD vigorous heating (dose IV) via inductive diplode applicator to right calf, 20 min/day, 5 days/week for 2 weeks.
- PSWD moderate heating to lumbar spine sympathetic ganglia with inductive drum, 20 min/day, 5 days/week for 2 weeks.
  Note: The first three choices are not appropriate due to impaired circulation of the right leg and foot.

TREATMENT GOALS/DESCRIPTION

- Improve blood perfusion to distal RLE.
- Improve patient's walking distance before onset of claudication pain.
- Position patient prone with 6-inch-diameter rolled towel supporting right ankle.
- Measure baseline temperature of skin on second through fifth toes or measure toe-skin blood flow with laser doppler.
- Cover RLE including ankle and foot with warm blanket.
- Apply PSWD drum applicator touching one layer of toweling over the lumbar spine area.
- Induce moderate heating (dose III) to lumbar sympathetic ganglia to reduce constrictor tone to distal RLE arterioles.
- Evaluate treatment outcome by measuring temperature of skin on second through fifth toes or measure toe-skin blood flow with laser doppler.

HOME PROGRAM

- Instruct patient to protect RLE from all trauma and only have podiatrist cut nails.

- Instruct patient to keep RLE warm with appropriate clothing.
- Instruct patient to avoid elevation of RLE and long periods of dependent positioning of RLE.
- Instruct patient to ambulate only to preclaudication pain tolerance.

PULSED RADIO FREQUENCY (NONTHERMAL) ENERGY (PRFE)

In 1934 Abraham Ginsberg,[58] a physician, in collaboration with Arthur Milinowski, a physicist, developed an ultra-shortwave device that delivered pulses of RF radiation. This device was described by Ginsberg as an athermal shortwave apparatus. In essence, this device took the continuous-high-frequency radio waves of CSWD and regularly interrupted them, producing short pulse trains or bursts of EM energy in the same way that continuous waves of ultrasound are interrupted to produce pulsed ultrasound and CSWD waves are interrupted to produce PSWD. Because Ginsberg described the maximum output of the device as being athermal below one's sensory heat perception threshold, the device has therefore been referred to by the biophysics community as a "pulsed nonthermal shortwave modality." However, in some instances it has also been called a "pulsed high-peak-power EM energy," "pulsed high-frequency current," "pulsed electromagnetic field" (PEMF), and "pulsed shortwave diathermy" (PSWD). If the device is truly athermal, then any of the above descriptions would be technically correct except PSWD, because the word diathermy means to "heat through." The term "pulsed high peak power EM energy" is not fully descriptive because it simply refers to the relative power (in watts) in a single high-frequency pulse, which describes only one of the pulse parameters. The acronym PEMF is really a generic term that may be used to describe a pulse modulation of any frequency in the nonionizing portion of the EM spectrum. However, since we are dealing with 27 MHz in the RF band of the EM spectrum, technically it would be most correct to refer to these devices as "pulsed radio frequency (nonthermal) energy" (PRFE).

With respect to the difference between the terms athermal and nonthermal, the biophysics community defines a nonthermal PRFE device as one that raises the temperature on the target tissue less than 1°C after exposure for 1 hour.[59] Reports by Markov and Pilla,[59] who measured the temperature rise in a saline phantom model and in rabbit muscle tissue, indicate that the rise in temperature produced by the sofPulse (Electropharmacology, Inc., 2301 N.W. 33rd Ct, Pompano Beach, FL 33069) was within the 0 to 1°C range.

A PRFE device called the Diapulse (Diapulse Corporation of America, 321 East Shore Road, Great Neck, NY 11023) began being marketed in 1959. Between 1959 and 1972 a few clinical and animal model studies with Diapulse gradually appeared in the literature. However, in 1972 the FDA required Diapulse Corporation to remove its device from the market because the FDA subsequently asserted that the studies were "not well-designed, were not quantifiable and were not otherwise conducted under applicable and essential principles of adequate and well-controlled investigations."[60] In 1987 the FDA allowed the Diapulse Corporation to begin marketing the device with a shortwave diathermy classification "b," which has led to some confusion. Neither the Diapulse Corporation nor Electropharmacology, Inc., the manufacturer of the MRT sofPulse (another PFR device deemed by the FDA to be substantially equivalent to Diapulse) make any claims indicating that heat is a mechanism of action. In 1992 Mayrovitz and Larsen[61] reported that the sofPulse PRFE device produced elevated skin temperature changes and a statistically significant increase in blood perfusion in forearm skin microvasculature of nine healthy subjects. The average 1.8°C rise in skin temperature occurred gradually during the first 30 minutes of a 40-minute treatment, whereas the 29 percent mean increase in perfusion was measured at 40 minutes of treatment. Note that the 1.8°C temperature increase was not detected at the subcutaneous target site. Although a thermal cutaneous response was recorded, the authors suggest that nonthermal mechanisms may have contributed to the increased blood flow because the largest increase in skin temperature occurred within 5 minutes of treatment, while the perfusion increase was not observed until 40 minutes into treatment. Interestingly, a 1991 report described arteriole dilatation in the frog web space following exposure to 10 MHz RF applied at 10,000 pps.[62] The generator provided 1 V, which induced a 7.3-milligauss (mG), 2.19-V cm EM field, which did not cause tissue heating. The authors attributed the vasodilatory effect to facilitation of Ca^{2+} outflow from the smooth-muscle plasma membrane and/or Ca^{2+} influx into the sarcoplasmic membrane. More about the purported effects of PRFE are discussed later in this chapter.

At the present time the FDA Center for Devices and Radiological Health categorizes "nonthermal" PRFE devices as class III, a classification that "regulates devices for which insufficient information exists to assure that general controls and performance standards provide reasonable assurance of safety and effectiveness."[63] On the other hand, PSWD and CSWD devices that induce significant levels of thermal energy in tissues are considered by the FDA as class II, a classification that "regulates devices for which general controls alone are insufficient to assure safety and effectiveness and for which existing information is sufficient to establish a performance standard that provides this assurance."[63] The parameters and characteristics that distinguish class II (thermal) from class III (athermal) devices are discussed next.

Generation of PRFE

Like PSWD, PRFE is produced by using a timing circuit to interrupt the 27 MHz RF waves so that the output is turned on and off at preset intervals, allowing bursts of pulse trains to be emitted from the PRFE treatment applicator. The pulse train duration, or "on time," is usually separated by a longer-lasting "off time" (see Fig. 8–12). Some PRFE devices allow the clinician some choice of pulse durations, while others provide a fixed pulse duration. The pulse frequency or the pulse repetition rate can be varied and determines the duration of the off time between pulses. Thus, within each burst or pulse train is a series of high-frequency sine-wave oscillations. At a continuous RF of 27.12 MHz, there are 27.12×10^6 cycles in 1 s and 27.12 cycles in 1 μs. Therefore, for class III PRFE devices with fixed 65-μs pulse durations like sofPulse and Diapulse, each burst or pulse train contains 1762.8 oscillations. At a maximum frequency of 600 pulses per second (pps), each complete period lasts 1,666.66 μs (1.7 ms); therefore, the interval between successive pulses would be 1601.66 μs. At 400 pps, each period lasts 2500 μs (2.5 ms) and the interval between successive pulses is 2435 μs. At 600 pps, the duty cycle is 65/1666 = 0.039, or less than 4 percent, while at 400 pps, the duty cycle is 65/2500 = 0.026, or less than 2.6 percent. Thus, with devices such as sofPulse and Diapulse, which have a fixed pulse duration, when the peak pulse power is preset, an increase in the pulse frequency from a minimum of 80 pps toward the maximum of 600 pps will increase the mean power accordingly.

As with PSWD devices, with PRFE devices, the power driving the applicator coil does not represent the level of absorbed power in the tissues. The power driving the applicator coil can be measured either as peak pulse power, which for Diapulse and sofPulse ranges from 185 to 975 W, or as mean power, which (for both devices) is much lower, ranging from 7.5 to 38 W. These values are determined by the settings of peak power and pulse frequency. Since 38 W or more of mean power is used as a measure of the heating effect for PSWD, less than 38 W mean power driving the coil applicator is used as an indicator of minimal or no heating effect for PRFE. Since both the sofPulse and Diapulse devices are described and categorized as class III, neither device (according to the FDA class III definition) is supposed to induce any significant tissue-heating effect, even at the highest peak power and pulse frequency settings. If transient, imperceptible heating with these devices does occur with each pulse, there should be no accumulative heating effect as long as perfusing blood dissipates the thermal energy.

As previously mentioned, the peak and mean power output from PSWD and PRFE generators is measured in watts and can be varied by adjusting the power output control on the device operation panel. Also, with a PRFE device like sofPulse, the pulse frequency can be varied between 80 and 600 times per second. Therefore, at 600 pps the maximum amount of time the EM signal is "on" and being delivered to the tissue is 4 percent of the total treatment time, which is generally between 15 and 45 minutes. Thus, in a typical tissue load being treated with a PRFE device like sofPulse, the dosage of the magnetic field is determined by settings of power amplitude, pulse frequency, and total daily exposure time. The manufacturers of sofPulse define the therapeutic input to the tissues as the magnetic field and associated electric field and current density in the tissues. Thus, for a PRFE device like sofPulse, the treatment applicator output in air does not represent the signals produced in the tissues. Figure 8–15 shows that the magnitude of the magnetic field is between approximately 1 and

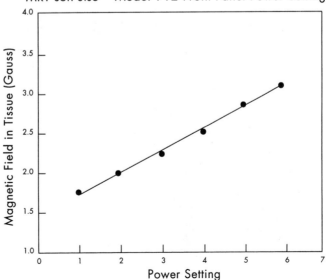

Dependence of Tissue Level Magnetic Field on
MRT sofPulse™ Model 912 Front Panel Power Setting

FIGURE 8–15. With the sof-Pulse PRFE device having a fixed-pulse duration (65 μ/s) and fixed-pulse frequency (600 pps), the level of the magnetic field in a tissue model (saline) increases linearly with successive increases in RMS pulse power.

4 G in a tissue model (saline) for the sofPulse 912 with successive increases in power output.[59] In comparison, the earth's magnetic field is approximately 0.4 G. In the saline tissue equivalent model, the maximum peak power density is approximately 1 W/cm^2 and the maximum average power density at 600 pps is 40 mW/cm^2. This level of power density is certainly less than the power density in nonhomogeneous tissue in which average resistivities are higher.

Transmitting Nonthermal Pulsed RF Energy to the Patient

PRFE is introduced into the tissues of the body with the inductive or magnetic field method of application using a drum-type applicator. Like the drum applicator used for PSWD, this applicator has a flat metal coil contained in a plastic-casing monode, which serves to space the drum surface away from the skin surface. This method of application induces oscillating electric "eddy" currents in tissues with the lowest impedance such as skin and superficial muscle. Since the mean power output is less than 38 W, there is little if any sensation of heat by the patient. Therefore, additional insulation with terry cloth is not necessary. However, for hygienic purposes it is good practice to cover the treatment drum prior to treatment with a clean elastic surgical cap (Fig. 8–16). The patient should be comfortably positioned and the purpose of the treatment explained. The surgical cap covering the drum is placed in light contact with the skin. The parameters for pulse power, pulse fre-

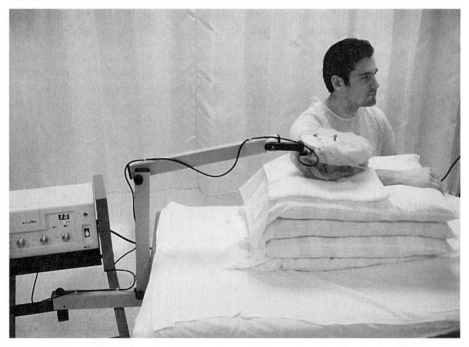

FIGURE 8–16. A PRF device (sofPulse) with surgical cap covering the drum treatment applicator.

quency, and treatment duration are set, and the device is activated to deliver the PRFE energy.

Putative Athermal Effects of PRFE

Most of the clinical reports related to athermal PRFE address its use in the treatment of wounds and soft-tissue injuries. Although reports on the efficacy of this form of RF energy in promoting tissue repair and resolution of the inflammatory reaction are conflicting, nevertheless, it seems that in theory, the explanation for the reported effects may occur at the cell membrane level. When cell injury occurs, there is some depolarization associated with cell dysfunction. It has been suggested that PRFE may help healing by repolarizing damaged cells. In addition, based on the proposition that the cell-membrane potential is involved in the control of cell division and cell proliferation, and that neurons and muscle cells (which have relatively high, stable membrane potentials) do not regenerate, perhaps such mechanisms could be favorably influenced by PRFE.[64] Barnothy[65] has noted that reactions of biologic materials following exposure to PRFE are delayed and, therefore, perhaps biologic changes are triggered. Another theory suggests that, during the inflammatory state, the action of the sodium pump is reduced, causing sodium to build up in the cell, which in turn causes a decrease in cell negativity. In this situation, it may be possible that under the influence of a magnetic field, the sodium pump is reactivated, which allows the cell to restore its own ionic balance.[66]

Thus, it is speculated that PRFE energy, through its specific waveform configuration, may modulate biologic processes by introducing a more accurate and effective dosage to injured tissues. Once the athermal RF signal reaches the target, the tissue response time and minimum amplitude requirements for nonthermal effects may be satisfied. In addition, the optimum modulation of biologic processes may depend on the biologic state of the target tissues. In any case, the electrochemical information transfer theory proposes a mechanism whereby the rate of ion or ligand binding to enzyme and/or receptor sites could be altered by high-frequency PRFE (3 to 30 MHz) or extremely low frequency PEMF (0 to 300 Hz), either or both acting to trigger the biochemical cascades necessary for cell function.[67,68] Indeed, within the high-frequency PRFE range, the primary frequency of 27.12 MHz is used in the treatment of pain and edema,[69-71] wound healing,[72] nerve regeneration,[73] and burns.[74] The primary PEMF frequency of 5 Hz is used to treat nonunion bone fractures,[75,76] avascular necrosis,[77] osteoporosis,[78] spinal fusions,[79] and tendinitis.[80] The 27.12 PRFE signal induces maximum electric fields in soft tissues in the volts per centimeter range, while the 5-Hz PEMF signal induces maximum electric fields in bone tissue in the millivolts per centimeter range. Comparison of the PRFE and PEMF signals shows that the PRF waveform is considerably broader band and therefore provides adequate amplitude over a wide frequency range, being detectable by both single cells (e.g., lymphocytes) and tissues like muscle and blood vessels. This suggests that PRFE signals may evoke a broader range of biologic and clinical effects than those elicited by PEMF signals.[81-83] PRFE and PEMF signals have been shown to have overlapping effects, as evidenced by their similar modulation of fibroblast cell activity in culture.[83,84]

Although the biophysical mechanism(s) is (are) are not completely understood, it seems that PRFE and PEMF athermal signals can have biologic effects that most likely occur at the cell membrane.[85]

Treatment and Dosage Considerations for PRFE

Recall that with thermal devices such as CSWD and PSWD, the dosage selected is based on using the patient's subjective heat-sensation response as a guide. Since patients with sensate skin do not experience heat sensation when they are treated with PRFE, heat sensation cannot be used as a guide based on patient response. With PRFE devices, all output setting combinations of pulse power and pulse frequency deliver energy that corresponds to dose I, that is, the lowest dose, just below the point of any sensation of heat. This dose is indicated for the treatment of acutely inflamed tissues that are painful and edematous. Later, when the condition resolves into the subacute phase, a low dose of very mild heat that is barely felt (dose II) would be indicated and could be applied with mean wattages from 38 to 80 using a PSWD device.

The scant amount of clinical research that deals with PRFE is not in agreement with the treatment parameters used with these devices. The following summaries of clinical trials bear this out.

Many scientific attempts have been made to demonstrate the efficacy of PRFE for therapeutic purposes. Some studies[86,87] have shown that the benefits of EM energy in deep tissues with PRFE and CSWD have similar therapeutic value. In one of these, Pasila and associates[86] compared two PRFE devices (1 hour/day for 3 days) with a placebo in the treatment of 300 ankle and foot sprains. In measurements of strength, joint range of motion, swelling, impairment of gait, and function of disability, they found little significant difference between the placebo group and those treated with PRFE. Barker and associates[88] also reported no significant differences between two groups of patients following PRFE treatment or placebo applications to acute ankle sprains with respect to range of motion, gait, pain, or swelling.

Wilson,[70,89] on the other hand, has demonstrated that PRFE reduced pain and disability in several acute ankle sprains significantly better than did CSWD treatment. In one study, Wilson[89] compared the nonthermal effects of PRFE with the placebo effects of PRFE. He assigned patients with recent inversion ankle sprains to two match-paired groups of 20. The treatment group received a 1-hour treatment of PRFE daily for 3 days. For these treatments, a PRFE device with a frequency of 27.12 MHz was set to provide a peak pulse power of 975 W for each 65-μs pulse. The off time interval between successive pulses was approximately 1600 μs. The control group received a 1-hour placebo treatment of PRFE daily for 3 days. Wilson reported that, statistically, symptoms of pain and disability were relieved more rapidly in the treatment than in the control group; however, there was no significant difference between the two groups regarding improvement in swelling. To assess the possibility that the beneficial effects observed in the treatment group might have resulted from an increase in blood flow owing to some small, transient degree of heating (which is the mode of action attributed to CSWD), a second clinical study was conducted to compare the effects of PRFE with CSWD.[70] The same number of patients with recent inversion ankle injuries were assigned in matched pairs to two groups and, depending on the group, received either a 1-hour treatment of PRFE or two 15-minute treatments within 1 hour of inductive CSWD daily for 3 days.

Analysis of the data revealed statistically significant differences—at the 1.0 percent level of confidence in reduction of swelling and at the 0.1 percent level in reduction of pain and disability—by PRFE compared with CSWD. In comparing total energy delivered to patients in the two groups, it was found that those treated with CSWD received approximately 22.5 watt-hours compared to 15 watt-hours received by patients treated with PRFE. The fact that better clinical responses were produced with less energy was interpreted by Wilson[89] as support for the idea that beneficial results occurred because of specific nonthermal effects. It is widely accepted, however, that heat applied in the early stages following soft-tissue trauma may exacerbate the inflammatory response to injury. Thus, it is possible that patients in this study who were treated with heat either did not improve or got worse, whereas those who received PRFE would have improved spontaneously without any treatment. This question could have been resolved if the design of the study had included a control group.

An improvement in the rate of soft-tissue healing has also been reported following studies with PRFE in the treatment of surgical wounds from dental and podiatric procedures. In 90 patients who had had dental surgery, Aronofsky[90] treated 30 with PRFE preoperatively and postoperatively, 30 others only postoperatively, and 30 served as controls. Patients in both treatment groups reportedly exhibited substantially less time for their wounds to heal compared to wounds of patients in the control group. In a double-blind study of 100 patients who received a variety of podiatric surgical procedures, Kaplan and Weinstock[91] randomly applied placebo or actual PRFE treatments to the surgical site. They anecdotally reported significant reductions in postoperative edema, erythema, and pain in patients who received real PRFE treatments, compared to those who received placebo. More recently, in a randomized, prospective, double-blind study of 50 grade I and II sprained ankles, Pennington and coworkers[69] reported finding a statistically significant decrease in edema following one treatment with a PRFE device.

Golden and associates[92] conducted a controlled double-blind clinical study, which compared treatment of donor sites of medium-thickness split grafts with PRFE versus control-donor sites treated with a placebo of PRFE. Patients in both groups received one 30-minute treatment before receiving medication before surgery and then received a 1-hour treatment daily for 7 days after surgery. The group treated with the real PRFE device was treated at a peak generated power output of 975 W and a frequency of 400 pps. With a pulse duration of 65 μs, the mean power output was 25.3 W. Wounds were evaluated daily by medical staff who were unaware of the patients' grouping. On the seventh postoperative day, dressings were removed and the percentage of wound area healed was determined. In the real PRFE treatment group, 17 of 29 patients had wounds that were healed 90 percent or more, compared with only 11 of 38 patients in the placebo group. Data analysis revealed that this difference was statistically significant. Cameron[93] also reported favorable results in surgical wound healing during a double-blind clinical study in which 100 patients were assigned either to a PRFE placebo group or to a real PRFE treatment group. In addition, the effects of PRFE on healing of induced wounds in animals reportedly reduced edema faster in treated than control wounds[94] and significantly accelerated reabsorption of hematomas.[71,95] Other studies in which PRFE was used to treat induced full-thickness skin wounds or burn wounds in an animal model showed no significant difference in healing time or tissue strength between treatment and control wounds.[94]

Other studies related to PRFE have been published, especially those done with animal models.[96,97] PRFE applied to nerve-damaged rats resulted in quicker regeneration, as well as earlier wound healing, compared with results from a control group, according to Wilson and associates.[96] They also noted considerably more scarring and fibrosis around the nerve-suture site in the control group. Following injections of a myotoxic drug into the gastrocneumius muscle in rabbits, Brown and Baker[97] found no significant differences between a control group and a group treated with PRFE.

Despite the positive clinical outcomes reported in the literature for PRFE, additional controlled clinical studies are needed to establish the efficacy and effectiveness of this modality before it can be considered as a viable treatment for managing soft-tissue injury or enhancing pain relief.

In summary, the main effects reported following treatment with PRFE radiation include reduced inflammation, reabsorption of hematoma, reduced edema, increased rate of soft-tissue repair, increased nerve growth and repair, and reduced pain.

Contraindications and Precautions to Clinical Use of PRFE

Since there is no significant tissue-heating effect with PRFE devices, there is no danger of burning tissue because of a concentration of the EM field by metal or moisture on or in the tissues. Therefore, PRFE can be applied to tissues containing metal implants and to wounds with moist dressings. Keep in mind that this applies to PRFE devices having a mean generated power output that does not exceed 38 W. No adverse effects of any kind have been reported to date with PRFE. Nevertheless, because the nonthermal mechanism(s) by which PRFE acts on the cell membrane are not clearly delineated, it is considered prudent to avoid applying this form of EM energy over cancerous tissues and the pregnant uterus. Because these devices may cause electromagnetic interference of electromedical and/or electronic devices, as was discussed for diathermy, the therapist should avoid applying PRFE over or near externally worn or implanted electronic devices such as unshielded cardiac pacemakers/monitors, electrophrenic pacers, and cerebellar and urinary bladder stimulators.

CASE STUDY 3

A 20-year-old female college basketball player in good health sustained a left lateral ankle sprain 2 hours ago. She has no previous history of ankle sprain. Treatment included ice pack, elevation, and compression during last 2 hours. X-ray has ruled out fracture.

PROBLEM

1. Pain and swelling in left lateral ankle.
2. Unable to bear weight on left lower extremity (LLE).

DECISION MAKING/CHOICE OF TREATMENT

Consider the following choices:

1. Continue treatment with ice, elevation, compression.
2. Cold whirlpool 15 minutes followed by effleurage massage.
3. PRFE.

TREATMENT GOAL/DESCRIPTION

1. Reduce ankle swelling and pain and increase ankle function.
2. Position patient supine with LLE supported and elevated 30 degrees.
3. Apply PRFE drum applicator to within 0.5 cm from edematous ankle tissues.
4. Set PRFE controls at 585 W of peak pulse power, a pulse duration of 65 μs, a pulse frequency of 600 pps, giving a mean power output of 22.8 W.
5. Treat 30 minutes daily for 2 weeks or until volume displacement measurements show significant reduction in swelling and pain.

SUMMARY

Either CSWD or PSWD may be used to produce a rise in tissue temperature within the therapeutically desirable thermal range of 37.5°C to 44°C. The depth of penetration and extent of temperature rise depend on wave frequency, the electrical properties of the tissue(s) receiving the EM energy, and the type of applicator used. Either mild or vigorous heating may be produced. Mild heating is usually desired in acute musculoskeletal conditions, whereas vigorous heating may be needed in chronic conditions.[23] Non-thermal effects may be produced by PRFE when this form of EM energy is delivered to the body at mean power values less than 38 W. When PRFE is used at mean power values above 38 W mild to moderate heating occurs. This means that PRFR may be used either in acute or in subacute conditions, where minimal to moderate heat is desirable, or in conditions that require enhancement of tissue healing by nonthermal effects.

Various conditions for which CSWD, PSWD, and PRFE are beneficial are discussed. Contraindications for these types of RF energy are also presented.

Study Objectives

Having completed this chapter, the reader should now be able to:

1. Define diathermy.
2. Discuss magnetic field and electric field applications of diathermy.
3. Define dielectric and its relevance to diathermy.
4. Describe the electrodes used for diathermy application.
5. Describe how PRFR is generated.
6. Discuss the clinical uses of PRFR.
7. Define PRFE.
8. Describe contraindicators and precautions to the use of CSWD, PSWD, and PRFE.

REFERENCES

1. Schwan, HP and Piersol, GM: The absorption of electromagnetic energy in body tissues, Part I. Am J Phys Med 33:371, 1954.
2. Schwan, HP and Piersol, GM: The absorption of electromagnetic energy in body tissues, Part II. Am J Phys Med 34:425, 1995.
3. Wilkening, GM and Sutton, CH: Health effects of nonionizing radiation. Environ Med 74(2):489, 1990.

4. Yost, MG: Nonionizing Radiation Questions and Answers. San Francisco Press, Inc. San Francisco, 1993, p 2.
5. Diathermy Units, Microwave: Diathermy Units, Shortwave. In Product Comparison System. ECRI, Plymouth Meeting, PA, March, 1988, p 1–10.
6. van den Bouwhuijsen, F, et al: A Manual on Pulsed and Continuous Shortwave Diathermy: ENRAF-NONIUS, cat. no. 1419.762, Delft, Holland.
7. Millard, JB: Effect of high frequency currents and infra-red rays on the circulation of the lower limb in man. Ann Phys Med 6:45, 1961.
8. McNiven, DR and Wyper, DJ: Microwave therapy and muscle blood flow in man. J Microwave Power 11:168, 1976.
9. Harris, R: Effect of shortwave diathermy on radio-sodium clearance from the knee joint in the normal and in rheumatoid arthritis. Phys Med Rehabil 42:241, 1961.
10. Low, J and Reed, A (eds): Electrotherapy Explained: Principles and Practice. Butterworth/Heinemann, Oxford, 1992, p 230.
11. Ward, AR: Electricity Fields and Waves in Therapy. Science Press, Marrickville, NSW, Australia, 1986, p 166.
12. Schwan, HP: Biophysics of Diathermy. In Licht, S (ed): Therapeutic Heat and Cold. Waverly Press, Baltimore, 1965, p 116.
13. Scott, BO: Shortwave Diathermy. In Licht, S (ed): Therapeutic Heat and Cold. Waverly Press, Baltimore, 1965, p 295.
14. Guy, AW: Biophysics of High Frequency Currents and Electromagnetic Radiation. In Lehman, JF (ed): Therapeutic Heat and Cold. Williams & Wilkins, Baltimore, 1982, p 259.
15. Griffin, JE and Karselis, TC: Principles of Instrumentation. In Griffin, JE and Karselis, TC: Physical Agents for Physical Therapists, ed 2. Charles C Thomas, Springfield, IL, 1982, p 202.
16. Shortwave Diathermy Units. Health Devices, 175, June, 1979.
17. Lehmann, JF, et al: Review of evidence for indications, techniques of application, contraindications, hazards and clinical effectiveness for shortwave diathermy. DHEW/FDA HFA-510, Rockville, MD, 1974.
18. Thom, H: Introduction to Shortwave and Microwave Therapy, ed 3. Charles C Thomas, Springfield, IL, 1966, p 46.
19. Lehmann, JF, et al: Comparison of relative heating patterns produced in tissues by exposure to microwave energy at frequencies of 2450 and 900 megacycles. Arch Phys Med Rehabil 46:307, 1965.
20. Schliephake, E: Carrying out treatment. In Thom, H: Introduction to Shortwave and Microwave Therapy, ed 3. Charles C Thomas, Springfield, IL, 1966, p 65.
21. Hayne, CR: Pulsed high frequency energy: Its place in physiotherapy. Physiotherapy 70:459, 1984.
22. Warren, CG, Lehmann, JF, and Koblanski, NJ: Heat and stretch procedures: An evaluation using rat tail tendon. Arch Phys Med Rehabil 57:122, 1976.
23. Lehmann, JF: Therapeutic Heat and Cold, ed 4. Williams & Wilkins, Baltimore, 1990, p 470.
24. Lehmann, JF, Warren, CG, and Scham, SM: Therapeutic heat and cold. Clin Orthop 99:207, 1974.
25. Fischer, C and Solomon, S: Physiological responses to heat and cold. In Licht, S (ed): Therapeutic Heat and Cold. Elizabeth Licht, New Haven, 1965, p 127.
26. Abramson, DI: Physiologic basis for the use of physical agents in peripheral vascular disorders. Arch Phys Med Rehabil 46:216, 1965.
27. Wise, CS: The effect of diathermy on blood flow. Arch Phys Med Rehabil 29:17, 1948.
28. Allberry, J: Shortwave diathermy for herpes zoster. Physiotherapy 60:386, 1974.
29. Barnett, M: SWD for herpes zoster. Physiotherapy 61:217, 1975.
30. Sandler, B: Heat and the U.U.C.D. Br Med J 25:458, 1973.
31. Nielsen, NC, et al: Heat induction in copper-bearing IUD's during shortwave diathermy. Acta Obstet Gynecol Scand 58:495, 1979.
32. Jones, SL: Electromagnetic field interference and cardiac pacemakers. Phys Ther 56:1013, 1976.
33. Smyth, H: The pacemaker patient and the electromagnetic environment. JAMA 227:1412, 1974.
34. Konarska, I and Michniewicz, L: Shortwave therapy of diseases of the anterior portion of the eye. Klin Oczna 25:185, 1955.
35. Daily, L, et al: The effects of microwave diathermy on the eye. Am J Ophthalmol 33:1241, 1950.
36. Daily, L, Jr, et al: Influence of microwaves on certain enzyme systems in the eye. Am J Ophthalmol 34:1301, 1951.
37. Richardson, AW, Duane, TH, and Haines, HM: Experimental lenticular opacities produced by microwave irradiation. Arch Phys Med 29:765, 1948.
38. Richardson, AW, et al: The role of energy, pupillary diameter and alloxan diabetes in the production of ocular damage by microwave irradiations. Am J Ophthalmol 35:993, 1952.
39. Scott, BO: Effect of contact lenses on shortwave field distribution. Br J Ophthalmol 40:696, 1956.
40. Hollander, JL, et al: Joint temperature measurement in evaluation of antiarthritic agents. J Clin Invest 30:701, 1951.
41. Harris, E, Jr and McCroskery, PA: Influence of temperature and fibril stability on degradation of cartilage collagen by rheumatoid synovial collagenase. N Engl J Med 290:1, 1974.
42. Harris, ED (ed): Rheumatoid Arthritis. MEDCOM Press, New York, 1974.

43. Feibel, H and Fast, H: Deep heating of joints: A reconsideration. Arch Phys Med Rehabil 57:513, 1976.
44. Ely, TS, et al: Heating characteristics of laboratory animals exposed to ten centimeter microwaves. US Navy Med Res Inst (Res Rep Proj NM 001-156.1302) IEEE Tran Biomed Eng 11:123, 1964.
45. Gorodetskaya, SF: The effect of centimeter radio waves on mouse fertility. Fiziol Zh 9:394, 1963.
46. Imig, CJ and Free, JR: Testicular degeneration as a result of microwave irradiation. Proc Soc Exp Biol Med 69:382, 1948.
47. Van Demark, NL and Free, MJ: Temperature effects. In Johnson, AD, et al (eds): The Testis, Vol 3. Academic Press, New York, 1973, p 254.
48. Smith, DW, Clarren, SK, and Harvey, MAS: Hyperthermia as a possible teratogenic agent. J Pediatr 92:878, 1978.
49. Dietzel, F: Effects of non-ionizing electromagnetic radiation on the development and intrauterine implantation of the rat. In Tyler, AE (ed): Biological Effects of Nonionizing Radiation. Ann NY Acad Sci 247:367, 1975.
50. Ouellet-Hellstrom, R and Stewart, WF: Miscarriages among female physical therapists who report using radio- and microwave-frequency electromagnetic radiation. Am J Epidemiology 138(10):775, 1993.
51. Havey, MAS, McRorie, MM, and Smith, DW: Suggested limits of exposure in the hot tub and sauna for the pregnant woman. Can Med Assoc J 125:50, 1981.
52. Paliwal, BR, et al: Heating patterns produced by 434 MHz erbotherm UHF69. Radiology 135:511, 1980.
53. Doyle, JR and Smart, BW: Stimulation of bone growth by shortwave diathermy. J Bone Joint Surg 45-A:15, 1963.
54. Hutchinson, WJ and Burdeaux, BD: The effects of shortwave diathermy on bone repair. J Bone Joint Surg 33-A:155, 1951.
55. Stuchly, MA, et al: Exposure to the operator and patient during shortwave diathermy treatments. Health Physics 42:341, 1982.
56. Progress Report. American Physical Therapy Association, June, 1980.
57. Kloth, LC, Morrison, M, and Ferguson, B: Therapeutic microwave and shortwave diathermy: A review of thermal effectiveness, safe use, and state-of-the-art, 1984. Center for Devices and Radiological Health, DHHS, FDA 85-8237, December, 1984.
58. Ginsberg, AJ: Ultra-short radio waves as a therapeutic agent. Med Rec 1:1, 1934.
59. Markov, M and Pilla, A: Personal communication, February, 1995.
60. Beardsley, DR: Division of Compliance Operations, Office of Medical Devices, National Center for Devices and Radiological Health. Letter to Solomon H. Friend (attorney for Diapulse Corporation, June 8, 1983).
61. Mayrovitz, HN and Larsen, PB: Effects of pulsed electromagnetic fields on skin microvascular blood perfusion. Wounds 4(5):197, 1992.
62. Miura, M and Okada, J: Nonthermal vasodilatation by radio frequency burst-type electromagnetic field radiation in the frog. J Physiol 435:257, 1991.
63. U.S. Department of Health and Human Services, FDA, Center for Devices and Radiological Health. Everything you always wanted to know about the medical devices amendments . . . and weren't afraid to ask, ed 3. HHS Pub 90-4173, 1990.
64. Low, JL: The nature and effects of pulsed electromagnetic radiations. NZ Physiother 6:18, 1978.
65. Barnothy, JM: Biological Effects of Magnetic Fields. Plenum Press, New York, 1964.
66. Sanseverino, EG: Membrane phenomena and cellular processes under action of pulsating magnetic fields. Presented at the Second International Congress for Magneto Medicine, Rome, November, 1980.
67. Pilla, AA: Electrochemical information transfer at living cell membranes. Ann NY Acad Sci 238:149, 1974.
68. Chiabrera, A, et al: Electric and magnetic field effects on ligand binding to the cell membrane. In Chiabrera, A, Nicolini, C, and Schwan, HP (eds.): Interactions between Electromagnetic Fields and Cells. Plenum, New York, 1985, p 253.
69. Pennington, GM, Danley, DL, and Sumko, MH: Pulsed, non-thermal, high-frequency electromagnetic energy (DIAPULSE) in the treatment of grade I and grade II ankle sprains. Milit Med 158:101, 1993.
70. Wilson DH: Comparison of short wave diathermy and pulsed electromagnetic energy in treatment of soft tissue injuries. Physiotherapy (Br) 60:309, 1974.
71. Sambasivan, M: Pulsed electromagnetic field in management of head injuries. Neurol India 41(suppl):56, 1993.
72. Itoh, M, Montemayor, JS, and Matsumoto, E: Accelerated wound healing of pressure ulcers by pulsed high peak power electromagnetic energy (Diapulse). Decubitus 2:24, 1991.
73. Raji, ARM, and Bowden, REM: Effects of high peak pulsed electromagnetic field on the degeneration and regeneration of the common peroneal nerve in rats. J Bone Joint Surg 65:478, 1983.
74. Ionescu, A, et al: Study of efficiency of diapulse therapy on the dynamics of enzymes in burned wound. Sixth Intl. Congress on Burns, San Francisco, 6:25, 1982.
75. Sharrard, WJW: A double-blind trial of pulsed electromagnetic fields for delayed union of tibial fractures. J Bone Joint Surg 72B:347, 1990.
76. Basset, CAL, Pilla, AA, and Pawluk, RJ: A non-surgical salvage of surgically-resistant pseudoarthroses and non-unions by pulsing electromagnetic fields. Clin Orthop 124:117, 1977.
77. Aaron, RK, et al: The conservative treatment of osteonecrosis of the femoral head. A comparison of core decompression and pulsing electromagnetic fields. Clin Orthop 249:209, 1989b.

78. Tabrah, F, et al: Bone density changes in osteoporosis-prone women exposed to pulsed electromagnetic fields. J Bone Min Res 5:437, 1990.
79. Mooney, V: A randomized double-blind prospective study of the efficacy of pulsed electromagnetic fields for interbody lumbar fusions. Spine 15:708, 1990.
80. Binder, A, et al: Pulsed electromagnetic field therapy of persistent rotator cuff tendinitis. Lancet 8379:695, 1984.
81. Pilla, AA, Sechaud, P, and McLeod, BR: Electrochemical and electromagnetic aspect of low frequency electromagnetic current induction in biological systems. J Biol Phys 11:51, 1983.
82. Conti, P, et al: A role for calcium in the effect of very low frequency electromagnetic fields on the blastogenesis of human lymphocytes. FEBS Lett 181:28, 1985.
83. Murray, JC and Farndale, RW: Modulation of collagen production in cultured fibroblasts by a low frequency, pulsed magnetic field. Biochim Biophys Acta 838:98, 1985.
84. Bourguignon, GJ and Bourguignon, LYW: Electric stimulation of protein and DNA synthesis in human fibroblasts. FASEB J 1:398, 1987.
85. Blank, M (ed): Electricity and Magnetism in Biology and Medicine, San Francisco Press, San Francisco, 1993.
86. Pasila, M, Visuri, T, and Sandholdm, A: Pulsating shortwave diathermy: Value in treatment of recent ankle and foot sprains. Arch Phys Med Rehabil 59:383, 1978.
87. Silverman, DR and Pendlton, L: A comparison of the effects of continuous and pulsed short-wave diathermy on peripheral circulation. Arch Phys Med Rehabil 49:429, 1968.
88. Barker, AT, et al: A double-blind clinical trial of lower power pulsed shortwave therapy in the treatment of a soft tissue injury. Physiotherapy 71(12):500, 1985.
89. Wilson, DH: Treatment of soft-tissue injuries by pulsed electrical energy. Br Med J 2:269, 1972.
90. Aronofsky, DH: Reduction of dental post-surgical symptoms using nonthermal pulsed high-peak power electromagnetic energy. Oral Surg 32(5):688, 1971.
91. Kaplan, EG and Weinstock, RE: Clinical evaluation of Diapulse as adjunctive therapy following foot surgery. J Am Podiatry Assoc 58(5):218, 1968.
92. Golden, JH, et al: The effects of Diapulse on the healing of wounds: A double-blind randomized controlled trial in man. Br J Plast Surg 34:267, 1981.
93. Cameron, BM: Experimental acceleration of wound healing. Am J Orthop 53:336, 1961.
94. Constable, JD, Scapicchio, AP, and Opitz, B: Studies of the effects of Diapulse treatment of various aspects of wound healing in experimental animals. J Surg Res 11(5):254, 1971.
95. Fenn, JE: Effect of pulsed electromagnetic energy (Diapulse) on experimental hematomas. Can Med Assoc J 100:251, 1969.
96. Wilson, DH, et al: The effects of pulsed electromagnetic energy on peripheral nerve regeneration. Ann NY Acad Sci 238:575, 1975.
97. Brown, M and Baker, RD: Effect of pulsed shortwave diathermy on skeletal muscle injury in rabbits. Phys Ther 67:208, 1987.

CHAPTER 9

Therapeutic Uses of Light in Rehabilitation

Lynn Snyder-Mackler, ScD, PT, SCS
Stacie L. Collender, PT

The healing properties of light have been described since ancient Roman times. Light has been used in physical therapy to treat many disorders. This chapter will discuss the use of two forms of light in rehabilitation: low-power laser and ultraviolet light.

LASER

Laser is an acronym for *l*ight *a*mplification by *s*timulated *e*mission of *r*adiation.[1] Radiation is the process by which energy is propagated through space.[2] The common characteristics of all forms of radiant energy are as follows: (1) They are produced by applying electrical or other forces to various forms of matter; (2) they all may be transmitted without the support of a sensible medium; and (3) their velocity of travel is equal in a vacuum, but may vary within different media. The direction of propagation is normally a straight line; they undergo reflection, deflection, and absorption by the media through which they travel. They are designated collectively as electromagnetic radiations. A laser is generally used as a source or generator of radiation.[3] The low-power laser is used in physical rehabilitation for pain control and soft-tissue healing.

The objectives of this section are to: (1) Establish a basic understanding of the physical principles of therapeutic laser; (2) delineate the differences between low- and high-power laser as therapeutic modalities; (3) present the clinical application of laser in physical therapy for wound healing and pain management; and (4) discuss the contraindications, precautions, and guidelines for the safe and proposed use of laser in physical therapy.

BACKGROUND ON LASER

The reader should understand how laser is produced and what makes it unique from other forms of light before its use as a therapeutic agent is discussed. Einstein proposed the concept of stimulated emission as it related to the atom and its component parts.[4,5] Einstein reasoned that a stimulus can cause the electron configuration of an atom to be momentarily rearranged. In returning to its original configuration, surplus energy will be released in the form of a photon, the basic unit of light. This massless particle, in turn, can release a photon from every pre-excited atom or molecule with which it collides. A chain reaction is initiated, and the stimulated emission of radiation occurs.[4]

Beginning in 1953, an interest in stimulated emission reappeared with the advent of microwave amplification.[5,6] Microwave radiations are wavelengths that possess optic properties; that is, they can be refracted, diffracted, and reflected, and can be focused by suitable lenses.[2] With the development of masers (*m*icrowave *a*mplifiers by the *s*timulated *e*mission of *r*adiation), speculation arose concerning the possibility of extending this principle into amplification and generation in the region of visible radiation.

Schawlaw and Townes reportedly presented the feasibility of producing stimulated emission in the microwave wavelength area near the optic regions of the spectrum.[7] Their work, considered to be the impetus for the initial discoveries of all types of lasers, turned out to be surprisingly accurate in predicting the size, wavelength range, and output power for typical gas lasers having moderate input-power-excitation requirements.[8] (However, it did not propose the use of a gas discharge for excitation of atomic components.[9])

Two years later, Maiman successfully produced the first working model of the ruby laser.[6] Javan, Bennett, and Herriott discovered the helium-neon (HeNe) laser in the fall of 1960.[6] The discovery of visible red laser output at 623.8 nanometers (nm) by White and Rigden occurred in early 1962.[10] This work generated interest in other possible applications for the laser that were in the infrared, noninvisible emission range.[9]

PHYSICAL PRINCIPLES OF LASER

When a photon, or energy particle of light, is directed at an atom, it may be absorbed, reflected, or transmitted. If the particle is reflected or transmitted, no light-energy change occurs. If the photon is absorbed, however, energy in the orbital electrons is increased. One or more electrons undergo a positional change from an inner orbit to a more peripheral orbit. The affected atom will have gained energy and is then said to be "excited."[9]

Excited atoms are unstable and will seek their ground state in random fashion, after a short time, without further external stimulation. This phenomenon produces spontaneous emission of light. If allowed to reach its end, this process will prevent the energy-transfer level necessary for laser radiation. If, however, a photon of appropriate energy strikes an atom while it is maintained in an excited state, the atom is immedi-

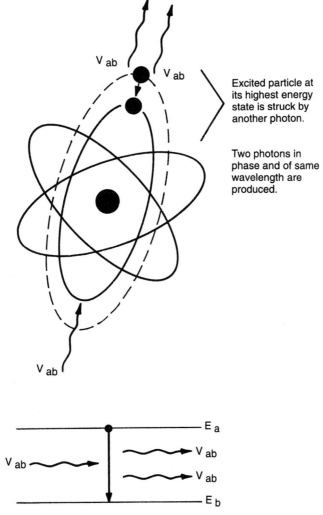

FIGURE 9–1. The principle of stimulated emission. Two photons are emitted from orbit when another photon strikes (E_a, E_b = electrons; V_{ab} = energy photons.)

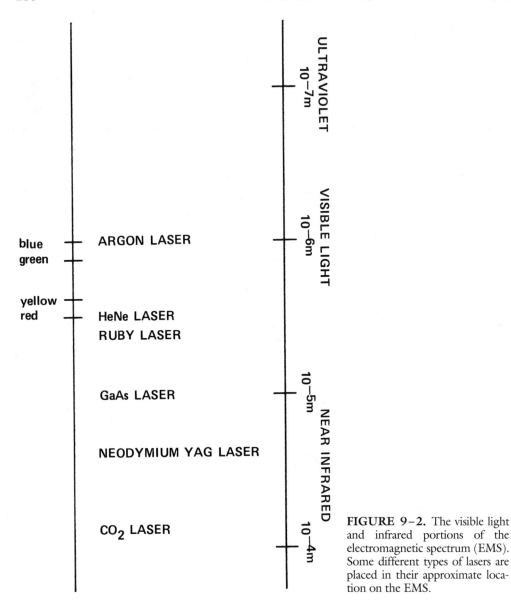

FIGURE 9–2. The visible light and infrared portions of the electromagnetic spectrum (EMS). Some different types of lasers are placed in their approximate location on the EMS.

ately stimulated to emit its excess energy and make its transition to the ground state. This process is called *stimulated emission*. The emitted photon is an amplification of stimulating radiation[9] (Fig. 9–1). Laser is a special form of electromagnetic energy that is within the visible or infrared regions of the electromagnetic spectrum (Fig. 9–2).

In a laser, when electrons are stimulated by an external power source at a rapid rate, resultant photons are aligned in a reflecting chamber. When they hit a semipermeable silver resonating mirror, photons are reflected back to a reflecting mirror. The back-and-forth reflection of photons between two mirrors through the laser medium further amplifies that light (Fig. 9–3). This process continues as more and more photons are stimulated, until the chamber cannot contain the energy level. Photons are then ejected through the semipermeable mirror and out a fiber-optic cable. The fiber optic is a threadlike filament composed of glass that guides the stimulated photons by directing them to the surface to

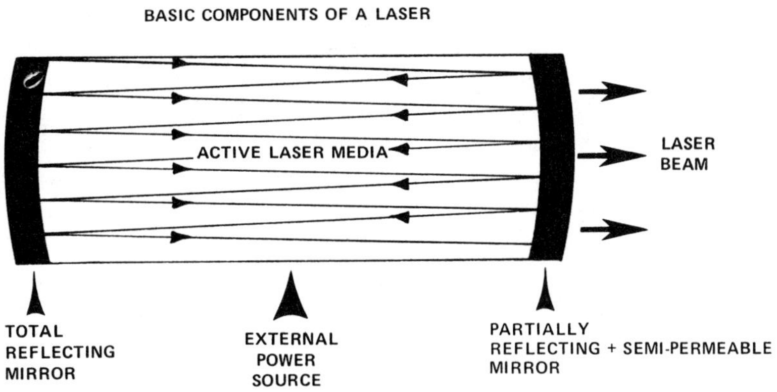

BASIC COMPONENTS OF A LASER

ACTIVE LASER MEDIA

LASER
BEAM

TOTAL
REFLECTING
MIRROR

EXTERNAL
POWER
SOURCE

PARTIALLY
REFLECTING + SEMI-PERMEABLE
MIRROR

FIGURE 9–3. Basic components of laser.

be treated. As photons pass through the cylindric stylus, some of the excited atoms in the reflecting chamber begin to revert back to their ground state. This previously mentioned process of spontaneous emissions creates a lower intensity of emitted photons to the tissue. Another type of laser uses a diode in the applicator tip rather than a fiber optic.

Basic Components of Laser

There are three properties of the laser that distinguish it from incandescent and fluorescent light sources: coherence, monochromaticity, and a collimated beam.

The property of coherence denotes several things. All of the photons of light emitted from individual gas molecules are of the same wavelength. The individual light waves are locked in step with another. Having the same phase, waves are said to be temporally coherent. Also, they are all traveling in the same direction; this is called *spatial coherence* (Fig. 9–4).

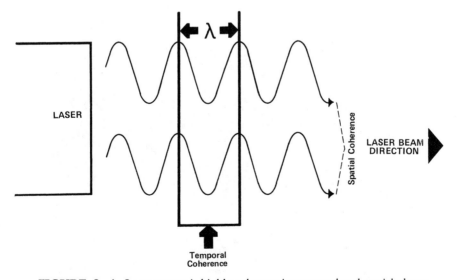

FIGURE 9–4. Laser energy is highly coherent in temporal and spatial planes.

When light is spatially coherent, it can be focused to a very small spot by a lens. Since light from a laser is similarly coherent, possible damage to the eyes can occur if that light is focused by the lens of the eye onto a small retinal spot.[11]

Monochromaticity refers to the specificity of light in a single, defined wavelength, which gives it added purity not found in most light sources. If this specificity is in the visible spectrum, it is of a single color. For example, HeNe produces a red light. A laser is one of the few light sources that produces a specific wavelength. The shorter the wavelength, the greater the purity of the light. HeNe has a 632.8-nm wavelength. Gallium arsenide (GaAs) has a wavelength of 910 nm.

The laser beam is well collimated. There is minimal divergence or moving apart of the photons.

Power is the rate at which energy is being produced and is measured in watts (joules per second [J/s]) or as a smaller unit, such as the milliwatt (mW) or 10^{-3} watts (W). If the laser produces one pulse per second, its average power, the amount of energy transferred in 1 second would be 0.001 J/1 s = 0.001 W, or 1 mW. When the average power of a laser is below that which causes tissue heating, it is called a low-power or "cold" laser.[12] It also may be referred to as a low-energy or "soft" laser.

Dosage is equal to the total energy delivered. Therefore, it is equal to the average power multiplied by the time of treatment. When using an HeNe laser (Fig. 9–5) in a chopped or pulsed mode, average power is approximately 0.45 mW.

Power density describes the concentration of power in a particular area. It is determined by power divided by area. A 1-mW laser source distributed over a 1-cm^2 area, therefore, has a power density of 1 milliwatt per square centimeter (1 mW/cm^2).

When the laser is focused on the epidermis, the amount of energy absorbed is proportional to the absorption quality of the tissue. Human epidermis absorbs approximately 99 percent of the laser radiation.[12] Laser energy absorption is greater with darker or pigmented tissues. As tissues are not homogenous, the quality of each structure produces a varying absorption of laser energy. The physiologic variability of the effect on the tissue also depends upon wavelength, energy, and exposure time. This will be elaborated on throughout the chapter.

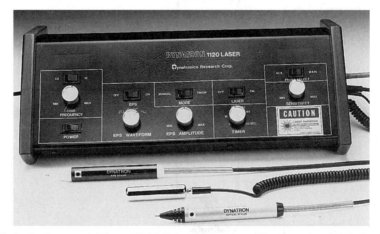

FIGURE 9–5. Dynatron 0.9 nm HeNe laser. (Courtesy of Dynatronics, Salt Lake City, UT.)

Classification of Laser

Laser can be classified as high-power or low-power (cold). At present, the most common image of laser radiation and its biologic effects is associated with damaging changes to cells and tissues through its thermal effects. This concept probably originated and was exaggerated by science fiction literature and movies. With the advent of the surgical laser, controlled heating and cutting have become more realistically associated with the device.

The different intensities of lasers are represented by different wavelengths. Tissue responses produced by a high-intensity laser are directly linked to intensity and include five effects: (1) elevation of tissue temperature; (2) dehydration of tissue; (3) coagulation of protein; (4) thermolysis; and (5) evaporation.

The magnitude of thermal reactions produced by high-intensity lasers depends on: (1) the absorption, reflection, and transmission of the tissues at the laser wavelength; (2) the power density of the laser beam; (3) the speed of incision or time of exposure; (4) the volume and the velocity of blood flow of local blood vessels; and (5) the degree of tension at the area of incision when cutting is used.

Lasers with powers less than 60 mW (a low-power laser) will cause minimal to no thermal response. Total optic illumination in most cases is limited to less than 50 mW at a total peak power or to less than 10 mW in a pulsed mode. At this low milliwattage, the laser beam does not even warm the tissues.

Effects of low-power laser are direct effects of irradiation rather than secondary effects of tissue heating. Low-energy laser systems have been used experimentally and have been suggested clinically to stimulate wound and fracture healing and to obtain analgesic effects. The low-energy systems used include HeNe and GaAs.

HELIUM-NEON (HeNe) LASER

Helium-neon laser is produced by a tube containing atoms of these two gases (see Fig. 9–5). The helium gas is elevated from the ground state to one of two excited states by electrical excitation. These states are a direct result of either stimulated or spontaneous emission. The atoms of the gas are in a vacuum chamber and are stimulated with a special light called a flash gun. The excited levels of the helium atom very closely approximate ground-state levels of the neon atom. When an excited helium atom collides with a ground-state neon atom, the energy produced is transferred to the latter, and the helium reverts to the ground state.

The wavelength of helium-neon laser is 632.8 nm (within the red band of visible light). It is directed toward the tissue in a pulsed or continuous mode by a fiber optic.[5] The helium-neon depth of penetration is up to 0.8 mm directly and from 10 to 15 mm indirectly. Direct penetration refers to the characteristic properties of laser that have not been altered. In indirect penetration, the light is transmitted into the deeper tissues through hyperscopic absorption properties of the surrounding tissue. Once this occurs, the coherent and collimated properties of laser are altered. Therefore, the difference between the two depths may be due to the dispersion of light in tissue.

GALLIUM ARSENIDE (GaAs) LASER

The first "semiconductor" laser, used in 1962, was the gallium arsenide laser. This laser is housed in a diode (Fig. 9–6). A diode is an electrical component that allows

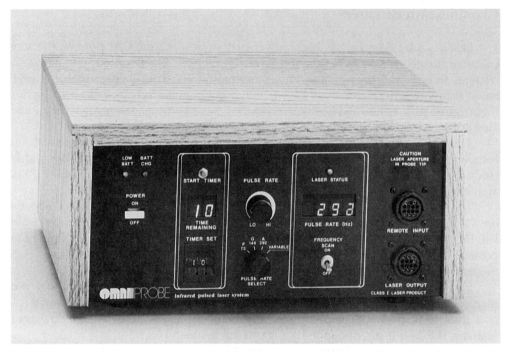

FIGURE 9–6. Omniprobe 0.9 mW infrared laser. (Courtesy of Physio Technology, Inc., Topeka, KS.)

electric current to pass in one direction through the device, offering high electrical resistance in the reverse direction. Using GaAs, upon which has been deposited a thin coating of zinc, a junction diode may be formed. This design allows the current to flow more readily in the direction from the zinc to the GaAs. The laser reaction occurs in this junction region. The energy is delivered in the pulsed mode.

One further difference between the two low-powered lasers is that the indirect depth of tissue penetration of the GaAs output is 5 cm, compared with that of the HeNe laser, which is 10 to 15 mm. At a wavelength of 910 nm, GaAs is within the infrared for invisible spectrum.

COMBINATION LASERS

Combination lasers have also been developed. An example is one where five GaAs emitters surround a HeNe source. The GaAs output has a peak power of 10 W pulsed at a frequency of 3800 Hz for an average power of 4 mW. The HeNe output is continuous at a peak output of 5 mW. As one would expect, the applicator is quite a bit larger for the combination laser than for the single-source types.

BIOPHYSICAL EFFECTS OF LASER

The investigation into the biologic and physical effects of cold laser radiation is still in its early stages. Some of the *preliminary proposed* physiologic effects attributed to low-power laser energy include an acceleration in collagen synthesis, an increase in vascularization of healing tissue, a decrease in microorganisms, and pain reduction. Much of the work reported to date is empirical observation, which can serve as a foundation for the design of well-controlled laboratory and clinical studies on the bioeffects of laser irradiation.

Tissue Healing

In laboratory studies with animal models, exposure to low-power laser was reported to accelerate phagocytosis, facilitate collagen synthesis, and increase wound closure and contracture. Mester and colleagues[16] studied the effect of ruby laser on *Staphylococcus aureus*, a gram-positive bacteria. Blood was obtained from human subjects and rats. The rate of phagocytosis of the bacteria was accelerated by the application of the laser.

Mester and Jaszsagi-Nagy[17] examined the effects of nonthermal laser on collagen synthesis in induced wounds in rats. Bilateral symmetric wounds were induced in the hindquarters of Wistar rats. One wound of each pair was irradiated. Analysis was completed 72 hours after surgery. The authors reported greater collagen synthesis in the laser-irradiated wounds than in the untreated site.

Cummings[18] studied the effect of HeNe laser irradiation on induced hindlimb wounds in rats. Rats were divided into three groups: daily laser treatment, every-other-day treatment, and sham laser. The rats that received laser achieved wound closure before those that received sham laser. The rats that received every-other-day treatment healed the most rapidly. The result of this study suggests that there might be an optimal dosage.

Kana and associates[19] examined the effect of HeNe and argon laser on wound healing in rats. An acceleration of wound healing was noted in the 4 per cm^2 per day groups, as compared to the higher-power laser group or controls.

Dyson and Young[20] studied the effects of varying frequencies of laser stimulation on wound contracture in mice. Treatment with 700-Hz laser increased the rate of wound contracture, total cell count, and the number of fibroblasts, as compared to 1200-Hz laser and a control group.

Braverman and associates[21] studied the effect of HeNe, infrared, and combined HeNe and infrared laser irradiation on wound healing in rabbits. All three experimental groups' wounds demonstrated greater tensile strength than the wounds of nonirradiated control rabbits.

In a quantitative review of the literature (a meta-analysis), Beckerman and associates[22] concluded that because the methodologic quality of the studies of laser and skin disorders was relatively poor, no conclusions can be drawn about the effectiveness of laser for these problems. Although animal studies have been largely encouraging, no large-scale prospective, randomized, controlled clinical trials have been performed.

Pain Modulation

Walker[23] investigated the effect of HeNe-laser irradiation on serum serotonin levels in patients with chronic pain. An increase in serotonin metabolism was noted in laser-treated patients. Serotonin has been implicated as an endorphin precursor.

Ponnudurai and coworkers[24,25] have studied the effect of low-power laser on pain threshold in rats in two studies. In the first, 1-mW HeNe laser was applied to the rats' tails at either 4, 60, or 200 Hz for 15 seconds. The 4-Hz frequency resulted in a 50 percent increase in pain threshold, as measured by the rat-tail-flick test. In the second study, 1-mW HeNe laser applied at a frequency of 4 Hz to the base of the tail produced an increased pain tolerance to rat-tail-flick and hot-plate tests. Pretreatment with low-dose naloxone, an opiate antagonist (2 mg/kg), did not reverse the effects. High-dose naloxone (20 mg/kg) reversed the laser's analgesic effect, as measured by the hot-plate technique, but not by the tail-flick test.

Greathouse and colleagues[13] studied the effect of 1-mW GaAs laser on the latency of superficial radial nerve in human subjects. No change in latency was noted when laser-treated subjects were compared with sham-irradiated controls. Conversely, using an identical protocol, Snyder-Mackler and coworkers[26] found a slight but statistically significant increase in the distal latency of the superficial radial nerve in HeNe laser-irradiated subjects as compared to sham-irradiated controls. Jarvis, MacIver, and Tanelian[27] studied the effect of low-power (0.1 to 5 mW) HeNe laser on A-delta and C-fiber responses to mechanical, thermal, and chemical stimulation and found that it did not alter spontaneous or evoked neural activity.

INDICATIONS AND CLINICAL APPLICATION OF LASER

The purported indications for the therapeutic use of cold, or low-intensity, laser are typically separated into categories of tissue healing and pain management (acute or chronic). This section will discuss proposed clinical applications for laser.

Tissue Healing

Animal studies and anecdotal reports strongly suggest that low-power laser may accelerate healing rates of chronic open wounds and other soft-tissue injuries. Gogia and coworkers[28] reported positive results in two cases of patients who received HeNe laser and whirlpool to treat chronic open wounds. The wounds almost totally healed with this treatment.

Trelles and Mayayo[29] studied the effect of 2.4 J of HeNe laser every other day for 24 days on experimentally induced fractures in mice. Laser was applied through the skin. Histologic analysis revealed increased vascularization, more rapid formation of osseous tissue, and presence of a dense trabecular net in the treated animals as compared to controls.

Basically two different techniques for treating open wounds with laser have been reported in the literature: gridding the wound and surrounding the wound. To grid a wound, the clinician should imagine a grid or screen over the wound with 1- to 1½-cm^2 open squares. Irradiation of each square should take place for 20 seconds with the HeNe laser and 10 seconds with the use of the GaAs type (Seitz and Kleinkort, unpublished data). If indicated for cleansing and debridement, the whirlpool or saline cleansing should be introduced before laser application. One daily application of whirlpool is suggested. If there is eschar present, or if the wound is unusually large, the therapist may choose to surround the healthy tissue on the periphery of the wound. Stimulation is then applied every 2 cm^2 for 30 seconds using the HeNe laser and for 20 seconds using the GaAs. If the wound is closing from the outside, sterile saline or hydrogen peroxide can be poured into the wound. This fluid is then stimulated for 1 to 2 minutes with the laser. For wound healing, stimulation every other day at a frequency of 80 Hz, or continuously using the gridding or surrounding techniques is suggested by manufacturers of laser devices.

CASE STUDY 1

The patient is a 55-year-old woman with diabetes who has a persistent, 10-cm-diameter open wound over her right lateral malleolus. The wound has been treated with debridement and conventional wound management for 6 months. She has been referred for a trial of HeNe laser therapy.

Evaluation reveals a clean, dry wound with no evidence of re-epithelialization. No granulation tissue is apparent. The patient is anesthetic from the midcalf to the toes bilaterally. Her foot, calf, and anterior leg muscles are generally fair to fair + . She ambulates with a walker, partial weight bearing on the right. Reflexes are absent at the knees and ankles bilaterally. There is no evidence of other skin breakdown.

The wound is covered with a transparent paper and is traced. Laser treatment will be delivered using a circumferential technique: 20 seconds of continuous HeNe laser per cm^2 of wound edge. Treatment will be given daily with weekly tracings being made to monitor closure. Other treatment will include debridement, as necessary, and cleaning and dressing the wound.

Pain Management

In acute pain management, the manufacturers' recommended application techniques employed in the studies cited below are straightforward. After the area of pain is localized, the laser is applied for 20 seconds with the GaAs laser or 30 seconds with the HeNe unit. The GaAs laser is usually set at a frequency of 73 Hz, and the HeNe is usually used in the continuous setting. The use of trigger points, or other such body points, in conjunction with the painful site can be included when treating the acute patient.

Laser use has been suggested to reduce pain in the acute and chronic states. Many different protocols are used, including direct stimulation over the site of dysfunction or stimulation of associated acupuncture, trigger, or motor points. Some of the more commonly treated dysfunctions will be discussed in this section.

In most circumstances, the patient should require no more than 8 to 12 treatments. If pain reduction has occurred after 4 or 5 sessions, the use of laser is discontinued. This is prudent clinical decision making, as with other physical agents.

The effects of low-power laser irradiation on musculoskeletal pain have been the focus of two independent meta-analyses in the past 3 years.[22,30] Some, but not all, of the studies included in these two analyses were the same. Interestingly, the reports came to very different conclusions. Beckerman and coworkers concluded that, "For rheumatoid arthritis, post-traumatic joint disorders and myofascial pain, laser therapy seems to have a substantial therapeutic effect."[22] Conversely, Gam and colleagues, concluded that, "Low-level laser therapy has no effect on pain in musculoskeletal syndromes."[30] Randomized, controlled clinical trials published since these two analyses seem to support Gam's conclusions.

Although early reports were encouraging, most placebo controlled studies have failed to demonstrate any therapeutic effect of laser over placebo. In his editorial in a 1990 issue of the journal *Pain*, Devor[31] remarked that four studies in that particular issue of the journal reported "The lack of specific effect produced by a very expensive form of purported therapy (low power laser)." And further, he cautioned that if the major effect of laser was placebo, "There need[s] to be protection against financial exploitation."

BACK, HEAD, AND NECK DYSFUNCTION

There is some indication that neck and back pain may be affected by low-power laser. Snyder-Mackler and Bork[26] undertook a double-blind study to determine the effect of cold laser on musculoskeletal trigger points. They defined a trigger point as a site that elicits referred pain on deep palpation and demonstrates lowered skin resistance in comparison to surrounding tissue. Thirty patients with musculoskeletal pain were included in the study. Trigger points were treated for three successive treatments. Snyder-Mackler and Bork[26] noted that the patients who received the cold laser treatment demonstrated a significant increase in skin resistance when compared with the control. The difference was $p < 0.05$. They concluded that the results indicated that increases in skin resistance associated with the resolution of trigger points may be elicited by using cold laser therapy.

In a partial replication of the previous study, Snyder-Mackler and coworkers[33] found identical results in a second group of patients. They also found that laser significantly decreased pain, as recorded on a visual analogue scale, when compared to placebo laser.

Kreczi and Klinger[35] used a randomized single-blind crossover design to study the effects of HeNe laser on patients with radiating back and neck pain. Mean pain levels, as measured by visual analogue scales, were significantly lower after laser treatment. In the crossover portion of the study, laser gave a better result than placebo in all variables measured.

Hansen and Thoroe[32] studied the effect of GaAs laser at 78.9 mW/cm² on chronic orofacial pain in 40 patients. There was no difference between laser and placebo. Interestingly, they reported that the clinical impression was that placebo was superior to laser treatment. Incidentally, they reported that "During the study, the impression that probe A was the active one became evident, and six patients, not included in the study, were treated with this probe, which turned out to be the placebo probe." The authors offered this addendum as an example of "The enthusiastic anecdotal reports which . . . dominate . . . this field."

Arthritis

Clinical results with laser application to inflammatory joint conditions suggest that laser may be beneficial to these conditions. Treatment of osteoarthritis and rheumatoid arthritis is most practical when only one or two joints require radiation. The only exceptions to this observation are in the hand, the foot, and the cervical and lumbar areas. The treatment of a joint, as described in the articles below, is to approach it on all sides. The only time that circumferential exposure appears to be unproductive is when treating multiple joints in the foot or hand. In these cases, irradiation, both medially and laterally, are sufficient. The times remain the same as previously mentioned.

Goldman and associates[36] undertook a study using 30 people with classic or definite rheumatoid arthritis. They were classified by American Rheumatism Association criteria, 26 having classic, and 4 having definite, rheumatoid arthritis. There were 25 women and 5 men who ranged in age from 22 to 73 years. Twenty-one patients noted improvement of both their metacarpal phalangeal joints and proximal interphalangeal joints of both hands during laser therapy. Twenty-seven patients noted improvement of their proximal interphalangeal joints, and 26 noted improvement of their metacarpal phalangeal joints during therapy. The improvement was in both hand function and hand activity. The changes usually were bilateral, although more improvement in grip strength and tip pinch, and less erythema and pain, were noted on the side treated with laser perhaps explained in part by a placebo effect. Activity levels related to duration of morning stiffness and motion restricted by joint heat, erythema, tenderness, pain, and swelling.

Bliddal and colleagues[37] reported the effect of low-power laser on 17 patients with rheumatoid arthritis. One hand was irradiated with HeNe laser at 6 J/cm^2. The contralateral hand was treated with sham laser. When the hands were compared, there was a slight decrease in pain in the laser-irradiated hand, but there was no change in joint motion and morning stiffness.

Basford and coworkers[38] studied the effects of HeNe laser on range of motion, pain, joint tenderness, grip and pinch strength, activity level, and medication use in a blinded study of 81 patients with osteoarthritis of the thumb. The laser-treated group had a tendency for less tenderness of the treated MCP and interphalangeal (IP) joints, and an increase in three-finger-chuck-pinch strength in the treated hand as compared to the control hand. There was no statistical difference, however, between the groups in any of the variables tested.

Soft Tissue

The effects of low-power laser on soft tissue are equivocal. Investigators have used various strategies for assessing this effect. Lundeberg and associates[39] studied the effects of HeNe-laser irradiation to upper extremity acupuncture site on pain from lateral epicondylitis. No significant effect on pain was noted. In two distinct, randomized, controlled clinical trials of the effects of laser on lateral epicondylitis, Haker and Lundeberg found no effect of laser over placebo.[40,41] These studies complete a series of studies begun in 1987 by these investigators of the effects of low-power laser on this musculoskeletal problem.[39–41] They have used both GaAs and HeNe lasers at various doses and also a combination GaAs, HeNe laser. None showed any effect over placebo.

Seibert and coworkers[42] studied the effects of HeNe and GaAs laser on tendinitis. Patients were randomly assigned to a treatment or a placebo group (total = 64) and were treated for 10 consecutive days with low-power laser. All patients had a significant reduction in pain and symptoms during the course of the study and no difference was found between the two groups.

CASE STUDY 2

The patient is a 41-year-old woman with left lateral epicondylitis of 4 months' duration. She reports no history of specific trauma to the area.

Examination reveals a 9-cm^2 area of tenderness just distal to the left lateral epicondyle. There is some edema noted. She has pain with resisted isometric wrist extension and passive wrist flexion. There is a positive tennis-elbow test. Elbow and wrist range of motion and strength are within normal limits. There are no sensory changes. Her symptoms are consistent with pain and inflammation of the left-wrist extensor mass.

Plans for this patient, in addition to counterforce bracing and rest, include the use of low-power laser. HeNe laser will be delivered for 20 seconds to each cm^2 of painful area 3 times per week. Efficacy will be documented using a graphic rating scale and a log of medication usage.

DOCUMENTATION OF TREATMENT WITH LASER

Dosage is preferably described in joules per square centimeter. Laser power is given in watts, and the irradiating surface area is also usually provided. Joules can be determined by multiplying the number of watts by the treatment time in seconds. The rehabilitation professional should document the exact location treated, the total treatment time, the mode used (continuous or pulsed frequency), and the type of laser.

PRECAUTIONS AND CONTRAINDICATIONS FOR LASER

Research and safety criteria are necessary for any new therapeutic agent. Investigations on the safety and effectiveness of laser continue in Europe, Russia, and the United States.

Lasers less than 1 mW are classified by the Food and Drug Administration (FDA) as a class III medical device. The low-power laser, at the time of this writing, is still considered an investigational device, and the user should have an investigational-device exemption (IDE) under the abbreviated requirements of section 812.2(b)a of the FDA regulations before therapeutic intervention with laser. The FDA is concerned not only with safety, but also with therapeutic efficacy. The FDA's Center for Devices and Radiological Health now regulates the manufacture and safety of laser products in the United States (U.S. Department of Health, Education and Welfare, 1979). This regulation requires the manufacturer to classify the laser product.

Several other organizations have followed suit with safety standards that are comparable. The basic concepts of the classification schemes of the American National Safety Institute (ANSI), the American Conference of Governmental Industrial Hygienists (ACGIH), the World Health Organization (WHO), the International Electrotechnical Commissions (IEC), and the FDA are as follows:

Class I laser products are essentially safe and are typically enclosed systems that do not emit hazardous levels.

Class II laser products are limited to visible lasers that are safe for momentary viewing but should not be stared into continuously unless the exposure limits (ELs) and the dazzle of the brilliant visible light source would normally preclude staring into the course.[43]

Low-power lasers are class II or I laser devices. They are considered an insignificant risk to humans unless held close to the cornea of the eye.

The safety of these devices can further be evaluated by ANSI Standard 2-136.0. A review of the maximal permissible emission value of the lasers less than 1 mW shows a good margin of safety.[28]

The most prominent safety standard for laser was first produced in 1973 and has since been revised: ANSI Standard 2976, *Safe Use of Lasers*. A new edition of the ANSI standard was approved in 1980.

There are some contraindications for use of laser to which the clinician should adhere: Refrain from using laser in the pregnant woman; laser should not be used over the unclosed fontanels of children; the use of laser near cancerous lesions should be avoided; and laser should not be radiated directly into the cornea.

Ophthalmologic research has shown that, in rabbits, laser levels of 25 mW may produce retinal lesions in the continuous-wave HeNe laser mode. These lesions were obtained after 2.5 seconds, with a rise of temperature at the lesion site of 7.8°C. No lesions were present, however, with the use of 2- or 5-mW lasers.[44]

Lappin[45] has measured ocular damage threshold for the HeNe laser in the rhesus monkey. Exposure time of radiation was 2 ms to 10 seconds, with peak power of 50 mW. Mean values of the visible-damage threshold for power versus time were determined for each eye in the macula and in the extramacula. Approximately 500 exposures were made to determine mean-damage-threshold levels in 70 eyes for the macular, and an extramacula area between the optic disc and the macula. The macula was found to have a lower damage threshold than the extramacular area, the ratio of thresholds decreasing as exposure time increased. The macular-extramacular threshold ratio varied from about 2:1 at 5 ms to 1.3:1 at 1 second.

Ham and associates[46] studied the retinal-burn thresholds for the HeNe laser in the rhesus monkey. They concluded that the threshold power for irreversible burn damage in the monkey is about 7 mW at the cornea for the worst case of accidental exposure to HeNe lasers. For this exposure, the whole beam entered the eye and was focused on a minimal spot size. Available data indicate that the human retina is less susceptible to thermal damage than that of the monkey or the rabbit. Until more reliable data are available, the total power of the HeNe laser entering the human eye should be limited to 1 mW or less. This recommendation is based solely upon the chance of irreversible thermal damage to the retina.

ULTRAVIOLET

Ultraviolet (UV) light has been used in physical therapy for decades. Therapeutically, UV is not technically a thermal agent; treatment times are too short for substantial thermal effects to occur. Historically, UV has been used in the treatment of dermatologic problems, most notably psoriasis. Literature also describes the use of UV to treat pressure ulcers and other slow-healing wounds; however, the value of UV compared to other readily available modalities and treatments has been questioned. Although UV devices may still be present in some clinics, it has largely been dropped from the treatment regimens of rehabilitation clinics because of advancements in the pharmacologic treatment of skin disorders.

Ultraviolet radiation falls just below visible light on the electromagnetic spectrum. The ultraviolet portion of the spectrum can be further broken down into three types: UVA, UVB, and UVC. UVA, which has the longest wavelength—ranging from 320 to 400 nm, is a large part of the light delivered in tanning parlors and is associated with melanoma, one of the more virulent skin cancers. UVB lies in the middle of the UV spectrum with wavelengths ranging from 290 to 320 nm. UVB is directly associated with sunburn and premature aging of the skin. The therapeutic UV with the shortest wavelength, UVC, ranges from 180 to 290 nm. UVC is used for its bactericidal effects and causes the least amount of pigment change and skin damage.

Physical Principles of Ultraviolet

There are two laws of optic physics that are relevant to the UV application—the inverse square law and the law of cosines. The inverse square law ($E = I/D^2$, where E is the illumination intensity, I is the lamp intensity, and D is the distance from the source) states that the intensity of illumination varies with the square of the distance between the source and the treatment surface. This means that cutting the distance between the lamp and the patient by 50 percent will increase the dosage by 400 percent. The law of cosines states that the energy of illumination varies proportionally to the cosine of the degrees of deviation from the perpendicular. This means that as the area being irradiated becomes more oblique, the dose decreases.

Biophysical Effects

One of the primary purposes of therapeutic UV is to cause an erythemal response and, by doing so, to facilitate the healing process. This response usually occurs within 2 to 4 hours after treatment and usually peaks within 12 hours. Erythemal effectiveness peaks at 250 nm, which is found within the UVC spectrum, with a smaller peak noted at 297 nm, which is in the UVB spectrum.[47]

The second physiologic effect seen is thickening of the epidermis and pigmentation. This is more of a protective response of the skin that occurs to help shield the deeper skin layers from further UV exposure. This is not necessarily a desired response in rehabilitation treatments, but it explains why an increase in dosage is necessary for an effective amount of UV to be absorbed with repeated treatments. This effect applies to UVA and UVB treatments.

UV can also produce bactericidal effects. This effect is maximal at a wavelength of 253 nm, which is within UVC's spectrum.

Vitamin D production is also noted to be enhanced with UV exposure. This physiologic effect occurs at wavelengths from 270 to 300 nm.

Dosimetry for Ultraviolet

Erythemal doses are graded sub, minimal-, first-, second-, and third-degree erythema doses. The unit used to describe the dose is a unit of time (usually seconds to minutes). These doses are dependent upon age, skin color, and many other individual factors and, thus, cannot be generalized from patient to patient. This necessitates testing each patient before treatment. Testing is usually performed on the anterior aspect of the forearm, but probably should be performed in the area that is to be treated. A piece of UV-opaque material is windowed, as shown in Figure 9–7. Each of the four windows are cut to 1 to 2 cm^2 in area. The entire area in the UV

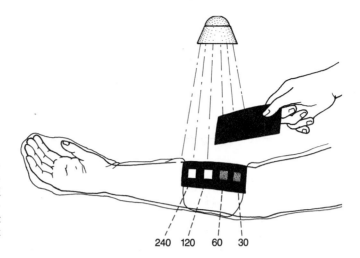

FIGURE 9–7. Determination of MED using a four-windowed shield. (Adapted from Stillwell, GK: Therapeutic Electricity and Ultraviolet Radiation, ed. 3. Williams & Wilkins, Baltimore, 1983).

field is draped except for the small testing area. The lamp is warmed up and placed so that the light is perpendicular to the test area. Traditionally, distances of 60 to 80 cm have been used for standard UVB dose testing. Times given here are for this distance. (Note that lamps may differ and manufacturers' recommendations for testing should be followed.) The first window is uncovered for 120 seconds, then the second is uncovered and both are irradiated for 60 seconds, the third is added for 30 seconds, and the final aperture is uncovered, and all four are exposed for an additional 30 seconds. Thus, the total exposure for the four windows is 240, 120, 60, and 30 seconds, respectively. Dosimetry cannot be immediately determined because of the latency period. Ideally, the skin should be examined 8 hours after exposure to inspect for the area where mild reddening of the skin has occurred. If the patient cannot be seen by medical personnel, self-reporting is acceptable with the reliable patient.

A suberythemal dose is a treatment time insufficient for perceptible reddening of the skin to occur. A minimal erythemal dose (MED) is the time required for mild reddening of the skin, which appears within 8 hours of treatment and disappears within 24 hours. Pigmentation changes occur only with repeated exposure, and exfoliation rarely, if ever, occurs at MED. First-degree erythema also appears after approximately 6 hours. This erythema is more pronounced, is similar to a mild sunburn, and lasts for several days. There may be associated discomfort, which is proportional to the surface area irradiated. This level of treatment may eventually be followed by slight exfoliation. A second-degree erythema occurs after a latency period of 2 hours or less and resembles a severe sunburn. The skin is angrily red, hot, tender, and may be accompanied by edema. This dose is always accompanied by significant exfoliation and prolonged pigmentation changes. A third-degree erythema is a second-degree burn where blistering occurs. Once the MED has been determined, all other doses may be calculated using the conversion formula in Table 9–1.

When using UVA and UVB, the amount of exposure to maintain a specific erythemal dose increases over time, much as tolerance to sunlight increases. It is necessary, therefore, to increase the time or to decrease the distance from the source in or-

TABLE 9-1 Ultraviolet: Conversion of Known Dose
to Desired Dose

Erythema degree	MED	1st	2nd	3rd
Factor	1	2.5	5	10
Equation				

$$\text{Desired dose} = \frac{\text{Known dose (sec)}}{\text{Factor (dose desired)}} \times \text{Factor (known dose)}$$

der to maintain therapeutic efficacy. The time required to maintain each level of ery-thema varies. MED usually is increased by 35 percent per treatment per day. First-degree requires an increase of 50 percent; second and third degree increases are from 75 percent to 100 percent per treatment. This progression is usually continued until exposure time reaches 5 minutes, at which time the distance is decreased to decrease the treatment time. The inverse square law is used to estimate an appropri-ate treatment time at the new distance. The equation for conversions is: $T = T_1 \times D^2)/D_1^2$, where T is the new time, D is the new distance, T_1 is the old time, and D_1 is the old distance.

It is not necessary to increase the dosage as described above when using UVC. Since the majority of the radiation is absorbed in the epidermis, very little reaches the dermis where tanning occurs. Repeated exposures to UVC, therefore, do not enhance tanning, which then does not interfere with the dosage of the radiation.

Therapeutic Applications of Ultraviolet

PSORIASIS

UV usually is used in one of two ways to treat this proliferative dermatosis: the Goeckerman regimen or psoralens UVA (PUVA). The Goeckerman regimen, developed at the Mayo Clinic, involves the use of a petroleum-based coal-tar mixture, which is used as a photosensitizing agent, followed by exposure to UVB. PUVA involves taking oral psoralens (photosensitizing agents) plus UVA. Although both of these treatments are effective for control of psoriasis, PUVA has been shown to be considerably more ef-fective and less messy. Unfortunately, PUVA therapy also results in an increased inci-dence of skin cancer.

Dosimetry

The dose is usually begun at the first-degree erythemal level. For the Goecker-man regimen, coal tar is applied and removed and an MED test is performed, as previously described. Treatment is delivered once or twice per day until the plaques clear. UVA has a longer latency until appearance of erythema. PUVA therapy usu-ally results in a longer lasting erythema that is more intense than with the Goecker-man regimen. Therefore, the initial dosage is usually determined by the referring dermatologist, who takes into consideration the patient's skin type and medication level. Ideally, the erythema should peak 48 hours after treatment as a first-degree dose. Because of the long latency of response, PUVA therapy is given at most every other day.

Instrumentation

Two types of generators may be used for UV treatment: "hot quartz" lamps and "cold quartz" lamps. The hot quartz lamps have a wide-spectrum emission that peaks at 273.7 nm, 280.0 nm, and 296.7 nm and may be applied to either general or localized treatment areas. The effects seen are mostly erythema and pigmentation. UV can be delivered by a single-bulb lamp (fog) or, more commonly, in a multibulb cabinet.

The cold quartz lamp is predominantly UVC at the wavelength of 253 nm. The effects seen with this generator are primarily bactericidal with minimal erythemal production. Pigmentation changes do not occur with this lamp. These lamps are usually portable and are used for local treatments.

CYSTIC ACNE

Ultraviolet is now used rarely for this disorder, because improved pharmacologic means are available for controlling cystic acne. The goal of UV treatment with this patient population was to dry out the skin and promote skin exfoliation.

Dosimetry

Dosage at the second-degree erythemal level was used, as significant exfoliation of skin was the desired response. Dosimetry was determined by the method described above.

CHRONIC WOUND MANAGEMENT

Chronic, infected wounds may be treated with UVC when traditional methods fail. Although UVB and UVA have also been used to treat these wounds, UVC produces the desired effect (reducing infection) with the fewest undesirable effects, and in the most advantageous time frame.[47]

Dosimetry

Since the blood supply to a chronically infected wound is poor, UV at second- and third-degree doses may be indicated to increase blood supply, kill bacteria, and stimulate a healing response. A "cold quartz" lamp is preferred. Although a MED test may need to be performed, a chart is often provided with the generator to guide dosage.

Adverse Effects and Treatment Precautions for Ultraviolet

Adverse effects of treatment include burns and redness of the skin acutely and premature aging and skin cancer chronically. Careful application of this physical agent should not result in burns. The patient should be informed of all risks and benefits of this type of therapy. Unfortunately, psoriasis often cannot be adequately controlled by pharmacologic therapy alone. In spite of its attendant risks, therefore, UV therapy is sometimes required.

The therapist and patient must take precautions during treatment. Polarized goggles should be worn at all times. Exposure times should be carefully monitored. Erythemal responses should be graded carefully. Treatment times should be carefully increased from visit to visit, so as to maintain therapeutic levels of treatment without causing burns. Areas of skin that are rarely exposed to light (breasts and genitalia) should be exposed to only ⅓ to ½ the dose for the rest of the body.

Caution must be taken when the patient is taking medications, that is, certain antibiotics or diuretics that photosensitize.

Reactions to the combination of UV and photosensitive medications may result in a general dermatitis and itching. Check with a pharmacist or the *Physicians' Desk Reference* when uncertain of a medication's photosensitivity.

Conditions such as pulmonary tuberculosis, lupus erythematosus, acute psoriasis, and acute eczema or dermatitis may be exacerbated by exposure to UV radiation. Patients with renal or hepatic insufficiencies, diabetes, or hyperthyroidism may not tolerate UV well. UV radiation should also be avoided in areas that are receiving radiation therapy because the skin is devitalized and, therefore, may be more susceptible to skin cancer.

Documentation of Treatment with Ultraviolet

Exposure in seconds, distance of the light source from the patient, and angle of incidence all figure into dosage and should be reported. Draping procedures should be documented for each treatment. The specific lamp used for treatment should be noted by its serial number. MED may vary from lamp to lamp due to varying outputs.

CASE STUDY 3

PATIENT HISTORY

The patient is a 38-year-old woman with a chronic, sacrococcygeal pressure ulcer. She is confined to a wheelchair as a result of a spinal-cord injury. The ulcer was discovered 5 months ago and treated with traditional care and debridement with little success.

EXAMINATION

The ulcer is infected and measures 3.7 cm wide by 4.1 cm long by 1.5 cm deep.

TREATMENT

UVC at a second-degree erythemal dose is required to stimulate healing and reduce the infection. A cold-quartz lamp is held perpendicular to the wound at a distance of 1 inch from the surface. An exposure time of 80 seconds was determined from a chart supplied by the manufacturer of the generator, taking the patient's "average" skin sensitivity into consideration. A 2-mm-thick layer of petroleum jelly was applied to the skin around the wound, and a layer of heavy paper toweling with a window cut in it to expose the wound was used to cover it. Treatment was repeated every other day for a total of 16 treatments. Other treatment included daily wound cleansing and patient positioning to avoid pressure on the ulcer. Treatment was ceased when wound closure occurred.

SUMMARY

The use of light in physical therapy has a long history. This chapter has described current practice using one of the older agents, ultraviolet, and one of the more recent, low-power laser. There is evidence that both agents can be used to effectively treat a number of conditions. Caution should be used in their application, and careful attention to details of indications for use, application time, and location should improve efficacy. The work supporting the efficacy of low-power laser in rehabilitation is preliminary and its use in the United States is restricted. The need for further well-controlled studies to support or refute its efficacy is apparent and required before it may be used to treat patients.

Study Objectives

Having read this chapter, the student will now be able to:

1. Describe the physical, biophysical, and physiologic effects of low-power laser.
2. Describe the common types of instruments used to deliver low-power laser.
3. Discuss the literature related to the use of low-power laser in rehabilitation.
4. Describe common problems for which low-power laser is used therapeutically and how dosimetry is determined.
5. Explain the physical and biophysical effects of ultraviolet radiation, including the application of the inverse square law and the law of cosines.
6. Describe the effects of UV radiation on human tissue.
7. Discuss the clinical uses for ultraviolet radiation in the rehabilitation setting.
8. Discuss the adverse effects of exposure to UV radiation.

REFERENCES

1. Kleinkort, JA and Roley, RA: Laser acupuncture: Its use in physical therapy. Am J Acupuncture 12:51, 1984.
2. Watkins, AL: A Manual of Electrotherapy. Lea & Febiger, Philadelphia, 1968, pp 12–15, 24–26, 197–199.
3. Bloom, AL: Gas Lasers. John Wiley & Sons, New York, 1971, pp. 1–24.
4. Calder, N: Einstein's Universe. Greenwich House, New York, 1982, pp. 29–30.
5. Goldman, L: Biomedical Aspects of the Laser. Springer-Verlag, New York, 1967, pp. 1–7.
6. Lengyell, BA: Lasers—Generation of Lightly Stimulated Emission. John Wiley & Sons, New York, 1962, pp 1–15, 22–23, 83–99.
7. Kroetlinger, M: On the use of laser in acupuncture. Int J Acupuncture Electrother Res 5:297, 1980.
8. Kovacs, L: Experimental investigation of photostimulation effect of low energy HeNe laser radiation. In Laser in Basic Biomedical Research, IV. Plenum, New York, 1977.
9. Litwin, MS and Glew, DH: The biological effects of laser radiation. JAMA 187:842, 1964.
10. Caspers, K: Laser stimulation therapy. Physikalilshe Medizin Rehabilitation 18:426, 1977.
11. Dynatronics: Dynatron 1120 Operators Manual. Dynatronics, Salt Lake City, UT, 1983.
12. Basford, JR: Low-energy laser therapy: Controversies and new research findings. Lasers Surg Med 9:101, 1989.

13. Greathouse, DG, Currier, DP, and Gilmore, RL: Effects of clinical infrared laser on superficial radial nerve conduction. Phys Ther 65:1184, 1985.
14. Lehmann, JF and DeLateur, B: Therapeutic heat. In Lehmann, JF and Basmajian, JV (eds): Therapeutic Heat and Cold, ed 3. Williams & Wilkins, Baltimore, 1982, p 404.
15. Fork RL: Laser stimulation of nerve cells in aplysia. Science 171:907, 1971.
16. Mester, E, Mester, AF, and Mester, A: The biomedical effects of laser application. Lasers Surg Med 5:31, 1985.
17. Mester, E and Jaszsagi-Nagy, E: The effects of laser radiation on wound healing and collagen synthesis. Studia Biophysica 35(3):227, 1973.
18. Cummings, JP: The effect of low energy (He-Ne) laser irradiation on healing dermal wounds in an animal model. Phys Ther 65:737, 1985.
19. Kana, JS, et al: Effect of low-power density laser radiation on healing of open skin wounds in rat. Arch Surg 116:293, 1981.
20. Dyson, M and Young, S: Effects of laser therapy on wound contraction and cellularity in mice. Lasers Surg Med 1:125, 1986.
21. Braverman, B, et al: Effect of helium-neon and infrared laser irradiation on wound healing in rabbits. Lasers Surg Med 9:50, 1989.
22. Beckerman, H, et al: The efficacy of laser therapy for musculoskeletal and skin disorders: A criteria-based meta-analysis of randomized clinical trials. Phys Ther 72:483, 1992.
23. Walker, J: Relief from chronic pain by low power laser irradiation. Neurosci Lett 43:339, 1983.
24. Ponnudura, RN, et al: Laser photobiostimulation-induced hypoalgesia in rats is not naloxone reversible. Acupunct Electrother Res 13:109, 1988.
25. Ponnudura, RN, Zbuzek, VK, and Wu, H-H: Hypoalgesic effect of laser photobiostimulation by rat tail flick test. Acupunct Electrother Res 12:93, 1987.
26. Snyder-Mackler, L and Bork, CE: Effect of helium-neon laser irradiation on peripheral sensory nerve latency. Phys Ther 68:223, 1989.
27. Jarvis, D, MacIver, MB, and Tanelian, DL: Electrophysiologic recording and thermodynamic modeling demonstrate that helium-neon laser irradiation does not affect peripheral A delta or C-fiber nociceptors. Pain 43:235, 1990.
28. Gogia, PP, Hurt, BS, and Zirn, TT: Wound management with whirlpool and infrared cold laser treatment: A clinical report. Phys Ther 68(8):1239, 1988.
29. Trelles, MA and Mayayo, E: Bone fracture consolidates faster with low-power laser. Lasers Surg Med 7:36, 1987.
30. Gam, AN, Thorsen, H, and Lonnberg, F: The efficacy of low-level laser therapy on musculoskeletal pain: A meta analysis. Pain 52:63, 1993.
31. Devor, M: What's in a laser beam for pain therapy. Pain 43:139, 1990.
32. Hansen, HJ and Thoroe, U: Low power laser biostimulation of chronic oro-facial pain: A double-blind placebo controlled cross-over study in 40 patients. Pain 43:169, 1990.
33. Snyder-Macker, L, et al: Effect of helium-neon laser on musculoskeletal trigger points. Phys Ther 66(7):1087, 1986.
34. Snyder-Macker, L, et al: Effects of helium-neon laser irradiation on skin resistance and pain in patients with trigger points in the neck or back. Phys Ther 69:336, 1989.
35. Kreczi, T and Klinger, D: A comparison of laser acupuncture versus placebo in radicular and pseudo-radicular pain syndromes as recorded by subjective responses of patients. Acupunct Electrother Res: 11:207, 1986.
36. Goldman, JA, et al: Laser therapy of rheumatoid arthritis. Lasers Surg Med 1:1, 1980.
37. Bliddal, H, et al: Soft-laser therapy of rheumatoid arthritis. Scand J Rheumatol 16:225, 1987.
38. Basford, JR, et al: Low-energy helium neon laser treatment of thumb osteoarthritis. Arch Phys Med Rehabil 68:794, 1987.
39. Lundeberg, T, Haker, E, and Thomas, M: Effects of laser versus placebo in tennis elbow. Scand J Rehabil Med 19:135, 1987.
40. Haker, HK and Lundeberg, TCM: Lateral epicondylalgia: Report of noneffective midlaser treatment. Arch Phys Med Rehabil 72:984, 1991.
41. Haker, E and Lundeberg, TCM: Laser treatment applied to acupuncture points in lateral humeral epicondylalgia. Pain 43:243–247, 1990.
42. Siebert, W, et al: What is the efficacy of "soft" and "mid" lasers in therapy of tendinopathies? A double-blind study. Arch Orthop Trauma Surg 106:358, 1987.
43. Goldman, L: Basic reactions in tissue. In Goldman, L (ed): The Biomedical Laser: Technology and Clinical Applications. Springer-Verlag, New York, 1981, 6.
44. Kohtiao, A, et al: Temperature rise and photocoagulation of rabbit retinas exposed the CW laser. Am J Ophthalmol 62:3, 1966.
45. Lappin, PW: Ocular damage thresholds for the helium-neon laser. Arch Environ Health 20:2, 1970.
46. Ham, WT, et al: Retinal burn threshold for the hellium-neon laser in the rhesus monkey. Arch Ophthalmol 84:6, 1970.
47. Nussbaum, EL, et al: Comparison of ultrasound, ultraviolet-C and laser for treatment of pressure ulcers in patients with spinal cord injury. Phys Ther 74:812, 1994.

SELECTED READINGS (UV)

1. Beckett, RH: Modern Actinotherapy. London, 1955.
2. Goeckerman, WH: The treatment of psoriasis. Northwest Med 24:229, 1925.
3. Hayes, KW: Manual for Physical Agents, ed 4. Appleton & Lange, Norwalk, CT, 1993, p 61.
4. McCulloch JM, Kloth, L, and Feedar, J: Wound Healing—Alternatives in Management. FA Davis, Philadelphia, 1995, p 354.
5. Sams, WM: Phototherapy of psoriasis. In TB Fitzpatrick (ed): Sunlight and Man. Tokyo University Press, Tokyo, 1974, p 793.
6. Stillwell, GK: Therapeutic Electricity and Ultraviolet Radiation (ed). Williams & Wilkins, Baltimore, 1983.
7. Stern, RS, et al: Photochemistry for psoriasis. NE to Med 300:809, 1979.
8. Sunlamp products: Performance standards, Federal/Register 44:65352, 1979.

Clinical Decision Making

CHAPTER **10**

Clinical Evaluation of Thermal Agents

Mary P. Watkins, MS, PT

Evaluation of the effectiveness and efficiency of therapeutic intervention is an essential function of every health-care professional. Participation of each individual in this process can vary from critical reading of the medical and scientific literature to conducting sophisticated research projects. In order to participate at all, health-care professionals must have an understanding of the existing problems and questions about current practice and have the ability to incorporate into practice those therapeutic advances that have been demonstrated to be effective by sound critical analysis. Acquisition of such understanding and ability depends upon a working knowledge of the aims, uses, and limitations of clinical investigation.

This book presents a comprehensive review of the physical and physiologic mechanisms that serve as the basis for the characteristics of energy delivered and the potential applications of thermal agents. From the physical sciences, for example, we have gained knowledge of heat-transfer mechanisms. From the biologic sciences, we have gained information about the responses of cells, tissues, and organs to thermal agents. In vitro laboratory studies include the influence of temperature changes on the viscoelastic properties of collagen and changes in ion fluxes across cell membranes when temperature is altered. In vivo animal studies have examined such changes as blood flow, muscle-spindle activity, synaptic transmission, and induction and resolution of inflammation and edema. These kinds of information are useful for establishing a rationale for employing thermal agents in the treatment of patients. Throughout this book, current instrumentation and techniques are also described, which demonstrate clinical application of heat, cold, pulsed ultrasound, laser, ultraviolet, shortwave diathermy, and pulse radiofrequency energy (PRFE). In many instances, however, the therapeutic effects of these modalities are based on anecdotal reports or on empiric evidence of success in ameliorating patient problems.

Further clinical research is needed to accomplish our professional goal of providing high-quality patient care in an economically sound manner. Although findings based on normal subjects may help in understanding physiologic responses to therapeutic applications, they do not answer the important questions regarding clinical efficacy. Formal clinical studies that document the effects of treatment procedures applied to real clinical problems will help clinicians to: (1) Determine the appropriateness of current techniques; (2) develop new methods tested by scientific inquiry; and (3) discard methods that do not stand up to such scrutiny.

The purpose of this chapter is to examine selected elements of the research process applicable to the clinical evaluation of thermal agents and other physical agents such as laser. General principles, samples of methodology, and instrumentation are presented to highlight the uses and limitations of the clinical-research process. Examples of research questions concerning the application of thermal agents will be used.

GENERAL PRINCIPLES OF CLINICAL RESEARCH

Planning and Preparation

The basic process of conceiving, planning, and preparing to conduct research can be described in several well-defined steps. These preliminary steps are:

1. Definition of the research question.
2. Collection of the relevant information.
3. Statement of the hypothesis or the specific aims of the research activity.
4. Selection and development of the method of study.
5. Preparation of the written research proposal.

This process applies to all types of research design and involves careful planning, including the recognition of problems that potentially can invalidate the outcome of a study. Several general guidelines can be defined to ensure well-planned and well-executed clinical research projects.[1,2]

The Research Question

The research question or problem must be specific and delimited, identifying the research variables precisely. The first potential failure in the research process is posing a question that is diffuse or broad, containing confounding elements that make it impossible to derive a useful answer. For example, "What is the effect of cold on edema?" The two key elements of this research question can be identified as: (1) the independent variable, cold, which the investigator will control, manipulate, or apply; and (2) the dependent variable, edema, which will be observed or measured to determine the effect of applying the modality. The question, however, is unmanageable. Many confounding elements, or extraneous variables, have not been taken into account. What kind of cold is being questioned? How often will it be applied? In what setting? On what kind of patient? What specific outcome is relevant—range of motion, limb circumference, limb volume, or functional abilities? These kinds of questions must be addressed and resolved during the process of defining the research question.

Collection of the Relevant Information

Background information must be carefully accumulated and analyzed. Clinical observation and experience are valuable sources of background information; indeed, the question at hand is often derived from some clinical event. Although clinically derived knowledge is important, it is never thorough enough to substitute for a critical review of the current medical and scientific literature.

As the investigator defines the problem to be studied and formulates the specific elements of the research project, several pertinent pieces of information should be incorporated, or at least considered. The approach to the literature review begins with preparing a list of topics, including details about the independent variable, the dependent variable(s), and the pathologic condition or patient population to be studied. This list will be transposed into appropriate "key words," which will then be used by the investigator to retrieve reference citations from the bibliographic indexes in medical or university libraries.[2]

Regarding the illustrative question of cold and edema, the literature search would include both laboratory and clinical studies. From animal studies, the investigator will learn the mechanisms of edema formation and, as discussed in Chapter 4, that the intensity and duration of cold application may influence the tissue response, possibly adversely. This knowledge should lead to careful consideration of the method of cold application to be used. From clinical studies, there is evidence that the application of cold may control swelling. In at least one study, however, compression wraps were also part of the treatment. This problem suggests a more definitive series of questions than did the first, vaguely stated question. In general, the investigator needs to know if his or her question has been studied, how it has been studied, what has not been studied, and what constitutes the scientific rationale for the proposed study. This information is necessary to solidify the importance of the current problem and to develop an appropriate approach to the research question.

At this point, the investigator should be able to pose an important, clinically relevant, sensible research question. Taking the initially stated global question, for example, a more refined question may be asked: "Is cold, or cold plus intermittent compression, more effective in reducing edema following ankle sprains in college athletes?" Then the question can be transposed into a working or research hypothesis.

Hypothesis or Specific Aims

Most research questions can and should be transposed into hypotheses. Certainly, if the study compares two treatment methods, a prediction of the outcome can be made based on the available background information. The hypothesis must be stated to clearly identify the independent and dependent variables and proposes a relationship between the two. This statement can be made in two ways: nondirectional or directional.

A statement of difference declares that the application of the independent variable will result in a change in the dependent variable. If the investigator predicts a change, but not the direction of that change, the statement is referred to as a *nondirectional hypothesis*. For example, "There will be a difference in the amount of residual ankle edema when sprains are treated with cold alone, compared with cold plus intermittent compression." A *directional hypothesis* predicts not only a difference but also the direction of that difference: "The application of cold plus intermittent compression will be more effective in reducing edema following ankle sprains than the application of cold alone."

Occasionally, a research hypothesis may be that "treatment *X* will be as effective as treatment *Y*." This statement should not be confused with the *null hypothesis*. The null hypothesis is a statistical statement of "no difference" that is used in the application of statistical procedures to determine significance of the research data.

In studies of a descriptive or correlational nature, when the purpose is to describe a particular phenomenon, a predictive hypothesis may not be appropriate. In this case, a clear statement of the specific aims of the study should be made.

Method

In order to answer the question or test the hypothesis, a method of study must be carefully selected and specifically described. The purpose of this major task is to make certain that: (1) all extraneous variables (factors other than the independent variable that could effect the outcome) are controlled for or eliminated; and (2) the kind and use of the measurement tools are appropriate.

An explicit written description of the method must be prepared and must include the following details: (1) the specific conditions of the study must be stated, such as the age, sex, and health status of subjects and the setting in which the study is to be conducted; (2) the testing instruments and their application are specifically defined to answer: what test, when used, how used, and by whom?; (3) the procedure for applying the independent variable is defined in order to outline, using our example, such details as: What type of cold?, How frequently administered?, How will the subject be positioned?, and What kind of supervision or monitoring?; and (4) statistical procedures or other techniques that will be used to analyze the data are outlined. Through this protocol, operational definitions will be stated: The meaning of cold and the meaning of edema should become clear.

At this point in preparing to conduct a research study, the investigator must analyze the proposed method to ensure that the design is correct and meets certain criteria. This process may require consultation with other investigators and clinicians, as well as a pretrial pilot study. Three important criteria should be met: reliability, validity, and objectivity.[3]

Reliability is synonymous with dependability, stability, consistency, predictability, and accuracy. If the same set of objects are measured again and again with the same or comparable instruments under the same conditions, will the results be the same? There are statistical techniques to estimate the degree of reliability of a testing situation.[4,5] (These techniques, in many cases, simply serve to confirm the investigator's good common sense.)

Validity refers to the soundness, logic, and appropriateness of the study design.[6] The *internal validity* of a study depends upon the extent to which the method controls extraneous factors that interfere with the true relationship between the stated independent and dependent variables. Is the investigator measuring what he or she thinks is being measured? In addition to the application of cold alone or cold and compression, what factors are important: weight bearing, elevation of the limb, anti-inflammatory medication? *External validity* refers to the extent to which the results can be generalized to other subjects, settings, or conditions. How representative are the findings to the "outside" world? Will cold-gel packs have the same effect as the application of chipped ice? Will the response of an athlete, anxious to return to competition, be the same as the response of a sedentary executive?

Objectivity means the extent to which the testing situation and the measurement tools control for the biggest kind of extraneous variable: the biases, subjective impressions, and feelings of the investigators and subjects.

The Research Proposal

At this point, the investigator prepares a written research proposal. This document reflects all of the preceding steps: identification of the research question, definition of the need and importance of the proposed study, relevant background from the literature review, and description of the specific protocol (method) to be followed. It, along with a written informed-consent form, will be reviewed by an appropriate institutional review board, which must approve the project.[1,7] The written protocol becomes the guide that must be strictly followed during every phase of the study.

Dissemination of Results

When data collection is complete and the results are analyzed according to plan, the investigator has one more responsibility—to share results with professional colleagues. The results of clinical studies may also be useful to the engineers and manufacturers responsible for the design, construction, and safety of therapeutic devices.

The information in the final report must be accurate and detailed enough so that the reader or listener can identify the question asked, assess the appropriateness of the method, replicate the study, and evaluate the strength and veracity of the conclusions.

The primary goal of any research is to improve or increase the body of knowledge in the relevant clinical or scientific arena. This can best be done by gathering and disseminating sound, reliable, accurate information.

TYPES OF CLINICAL RESEARCH

Some types of research are more rigorous than others, but all carefully planned and executed projects that follow the principles previously outlined will make a contribution to the existing body of knowledge. An understanding of the purposes and limitations of various research approaches will permit appropriate interpretation and analysis of information in the proper perspective. The research designs discussed here are those that seem most applicable to the clinical evaluation of thermal agents. Real and hypothetic examples will be cited.

The Single-Case Study

Many will argue that the report of a single-case study does not fulfill the criteria for research. On the other hand, the description of a single case can provide useful information, particularly if questions exist about the applicability of a known method of treatment in an unusual circumstance, or to elucidate a new approach to an old clinical problem. An innovative case report may be a stimulus for the author and others to investigate a topic in greater depth.

A report by Wing[8] illustrates that a well-planned, well-documented single case will contain several elements of the research process. The question asked was "What is the effect of phonophoretically driven hydrocortisone on the range of motion (ROM) of the temporomandibular joint (TMJ) and pain level in a patient with TMJ dysfunction?" Supportive rationale was provided in the introductory paragraph. The methods for assessment of ROM and pain were presented and conducted before and after treatment. The specific treatment protocol was described. The conclusion was stated clearly and appropriately: Phonophoresis with hydrocortisone "was influential in reducing pain and increasing ROM in this case." This statement, as written, acknowledges the most distinct disadvantage of the single-case study, which is the inability to generalize the result to a broader population. There is an inherent lack of control over extraneous variables, such as the effect of the passage of time, the patient's attitude toward treatment or, in this case, his desire to eat more heartily.

Single-Group Study

The same problems of lack of control and inability to generalize results exist in the single-group pretest, post-test design, whereby a number of subjects are tested before and after the application of a specific treatment regimen. Quillen and Rouillier[9] presented such a single-group study. The purpose of their project was to evaluate the effect of rapid pulsed-pneumatic compression, in conjunction with cold, on acute grade I sprains. Their conclusion, based primarily on edema reduction as measured by volumetric displacement, was that this form of compression was effective. A comparison of the pretreatment and post-treatment volumetric measurements was presented to support their conclusion. There can be more confidence in the effectiveness of treatment when the same or similar results are obtained in a group of individuals, in contrast to the single case.

The important questions, however, remain unanswered. Is the change in measurement caused by the treatment alone, or do other factors (i.e., time, bed rest, medication, or daily activities) contribute to the outcome? Is this group of patients different in some way from other patients with a similar clinical problem?

Campbell and Stanley[6] categorize these kinds of studies as "pre-experimental." The implication is that more rigor and control are needed to increase the value of the findings.

Comparative-Research Designs

Several approaches to comparative research can be used to study clinical questions. A common factor among them is that at least two carefully defined circumstances are compared. The choice of the approach to a specific research problem is based on: (1) the nature and content of the question to be studied, and (2) a number of pragmatic details, such as the availability of subjects, the support of patients, their families, and other health-care providers whose intervention may have an effect on the study, and whether or not withholding treatment from some subjects is ethically sound.

GROUP STUDIES

Two traditional methods for comparison are the two-group pretest, posttest design and the two-group post-test-only design.[6] Both require a rigorous control of patient selection and group assignment. Both will test the effect of a treatment scheme imposed on one group, but not on the second. The difference between these two designs is that to use a pretest determination, there must be a common pre-existing condition that can be measured and remeasured after the experimental period. For example, the question, "Is cold or cold plus intermittent compression more effective in reducing edema following ankle sprains?" presupposes that edema is present and measurable before administrating the two treatment regimens. Measured pretreatment edema becomes one criterion for patient selection, and a change in that edema becomes a determination of effectiveness. In contrast, the post-test-only design applies when the condition to be measured (the dependent variable) does not exist before treatment. If the question were, "Does the application of cold packs prevent edema following arthroscopic meniscectomy?", the preoperative condition would not necessarily include edema and, therefore, a pretreatment measurement would be irrelevant and noncontributory to answering the research question.

Both of these traditional experimental designs customarily require the most rigorous control of subject selection and assignment to treatment or control groups. The designs, for example, by classic definition require that subjects for study be drawn randomly from some defined, existing population. This requirement assumes that such a population is available to the investigator at the time a study sample is to be selected. In the case of studying the effect of cold on edema in college athletes, the investigator could hope that a huge number of athletes will suffer ankle sprains at 4 PM on a particular Wednesday. Of course, such an event is unrealistic. Furthermore, if that should happen and if the study sample could be randomly drawn from that number, would the investigator have adequate manpower, equipment, and facilities to conduct the evaluations and treatments outlined in the research protocol in a timely manner? This is highly unlikely and suggests one of the serious practical problems in performing traditional experimental research in the real clinical world.

Traditional designs can and are employed in the clinical setting despite such problems, although compromises are usually made. The study sample is often derived by the method of sequential assignment, rather than by random selection. In a two-group comparative study requiring 15 patients per group, for example, 30 slips of paper (15 with the number one, and 15 with the number two, written on them) can be placed in a hat and drawn out one by one. The order of the drawn numbers becomes the method of assigning the eligible patients as they appear to either group one or group two.

A second kind of adaptation or compromise can be made when the investigator believes that certain characteristics of subjects must be controlled by the process of group assignment. A common variable in clinical studies is the age of the subjects. In this case, an investigator who believes that healing time or functional recovery, or any element of the dependent variable, may be affected by age may choose to match the subjects according to this criterion and may assign subjects to groups in pairs, according to age.

TIME-SERIES DESIGNS

Research questions about treatment effectiveness and efficiency focus on the patient and on the management of the patient's problem in the clinic. In the clinical setting, practical issues such as time, numbers of patients with specific disorders, space and, at times, ethical considerations make it difficult to conduct two-group or multi-group studies with random samples. Procedures for conducting research have been described that may apply when the clinic is the "laboratory," the clinician is the "investigator," and the patient referred for treatment is the "subject." Of particular relevance in this clinical setting is that the time-series designs presented here can be applied to a single subject, as well as to groups of subjects. As the phrase "time series" implies, these methods of evaluation are based on serial assessment of the dependent variable over time. Depending upon the question, this may mean repeated measures over a period of hours, days, or weeks. The most important factor is that decisions about the measured variable are based not on a single assessment, but on a series of assessments.[10-13]

The simplest time-series model is the simple baseline design (A–B), in which A is a period of baseline measurement, and B is a period of measurement while treatment is being administered. In this, and in all time-series designs, the baseline period continues until the measured values are stable over repeated measures.[10,13] Figure 10–1 (top) represents a hypothetic example of the use of the A–B design to investigate the effect of ultrasound on range of motion of the shoulder in a patient with frozen shoulder. The results of this study would be less than convincing, because there is no way to be sure that some confounding variable is not responsible for the effect during phase B.

The investigator may have more confidence in the effect of treatment during phase B, if the treatment can be withdrawn for a period of time while baseline measurements are made again. If, during the second baseline period, the treatment effect is reversed toward the original baseline, and all other activities or aspects of management of the patient are unchanged, the evidence is strengthened that the treatment administered during phase B was responsible for the change in measurement values. The A–B–A, or even an A–B–A–B, time design can be used to evaluate treatment of conditions in which a return to baseline values might be expected, such as in the chronic inflammatory states of rheumatoid joints or limitations of motion secondary to long-term changes in joint structure (Fig. 10–1, bottom). These designs will not work when return

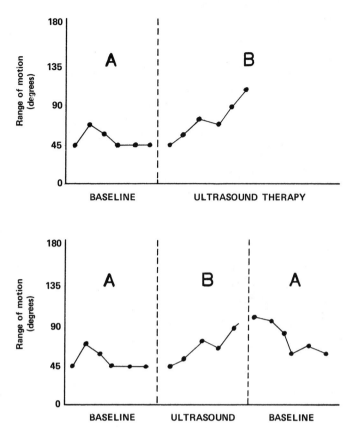

FIGURE 10–1. Hypothetical record representing the time-series designs.

to baseline is not expected. For example, when a patient is treated following a temporary period of immobilization and resumes normal activity, a return of limited motion or weakness should not happen. In this case, the A–B–A design is inappropriate.

A variation of time-series research is the *multiple-baseline design*, in which more than one measurement is obtained and evaluated. Two or more baseline measures can be derived in several ways: (1) within a single subject, studying multiple joints, limbs, or muscle groups; (2) across subjects, whereby the same method is applied to several subjects over a staggered time course; or (3) across setting, whereby a single subject is studied in different treatment settings introduced sequentially.[2,12]

SEQUENTIAL MEDICAL TRIALS

The sequential-medical-trials model is a comparative experimental system in which the results of each pair of observations, as they are obtained, determine if the experiment must continue in order to reach a definitive answer or if the experiment is to be terminated.[2,14,16] This system is based on alternative treatments randomly administered to individuals or to paired subjects. Subjects are admitted to the study until a decision is made about which of two treatments is superior. That decision is determined by the sequential plan, chosen in advance, based on the selected probability of obtaining a statistically significant result.

Formulas and calculations for these determinations have been presented by Bross[14] and Armitage.[15] Using the Bross model at a significance level of 0.05, for example, a grid is constructed. This grid, with a hypothetic set of data, is illustrated in Figure 10–2. When a preference for one treatment over the other is made for each pair of observations, an X is placed in the direction (vertical or horizontal) of that preference. As soon as the path of Xs crosses one of the bold lines, indicating a decision in favor of one of the two treatments (or in favor of neither, if the central portion lines are crossed), the study is terminated. In order for the Xs to progress, a clear decision within each pair must be made—preference for one or the other treatment must be achieved in each pair. If there is no preference (that is, if neither achieves, or if both achieve, the selected goal for success), then no X is recorded for that pair. This represents a potential fault with the design in that data are lost from the total evaluation of the comparison, unless the investigator reports this occurrence separately.

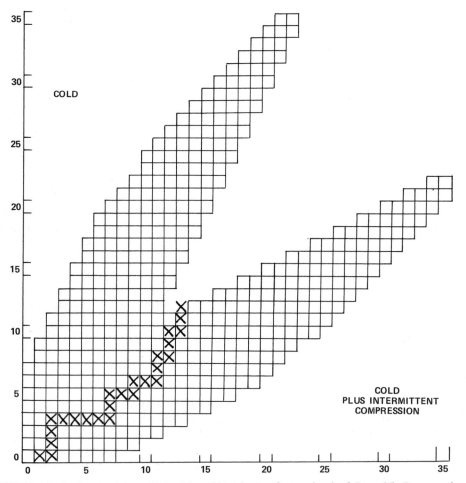

FIGURE 10–2. Sequential medical trials grid with significance level of $P \leq .05$. Data are hypothetical, comparing cold alone with cold plus intermittent compression in the treatment of ankle sprains.

The essential requirements for employing the sequential-medical-trials model include those that apply to all research designs: The alternative treatments and the measurement procedure must be specifically defined, and the criteria for subjects to be included in the study must be established in advance. Two other important requirements must be fulfilled. First, observations are made in pairs, one for each treatment. If the comparison is between two treatments in the same subject (within-subject comparison), then the order of presentation or administration of each of the treatments is random. Second, because the decision to place the Xs is based on a preference (i.e., treatment A or B or neither is better), the criterion or definition of "better" must be specified. For example, if the dependent variable is passive range of motion, what value will indicate "better": an increase of 15 degrees over the initial value; some percentage of the initial value; or a value relative to a normal value, perhaps of the uninvolved extremity?

Using the sample question, "Is cold, or cold plus intermittent compression, more effective in reducing edema following ankle sprains in college athletes?", this research model can be illustrated. The investigator will define "ankle sprain," perhaps limiting the sample to grade 2 sprains, and will determine the exact methods of applying the two treatments. The management of all subjects should be the same in all respects, except for the application of intermittent compression in one group. The number of treatments and treatment days should be specified. The daily activities of the subjects during the experimental period should be specified to control for such variables as weight bearing on the involved ankle. The criterion measured should be defined, perhaps a 50% reduction in foot and ankle edema measured volumetrically on the 4th day postinjury.

Hypothetically, 50 athletes suffered grade 2 sprains during an academic year. The effect of the two treatments was determined on each of 25 pairs and recorded on the grid (Fig. 10–2). With these 25 pairs, the central bold line was crossed, thereby indicating that neither method was better. In 13 pairs, cold plus intermittent compression resulted in a 50% reduction in edema on the 4th day and, in 12 pairs, cold alone resulted in achieving that criterion. Furthermore, the opposite member of each pair had not achieved the criterion measure. It can be noted, however, that, with the results obtained from the 20th pair, cold alone would not be found to be better. At that point, however, it was not known if cold plus compression would be determined to be superior or, as happened, if neither could be considered significantly better.

The efficiency of a sequential medical trial is a major advantage for the clinical investigator. Patients who meet the defined criteria are admitted to the study as they appear. This process is easily adapted to the clinical setting, where the ongoing clinical service cannot be disrupted in a major way, and where it is unlikely that a large number of patients are available at any one time to be randomly assigned to treatment groups. The recording of results on each pair is immediate. This process means three things: (1) data analysis is simple; (2) the study is terminated as soon as a preference is determined; and (3) when there is a clear demonstration of superiority, the impact on clinical decision making can be immediate.

The major argument against sequential trials is that an answer may be obtained after a small number of observations, or it may require a relatively large number of observations—as many as 58 pairs to reach either favorable choice, using the Bross model.[2] Numbers are of concern in interpreting the roles of chance and traditional statistical significance.[17]

This design is certainly more rigorous than the single-case study or the single-group design. It is economical and practical as a research approach in the setting of a busy clinical practice. As an example, Light and coworkers[18] have employed this model to compare two methods of stretching in patients with chronic knee-flexion contractures.

The approaches to research presented here are not all-inclusive, but rather were selected to exemplify the kind of options and some of the constraints that must be considered in order to answer any question about the value of a therapeutic regimen.

INSTRUMENTATION FOR CLINICAL EVALUATION

Clinical evaluation of thermal agents depends upon the use of measurement techniques that will provide accurate documentation of therapeutic effectiveness. Selecting appropriate measuring tools must be based on: (1) the therapeutic aims of treatment; (2) the reliability, validity, and objectivity of the measurement procedures; and (3) the value of the evaluation to the advancement of knowledge and practice of the clinician. Throughout this book, a number of clinical signs and symptoms have been discussed repeatedly: pain, edema, limitation of motion, and interference with normal muscular function. Each problem means something special to the patient and should be of major concern to the clinician. Appropriate evaluation procedures, therefore, should accurately document changes in the clinical conditions.

Many clinical characteristics are measurable in quantitative terms, for example, temperature, limb volume, muscle force, range of motion, and recovery time. Some values are qualitative in nature, for example, pain assessment and manual muscle-test grades. The importance of this distinction is that the approach to statistical analysis of data depends on an understanding of the measurement values.[2]

The following discussion will be limited to a review of the instrumentation that is currently available to the clinician or that is economically feasible to acquire and useful for measurement of the clinical problems enumerated above.

Pain Assessment

The presence of pain for many patients is a most debilitating problem. Pain relief, therefore, becomes a priority in clinical management. For this reason alone, the evaluation of pain is important. In addition, the comprehensiveness of the evaluation may also provide information about the causes of pain.

The complexities of the pain experience include not only the sensation itself, but also the impact of the patient's past experience, emotional state, and cultural attitudes on the interpretation of the quality and magnitude of the symptom. Herein lies one of the difficulties, for both the patient and the clinical investigator, in determining pain levels and changes in the pain state.

Many methods of approaching documentation of the pain experience have been described and evaluated for applicability, reliability, and validity.[19] The need for pain-assessment methods has been recognized, as the development of clinics to specifically treat patients with chronic pain has grown over the past 2 decades.[20]

McGILL PAIN QUESTIONNAIRE

In 1975, Melzack introduced the McGill pain questionnaire (MPQ).[21] This assessment tool is considered comprehensive in that it records information about sensory, affective, and evaluative dimensions of the patient's pain experience. One section of the MPQ consists of work descriptors, divided into three major categories and 20 subcategories. The sensory category (see Fig. 2–9, columns 1–10) is subdivided into groupings that describe spatial (shooting), temporal (flickering), pressure (stabbing), thermal (burning), and sharp-dull aspects of pain. The affective category (columns 11–15) includes words such as "exhausting," "vicious," and "terrifying." The evaluative words (column 16) relate to the patient's view of the total pain experience. Columns 17 to 20 consist of miscellaneous words, which represent a mixture of the three major categories. The patient is asked to select one word from each subcategory that applies to his pain and to skip a section if no word applies.

The scores obtained from this section of the questionnaire are the number of words chosen (NWC) and the pain-rating index (PRI). The PRI is derived by ranking each word per subcategory by its position in the list and summing the ranked values.

The questionnaire also includes an index of present pain intensity (PPI), which is derived from an ascending, ranked list of words: 0 = no pain to 5 = excruciating.

An abbreviated form of the MPQ has been described, which consists of 15 descriptive words (11 representing sensory qualities, and 5 representing affective qualities).[22] Each word is scored on an intensity scale from 0 = no pain to 3 = severe pain. The short form appears to be sensitive to changes in pain state and can be administered in 2 to 5 minutes, as compared to the 5 to 10 minutes required to complete the standard MPQ.

RATING SCALES

Several kinds of pain-rating scales have been described. *Verbal rating scales* (VRS) consist of word descriptors presented in ascending order, such as: "mild," "discomforting," "distressing," "horrible," and "excruciating." This example is incorporated in the McGill pain questionnaire. This descriptive scale implies a rank ordering, but should not imply equal intervals between ratings and may lack adequate sensitivity to small changes.[23]

A standard *visual analog scale* (VAS) consists of a 10-cm line labeled at the extreme ends: "No pain" at one end, and "pain as bad as it can be" at the other.[24] The VAS asks the patient to report pain intensity. The extreme case may state "as bad as it can be," which would indicate an affective quality of the assessment. In either case—"no pain" or "as bad as it can be"—the VAS measures only a unidimensional aspect of the pain experience. Using this scale, the patient is asked to make a mark along the line, which represents the level of pain. The distance from the "no pain" end of the scale to the patient's mark is the pain score.[25] When patients are assessed repeatedly using the VAS, they are usually presented with the line on a fresh piece of paper and do not see their previous markings, as suggested by Jacobsen.[26] Scott and Huskisson,[27] however, reported increasing errors in pain estimates, as time increased between assessments, when patients did not see their previous records.

Another pain-rating method is the *numerical rating scale* (NRS), on which numbers 0 to 10 (or some greater range) are aligned, and the patient is asked to circle the number that applies to his or her pain intensity. Downie and coworkers[28] found good correlation between VRS, NRS, and VAS in patients with various rheumatic disorders. They concluded that the NRS is a good compromise between the VRS, which provides only a few choices, and the VAS, where the freedom to mark anywhere along the line may be confusing to patients.

Other behavioral measures may be useful in clinical investigation to define or interpret the impact of pain.[19] For example, "up-time" versus "down-time" may be documented by asking the patient how long each day he or she spends lying down or sleeping. Records of medication intake also may indicate changes in pain levels.

When pain scales or questionnaires are used to generate research data, every possible precaution must be taken. For example, some patients have difficulty with the vocabulary used in the MPQ. If the test is too demanding, patients may not complete the test, as designed.[23] Melzack[21] discussed this potential problem regarding the reliability of the MPQ. He suggested that instructions be read aloud and that the researcher or an assistant may need to help patients comprehend the words presented. Jensen and colleagues[25] have suggested that supervision may result in fewer errors in using other rating scales, as well. Of course, the ability of the researcher or assistant to interact with a patient without bias is another potential source of variability.

PRESSURE ALGOMETER

In 1986, Fischer[29,30] described the use of a pressure gauge attached to a rubber disk (1 cm^2) for measuring pressure threshold and pressure tolerance (Fig. 10–3). This instrument has been used to document trigger-point sensitivity and responses to therapeutic intervention when pain, especially myofascial pain, is an important problem.[31] The advantage of this instrument is that it provides objective, quantitative data. When

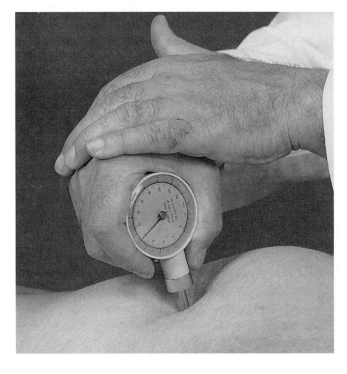

FIGURE 10–3. Pressure algometer. (Courtesy of Pain Diagnostics and Thermography Corp., Great Neck, New York.)

tested for intrarater and interrater reliability, the pressure threshold meter was demonstrated to be a highly reliable device for measuring trigger-point sensitivity.[32]

The disk is placed on the skin, and increasing pressure is applied at a 90-degree angle by the examiner. *Pressure threshold* is defined as the minimal pressure that induces discomfort, as reported by the subject. The gauge reading in kilograms or newtons, at the time the subject so indicates, is the pressure-threshold value. *Pressure tolerance* is defined as the maximal pressure the subject can tolerate. The gauge reading at the time the subject says "stop" is the pressure-tolerance value.

Fischer[33] studied 50 normal adult volunteers to document pain-threshold values over nine muscles of the shoulder, trunk, and hip. The results indicated that values were higher for men than women, that there were few differences in values between sides of the body, and that values differed from muscle to muscle. In a three-part study, Reeves and coworkers[34] documented intrarater and interrater reliability, using patients with myofascial pain as subjects. Their results showed good correlation between trials (generally, r = .70 or above) and that there was a significant difference in algometer values taken over trigger points, as compared to nearby non–trigger-point locations.

Two clinical studies using the pressure algometer have been reported. Jimeniez and Lane[35] documented increases in both pain threshold and pain-tolerance values, following a 21-day multidisciplinary treatment program, in patients with chronic pain. Jaeger and Reeves[36] studied the effect of a spray-and-stretch procedure on symptoms of myofascial pain in patients with chronic head and neck pain. They documented a significant increase in threshold values following treatment. During this study, patients also were asked to rate their pain intensity using a VAS. Although there was a significant decrease in VAS scores following treatment, there was a poor correlation between the VAS scores and algometer readings. This finding suggests that, at least in patients with chronic pain problems, the algometer data may be limited. Apparently, it does not reflect the complexity of the pain experience in chronic conditions.

OTHER CONSIDERATIONS

When pain assessment measures are used to evaluate the effects of thermal agents (or any other physical-therapy procedure), the investigator must take into account other aspects of the patient's management. Of particular importance is the administration of analgesics and anti-inflammatory drugs, which will undoubtedly influence the pain state. Cooperation between the patient, physician, and physical-therapy investigator is mandatory during a clinical trial. Clinical judgment will determine the reasonable course to follow in this case. Occasionally, stopping or withholding medication may be possible. If not, as is likely, medication administration may be regulated to ensure that no new medication is introduced and that the dosage schedule remains constant during the trial. At the very least, a record of drug intake should be maintained, as it will be if the patient is hospitalized. Control of compliance[37,38] by an outpatient is more difficult to regulate, but every attempt should be made to document the extent of this important extraneous variable.

The presence and magnitude of pain often accompanies or results in other physiologic changes. Concurrent muscle spasm or muscle guarding may interfere with range of motion. Pain may be the limiting factor in the patient's performance of daily activities. The converse may also occur if, for example, the patient has no pain at rest but, because of muscle tightness, has pain on motion. Many times, therefore, other measures of clinical effectiveness may be, and should be, obtained concurrent with the assessment of pain.

Range of Motion

Techniques of goniometry are well known to physical therapists. When these techniques are used accurately, they provide quantitative data about limitation in joint range of motion (ROM).

For research purposes, a specific protocol must be selected and defined to include such details as the type of goniometer, placement landmarks, patient position, and patient participation. The last consideration may seriously affect the validity of testing. The choice is whether to measure passive, active-assisted, or active ROM. The results may be quite different, depending upon muscle guarding, spasm, segmental-reflex interactions, or the patient's ability to follow instructions.

Common methods have been described[39,40] and are used as guides throughout the United States. Reliability of these methods has been evaluated.[41,42] Accurate goniometry requires skill and consistent performance of the examiner. These attributes may be assessed by determining intrarater reliability on repeated trials. Each investigator is obliged to determine his own reliability before initiating a study, using as a sample the same kind of patient and clinical problem that will be studied.[43] Knowledge of intrarater variability for specific measurements should be used to establish criteria for a change in patient status. Based on Boone's[42] data, for example, a change of greater than 5 degrees in the upper extremity, and 6 degrees in the lower extremity, must occur to state an improvement or a decline in ROM. Because of the documented differences between testers, it seems appropriate to use only one examiner in a given study.

Volumetric and Girth Measurements

Edema is a common problem in several of the clinical conditions for which thermal agents are employed and may be a major cause of pain, limitation of motion, and decreased functional ability. Reduction of swelling, therefore, becomes another important therapeutic goal. Two relatively inexpensive and efficient methods for obtaining quantitative data about limb edema are volumetric measurement and girth measurement.

Volume of an entire limb or a distal-limb segment can be estimated using a water displacement system,[44,45] in which the part to be evaluated is submerged in a water tank with an outflow spout from which the water displaced by the limb is collected in a graduated cylinder. The indicator of limb volume is the quantity of displaced water, measured in milliliters. The accuracy of this method depends upon (1) the initial level of water in the tank relative to the outflow spout; (2) the position of the limb in the tank, particularly depth of submersion; and (3) the state of relaxation of the patient's limb. Tanks made of clear material such as Plexiglas (Volumeters Unlimited, 524 Double View Drive, P.O. Box 145, Idyllwild, CA) are probably best to permit the examiner to observe the position of the limb within the tank (Fig. 10–4).

Smyth and associates[46] investigated the reproducibility of volumetric measurement in both normal subjects and patients with acute joint inflammation. The variability in repeated measures, taken several times in succession, was less than 1 percent for

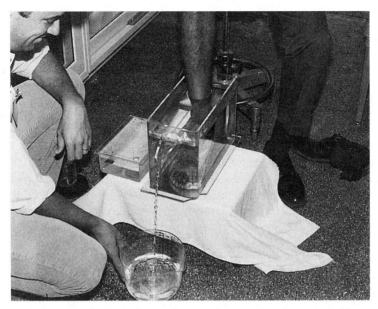

FIGURE 10-4. Foot and ankle volume is being measured using a volumeter.

hands and a maximum of 0.6 percent for feet in normal subjects. When measurements were taken at 8:30 AM and 3:30 PM, changes (both increases and decreases) were noted. The greatest change was a 1.7% decrease in the left hands of female subjects. Throughout 5 days of repeated measures, the maximal coefficient of variation was 2.3% for hand measurements and 1.5% for foot measurements. Two case studies were presented, both employing anti-inflammatory medications. In both cases, volumetric measures documented a marked decrease in volume in response to treatment: an 11% decrease in the hand measurement of the patient with rheumatoid arthritis, and a 7.4% decrease in the foot measurement of the patient with gout.

This method of volumetric measurement is appropriate when the swelling is distally located (i.e., hand and wrist or foot and ankle), or when swelling involves a large area from distal to proximal. If swelling is limited to a more proximal site (i.e., knee, thigh, or upper arm), this measurement method may not be sensitive enough to detect a change in such a delimited location, because the entire limb must be immersed. In that case, girth (or circumferential) limb measurements may be more appropriate. The only equipment required is a measuring tape; one made of flexible steel or fiberglass is probably preferred to one of cloth or plastic, which may change in length over time by stretching. Because examiner skill is required in placing and reading the tape, intrarater reliability should be evaluated before using this procedure. Limb posture and relaxation of the part to be measured may be confounding variables. Careful instructions to the patient, therefore, are necessary.

Evaluation of Muscle Performance

Muscle strength may not be of primary concern during the acute stage of injury or illness; however, restoration of normal muscle performance is usually found on any list of long-term therapeutic goals. The direct effects of cold on muscle strength have been discussed in Chapter 4. In addition, skeletal-muscle performance may be altered secondary to the demonstrated effects of thermal agents on nerve-conduction velocity, muscle-spindle activity, and synaptic transmission. For these reasons, muscle strength may be an important dependent variable in evaluating the long-term effects of applying thermal agents.

If so, the investigator must make a series of decisions in selecting the appropriate test instrument. The first problems to solve are the *operational definitions* of strength and the selection of criteria for determining whether strength is improving or declining. None of the currently used terms (such as force, tension, work, and power) are synonymous, although all can be used to describe a quality of being "strong" or "weak." Criteria for improvement or decline should be based on knowledge of the reliability or reproducibility of the selected test procedure. The second important consideration must be both the local and systemic *conditions* of the patients who will be studied. For example, testing procedures that require patients to generate high levels of force may be impractical and inappropriate in the presence of acute inflammation or serious debilitation secondary to prolonged bed rest. A third factor relates to the nature of the *research question*. If it is one in which the muscle testing should be correlated with functional activity, a determination of the functional requirements of the muscles to be tested will have to be made. Then, the investigator can select a test condition, such as isometric or dynamic, at low or high speed, that most closely relates to those functional requirements.

There is an imposing array of testing instruments for the measurement of muscle strength. Only four of the choices will be mentioned, to illustrate the available spectrum: the manual muscle test, the cable tensiometer, the hand-held dynamometer, and the isokinetic dynamometer. These instruments represent the diversity of information that can be obtained under the category of "strength" testing.

The manual muscle test[47] was developed by Lovett and Merrill in 1912 and, since that time, it has periodically fallen in and out of favor without careful analysis of the attendant reasons. One of the criticisms has been that it is not an "objective test." The objectivity of this test very definitely depends on the skill and precision of the examiner and on the adherence to strict rules for grading. Under sensible, controlled conditions, the reliability of the manual muscle test was assessed by Lilienfeld and coworkers,[48] and, based on their study results, this test was effectively employed during the polio era. This study has been criticized, however, because muscle scores were weighted by a muscle-bulk factor, which makes it impossible to relate the data to current practices of muscle testing.[49] A more recent study of interrater reliability was presented by Silver and associates.[50] This study demonstrated 97% agreement within plus or minus a half grade between three examiners, testing patients with chronic renal disease. This study affirms that standardized procedures and practice are important.

The qualitative ranking of muscle strength by manual muscle testing can be used to determine change, particularly in muscles that cannot move through the complete arc of motion against an externally applied resistance. In fact, there may be no other measure in common usage to assess muscle strength in this circumstance. The arguments against the manual muscle test become more appropriate when the variable of the examiner's manual resistance is introduced, as in the range of grades above fair (50%). Not only is the examiner's resistance part of the determination, but also the grade of "normal" (100%) may be interpreted to mean full recovery and normal function, which is not necessarily so. Watkins and colleagues,[51] for example, documented deficits in isokinetic torque production in the so-called uninvolved thigh musculature of patients with hemiparesis whose manual-muscle-test grades for quadriceps and hamstrings muscles were graded "normal."

When the muscles under study are able to develop higher levels of force, the quantitative measures of that force can, and should, be employed.

The cable tensiometer measures *isometric* tension.[1] The recorded values are pounds of kilograms of force. A calibrated length of cable is placed within a fixed cable or chain system, which is attached to the subject's limb and against which the muscle or muscle group exerts force. The force, translated through the calibrated cable, is recorded using a tensiometer attached to that cable. The advantage of this instrument is that, with the versatility of hardware attachments, the subject and tensiometer can be aligned to test a muscle at several points within the arc of motion.

A hand-held dynamometer is a device that measures the force exerted between the examiner's hand and the part being tested.[52,53] It is designed to test maximal voluntary isometric contraction. How accurate a reflection of maximal performance the dynamometer is may depend on whether a "make-test" or "break-test" protocol is used. In a make-test, the examiner holds the dynamometer in a fixed position and instructs the subjects to exert maximal force against the instrument. In a break-test, the subject holds the limb in a fixed position and the examiner exerts force through the instrument until the part gives way. Using a sample of 27 healthy women, Bohannon[54] found a significant difference in elbow-flexor forces between methods.

Good to excellent reliability of measures using a hand-held dynamometer have been documented in tests of normal children, children with Duchenne's muscular dystrophy, and patients with peripheral neuromuscular disorders.[53,55] This instrument should be considered when patients have weakness, but manual-muscle-test grades are above "fair," and when testing small muscle groups or children.[53] The magnitude of force that can be measured is limited by the range of the instrument (e.g., the Sparks' limit is 0 to 60 lb, or 27.2 kg) and the strength of the examiner, who must resist the patient's contraction.[52]

The capability of testing *dynamic* muscular performance requiring motion through an arc of motion is no longer limited to weightlifting and values such as the 10-repetition maximum of DeLorme and Watkins,[56] although this method may continue to be used if it suits the needs and criteria of a particular research question.

The concept of isokinetic exercise and the introduction of isokinetic dynamometers[57] interfaced with recording devices (such as the Cybex II, Lumex Corporation, Cybex Division, Ronkonkoma, NY) have expanded the choices of instrumentation for clinical measurement of strength. With isokinetic-exercise devices, which are based on the force-velocity principle, speed of motion can be preselected, and the instrument will prevent acceleration beyond that preset speed. Several measures of muscular performance, such as peak torque and joint angle at peak torque, can be obtained from the torque curves generated by the patient's attempt to accelerate. The Cybex II is designed to assess isometric or concentric contractions, whereas other devices (such as the KINCOM, Chattecx Corporation, Chattanooga, TN) permit assessment of eccentric contraction, as well. Assessment of performance over a range of speeds that may more closely simulate functional requirements is a potential advantage of these systems.[59] Further study, however, of both the reliability and validity is warranted, as related to functional performance.

Assessment of muscular performance can make an important contribution to the evaluation of long-term effects of thermal agents. There is, however, one final caution: All of these procedures designed to measure muscle strength depend on the *voluntary* participation and cooperation of the patients. Apprehension, inattention, lack of motivation, and the inability to follow instructions are factors that may interfere with the validity of these measures.

Functional Tests

In the course of therapeutic intervention, the question of the effectiveness and efficiency of treatment procedures eventually becomes: "How well does the patient function in carrying out the physical activities relevant to the patient's lifestyle?" In considering the efficacy of thermal agents and any comparison of specific modalities, the question may be: "How quickly does the patient return to his or her optimal level of function?" In this case, the measure is "recovery time." "Function," "recovery," and "time to recovery" then can become dependent variables in clinical studies. Again, the first necessary step is to define operationally those terms in a manner relevant to the specific research question.

The performance of functional tasks can be documented qualitatively or quantitatively. The system of noting whether a patient can perform a given activity independently, with an assistive device, or not at all can be translated into a qualitative rating scale for research purposes.

A number of quantitative measures are available or could be created. These are timed tests of functional performance in which the dependent variable is the time (usually in seconds) it takes to accomplish a defined task. An objective and standardized test of hand function by Jebsen[60] is an example of such a measure of upper-extremity function, including such items as writing a short sentence and stacking checkers. The time required to walk a fixed distance or climb a set of standard stairs[61] are other examples of timed tests.

Temporal and spatial characteristics of gait may also be quantitatively and reliably measured.[62,63] The basic implements of the method described by Boenig[62] are a mat or paper strip secured to the floor, inked tapes on the shoes of the subject, and a stop watch. Using this method, the data obtained include step length, stride length, step width, foot angle, and cadence. Using more sophisticated instrumentation, such as the computerized gait described by Wall and associates,[63] additional data can be collected, namely, stance time, double-support time, and velocity of walking.

All of the preceding examples of clinical instrumentation can be employed by physical-therapy clinicians for both the assessments of individual patients who are referred for treatment and, with careful planning and organization, the evaluation of therapeutic effectiveness or efficiency of thermal agents.

Related Evaluative Procedures

The practitioner and clinical investigator should be aware of other instruments relevant to the evaluation of thermal agents. Some have been cited elsewhere in this book. These measurements do not directly document *clinical* progress or outcomes. The information they provide, however, may be correlated with signs and symptoms that limit function. These techniques may be useful to draw attention to and further elucidate the underlying mechanisms of pathology or to document the nature and extent of a patient's problem.

Effects of thermal agents on blood flow and blood volume have been discussed in Chapters 4 through 8. Techniques to ascertain assessment of these functions include the ultrasonic Doppler flow meter,[64,65] plethysmography,[65,66] and ^{133}Xe washout studies.[67] Electromyography and nerve-conduction-velocity studies[67,68] have been cited elsewhere (see Chapters 4, 5, and 7) and may continue to provide insight regarding neuromuscular responses to thermal agents.

SUMMARY

This chapter has identified the need and selected methods for conducting clinical studies to evaluate the effectiveness and efficiency of applying thermal agents for ameliorating conditions of pain, swelling, limited motion, and functional limitations. Such evaluation cannot be done by informal opinions of practitioners whose private experiences are not tested in a well-organized manner. It must be done through sound, systematic research, most properly conducted in the clinical setting where the physical therapist and associates become the investigators, and the patients referred for treatment become the subjects of study.

The success of this kind of clinical research depends on multiple collaborations. Coordination and cooperation among physical therapists, physicians, other allied health professionals and, most certainly, the patients are important to ensure adequate control of extraneous variables. Consultation with a biostatistician during the process of establishing the appropriate research design will facilitate proper application of data-analysis procedures. In the case of thermal agent evaluation, the accuracy of energies delivered should be determined by the appropriate biomedical or electrical engineer. In summary, it is foolhardy to expect that clinical research can or should be done by a single individual.

The data derived from this kind of collaborative clinical investigation will contribute to the professional body of knowledge about therapeutic intervention and will enhance the process of clinical decision making to the benefit of both the practitioner and the patient.

Study Objectives

Having completed this chapter, the reader should now be able to:

1. Describe a research question related to the use of ultrasound in lateral epicondylitis.
2. Develop a nondirectional and a directional hypothesis regarding the use of heat and stretch for adhesive capsulitis of the shoulder.
3. List the types of clinical research available to study the effects of thermal agents in a treatment plan.
4. Explain the use of pain scales in assessing the results of treatment with thermal agents.
5. Discuss the use of volumetrics and girth measurements in assessing swelling in the extremities.

REFERENCES

1. Portney, LG, and Watkins, MP. Foundations of Clinical Research: Applications to Practice. Appleton & Lange, Norwalk, CT, 1993.
2. Payton, O: The Validation of Clinical Practice, ed 3. FA Davis, Philadelphia, 1994.
3. Rothstein, JM (ed): Measurement in Physical Therapy. Churchill-Livingstone, New York, 1985, p 5.
4. Colton, T: Statistics in Medicine. Little, Brown, Boston, 1974, p 39.
5. Fleiss, JL and Shrout, PE: The effects of measurement errors on some multivariate procedures. AJPH 67:1188, 1977.
6. Campbell, DT and Stanley, JC: Experimental and Quasi-Experimental Designs for Research. Rand McNally College Publishing, Chicago, 1963.
7. Code of Federal Regulations 45 CFR 46: Protection of human subjects (HHS). US Government Printing Office, Washington, 1983.
8. Wing, M: Phonophoresis with hydrocortisone in the treatment of temporomandibular joint dysfunction. Phys Ther 62:32, 1982.
9. Quillen, WS, et al: Initial management of acute ankle sprains with rapid pulsed pneumatic compression with cold. Journal of Orthopaedic and Sports Physical Therapy 4:39, 1982.
10. Ottenbacher, KJ: Evaluating Clinical Change Strategies for Occupational and Physical Therapists. Williams & Wilkins, Baltimore, 1986.
11. Barlow, DH and Hersen, M: Single-case experimental designs. Arch Gen Psychiatry 29:319, 1973.
12. Martin, JE and Epstein, LH: Evaluating treatment effectiveness in cerebral palsy. Phys Ther 56:285, 1976.
13. Wolery, M and Harris, SR: Interpreting results of single-subject research designs. Phys Ther 62:445, 1982.
14. Bross, I: Sequential medical plans. Biometrics 8:189, 1953.
15. Armitage, P: Sequential Methods in Medical Research. John Wiley & Sons, New York, 1971.
16. Gonella, C: Designs for clinical research. Phys Ther 53:1276, 1973.
17. Oldham, PD: Measurement in Medicine. JB Lippincott, Philadelphia, 1968.
18. Light, KE, et al: Low-load prolonged stretch vs. high-load brief stretch in treating knee contractures. Phys Ther 64:330, 1984.
19. Williams, RC: Toward a set of reliable and valid measures for chronic pain assessment and outcome research. Pain 35:239, 1988.
20. Schaefer, CA: The pain clinic approach. In Michel, TH (ed): International Perspectives in Physical Therapy, I: Pain. Churchill-Livingstone, New York, 1985, pp 233–258.
21. Melzack, R: The McGill pain questionnaire: Major properties and scoring method. Pain 1:277, 1975.
22. Melzack, R: The short-form McGill pain questionnaire. Pain 30:191, 1987.
23. Chapman, CR, et al: Pain measurement: An overview. Pain 22:1, 1985.
24. Huskisson, EC: Measurement of pain. Lancet 2:1127, 1974.
25. Jensen, MP, et al: The measurement of clinical pain intensity: A comparison of methods. Pain 27:117, 1986.
26. Jacobsen, M. The use of rating scales in clinical research. Br J Psychiat 111:545, 1965.
27. Scott, J, et al: Accuracy of subjective measurements made with or without previous scores: An important source of error in serial measurement of subjective states. Ann Rheum Dis 38:558, 1979.
28. Downie, WW, et al: Studies with pain rating scales. Ann Rheum Dis 37:378, 1978.
29. Fischer, AA: Pressure threshold meter: Its use for quantification of tender spots. Arch Phys Med Rehabil 67:836, 1986.
30. Fischer, AA: Pressure tolerance over muscles and bones in normal subjects. Arch Phys Med Rehabil 67:406, 1986.
31. Fischer, AA: Documentation of myofascial trigger points. Arch Phys Med Rehabil 69:386, 1988.
32. Delaney, GA and McKee, AC: Inter- and intra-rater reliability of the pressure threshold meter in measurement of myofascial trigger point sensitivity. Am J Phys Med 72:136, 1993.
33. Fischer, AA: Pressure algometry over normal muscles: Standard values, validity and reproducibility of pressure threshold. Pain 30:115, 1987.
34. Reeves, JL, et al: Reliability of the pressure algometer as a measure of myofascial trigger point sensitivity. Pain 24:313, 1986.
35. Jimeniez, AC, et al: Serial determinations of pressure threshold in chronic pain patients. Arch Phys Med Rehabil (abstr). 66:545, 1985.
36. Jaeger, B, et al: Quantification of changes in myofascial trigger point sensitivity with the pressure algometer following passive stretch. Pain 27:203, 1986.
37. Carpenter, J: Medical recommendations followed or ignored: Factors influencing compliance in arthritis. Arch Phys Med Rehabil 57:241, 1976.
38. Vincent, P: Factors influencing patient non-compliance. Nurs Res 20:509, 1971.
39. Moore, ML: The measurement of joint motion. Part II: The technic of goniometry. Phys Ther Rev 29:256, 1949.
40. Joint Motion: Method of Measuring and Recording. American Academy of Orthopaedic Surgery, Chicago, 1963.

41. Hellebrandt, FA, et al: The measurement of joint motion. Part III: Reliability of goniometry. Phys Ther Rev 29:302, 1949.
42. Boone, DC, et al: Reliability of goniometric measurement. Phys Ther 58:1355, 1978.
43. Miller, PJ: Assessment of joint motion. In Rothstein, J (ed): Measurement in Physical Therapy. Churchill-Livingstone, 1985, p 103.
44. Engler, HS and Sweat, RD: Volumetric arm measurements: Technique and results. Am Surg 28:465, 1952.
45. Devore, GL, et al: Volume measuring of the severely injured hand. AJOT 22:16, 1968.
46. Smyth, CJ: A method for measuring swelling of hands and feet. Acta Rheum Scand 9:293, 1963.
47. Daniels, L and Worthingham, C: Muscle Testing: Techniques of Manual Examination. WB Saunders, Philadelphia, 1980.
48. Lilienfeld, AM, Jacobs, M, and Willis, M: Study of reproducibility of muscle testing and certain other aspects of muscle scoring. Phys Ther Rev 34:279, 1954.
49. Lamb, RL: Manual muscle testing. In Rothstein, J (ed): Measurement in Physical Therapy. Churchill-Livingstone, 1985, pp 47–55.
50. Silver, M, et al: Further standardization of manual muscle testing for clinical study. Phys Ther 50:1456, 1970.
51. Watkins, MP, Harris, BA, and Kozlowski, BK: Isokinetic testing in patients with hemiparesis: A pilot study. Phys Ther, 64:184, 1984.
52. Edwards, RHT, et al: Hand-held dynamometer for evaluating voluntary-muscle functions. Lancet 2:757, 1974.
53. Stuberg, WA, et al: Reliability of quantitative muscle testing in healthy children and in children with Duchenne muscular dystrophy. Phys Ther 68:977, 1988.
54. Bohannon, RW: Make tests and break tests of elbow flexor muscle strength. Phys Ther 68:193, 1988.
55. Wiles, CM, et al: The measurement of muscle strength in patients with peripheral neuromuscular disorders. J Neurol Neurosurg Psychiat 46:1006, 1983.
56. DeLorme, TL and Watkins, AL: Progressive Resistance Exercise: Technic and Medical Application. Appleton-Century-Crofts, New York, 1951, p 23.
57. Thistle, HG, et al: Isokinetic contraction: A new concept of resistive exercise. Arch Phys Med Rehabil 48:279, 1967.
58. Farrell, M, et al: Analysis of the reliability and validity of the kinetic communicator exercise device. Med Sci Sport and Exercise 18:44, 1986.
59. Watkins, MP and Harris, BA: Evaluation of isokinetic muscle performance. Clinics in Sports Medicine 2:37, 1983.
60. Jebsen, RH: An objective and standardized test of hand function. Arch Phys Med Rehabil 50:311, 1969.
61. Vignos, PJ, Spencer, GE, and Archibald, KC: Management of progressive muscular dystrophy of childhood. JAMA 184:103, 1963.
62. Boenig, D: Evaluation of a clinical method of gait analysis. Phys Ther 57:795, 1977.
63. Wall, JC, Dhanendran, M, and Klenerman, L: A method of measuring the temporal/distance factors of gait. Biomed Eng 11:409, 1976.
64. Guyton, AC: Textbook of Medical Physiology, ed 8. WB Saunders, Philadelphia, 1991, p 153.
65. Hirsh, J: Noninvasive tests for thromboembolic disease. Hosp Pract (Sept) 1982, p 77.
66. Lasen, NA, Henriksen, O, and Sejrsen, P: Indicator methods for measurement of organ and tissue blood flow, Section 2. In Shepherd, JT and Abboud, FM (eds): Handbook of Physiology: The Cardiovascular System. American Physiological Society, Bethesda, 1983, p 40.
67. Goodgold, J and Eberstein, A: Electrodiagnosis of Neuromuscular Diseases, ed 3. Williams & Wilkins, Baltimore, 1983.
68. Kimura, J: Electrodiagnosis in Disease of Nerve and Muscle: Principles and Practice, ed 2. FA Davis, Philadelphia, 1989, p 227.

CHAPTER 11

The Application of Cold and Heat in the Treatment of Athletic Injuries

Kathryn Hemsley, MEd, ATC, PT, and
Wayne Smith, MEd, PT, ATC

CHAPTER OUTLINE

Kraus[1] has described athletic injuries as "those injuries produced by circumstances inherent in respective athletic performances." Musculoskeletal dysfunction incurred in such activity can vary from repetitive microtrauma-induced minor strains to sprains that disrupt joint ligamentous integrity to fractures. The healthcare practitioner faces a challenging goal in assisting the athlete in recovering the greatest level of protected function in the briefest period of time. Proper employment of therapeutic heat and cold modalities is contingent on understanding soft-tissue cellular and neuromuscular responses to injury. To determine the most efficacious and effective use of thermal agents in controlling the cellular responses to soft-tissue injury, the stage of inflammation and its functional sequelae (i.e., joint stiffness, loss of motion, the level of neuromuscular efficiency) must be evaluated by the treating therapist. To this end, a review of the literature is presented in this chapter, providing the rationale for use of thermal agents in management of specific pathologies commonly encountered in an athletically oriented practice.

COLD FOR EDEMA CONTROL

Management of initial swelling and control of its deleterious impact on neuromuscular function is critical to minimize recovery time from soft-tissue injury. Prompt use of cold is an integral tool for this purpose. The vasoconstriction it elicits is needed to control bleeding and to reduce the release of chemical mediators. Decelerating local cellular metabolic rate can minimize the damage caused by tissue hypoxia. The inflammatory response also evokes a pain response that inhibits normal neuromuscular function. This results in deficits in tissue extensibility, range of motion, and strength. The efficacious use of cold impairs conduction of afferent sensory input and decreases muscle-spindle sensitivity to stretch. The resultant reduction in pain and muscle spasm facilitates recovery of range of motion, allowing progressive strengthening and proprioceptive exercises to be undertaken. The potential morbidity following acute and subacute phases of injury recovery is thereby limited.[2-4]

Bennett[7] advocated the use of cold whirlpool baths (8°C) to control hemorrhage and edema, believing that this temperature would allow vasoconstriction but avoid the deleterious vasodilation response reported by Lewis.[8]

However, it was only after Hocutt and associates[9] compared cold with heat that any clinical documentation was formulated. Their study assessed patients recovering from ankle sprains. Patients who were treated with cold (i.e., whirlpool baths or ice packs applied 1 to 3 times daily, for 15 minutes each; from 1 to 36 hours or more than 36 hours after traumatic injury), returned to preinjury activities an average of 8 days sooner than did their counterparts, who were treated with heat (i.e., warm soaks or heating pads).[9] The significance of the study was threefold: (1) it was the first study of its kind reported in the literature; (2) it attempted to establish parameters with regard to temperature and duration of cold application; and (3) it was found that early cryotherapy allowed patients to return to full activities sooner than late cryotherapy or early heat treatments. Cote and coworkers[10] compared the effects of cold, heat, and contrast baths in minimizing edema in acute ankle sprains and concluded that cold therapy was the more appropriate of the three treatment regimens if the objective was to minimize swelling.

Cold and Compression

Cold has been reported to be effective when combined with other modalities in treating athletic injuries.[10-12] The addition of compression to cold application appears to enhance the effectiveness of treating sprains.[11-15] A basic cause of swelling is an increase in capillary-filtration pressure. Edema will occur when factors controlling the equilibrium between intravascular and extravascular fluids are disturbed. The use of a mechanical intermittent-compression device appears to help compensate for the body's own mechanisms to reduce interstitial fluid. With respect to osmotic pressures and hydrostatic pressures in the capillary beds, the homeostasis is maintained by encouraging lymphatic and venous return.[16] Results of clinical trials supported the use of a gradient pneumatic-pressure unit utilizing a three-celled compartmental sleeve.[16] This sleeve is inflated sequentially to facilitate movement of edema distally to proximally in the lower extremity. Several clinicians have sought to evaluate the efficiency of combining cold and intermittent compression in treating ankle sprains. Starkey[14] compared the simultaneous use of cold, elevation, and intermittent inflatable compression with that of cold, elevation, and compression wrapping. He concluded that 30 minutes of intermittent compression at a 15-second cycle, along with cold and elevation, proved to be more effective in edema reduction than were cold, elevation, and compression wrapping. In addition, time lost from practice was reduced with the former regimen by approximately 2 days. More recent research confirms earlier studies of the effectiveness of cold and compression. Merrick and coworkers[17] examined the intramuscular tissue temperature at various depths in an effort to evaluate the effectiveness of cryotherapy techniques. Ice only, when combined with compression, produced significant cooling at the surface, 1 and 2 cm below the subcutaneous fat layer. Sloan and associates[18] compared treatment of cold to cold and compression in the treatment of artificially induced acute inflammatory edema. They found that the most effective treatment was a combination of both modalities.

Another study was developed in an effort to minimize edema accumulation in the joint capsule and its resultant neural inhibition of dynamic stabilizers. Wilkerson and Horn-Kingery[19] examined three methods of applying compression in the management of acute grade II inversion ankle sprains: (1) use of elastic tape providing uniform compression; (2) focal compression achieved with a U-shaped device maintained at room temperature; and (3) compression utilizing this device when frozen. Application was to the soft tissues adjacent to the fibular malleolus. Each technique included subsequent application of an Aircast stirrup brace. All three treatment groups received a daily session of cryotherapy of 20 to 30 minutes' duration. The groups receiving focal compression attained their functional goals in 25% fewer days than the group receiving uniform compression. The authors credited the enhanced recovery rate to the focal compression. This compression facilitated the translocation of edema proximally to enhance its resolution via the lymphatic system. They suggested this minimized both the mechanical interference and the neural inhibition of dynamic stabilizers posed by the presence of edema. In their observations, however, the mode of external compression had a greater effect on restoration of function than the frequency or duration of cryotherapy.

Rucinski and coworkers[20] examined the efficacy of three treatment protocols in the edema management of grades I and II postacute ankle sprains. Each group received a 30-minute treatment of either intermittent or elastic wrap compression with limb elevation to 45 degrees. The control group that received elevation only had the least edema. The fluctuation in volume after compression demonstrated in this study invites further investigation. More information is needed to fully understand the mechanical and physiologic responses to compression management techniques for optimal integration with cold applications.

Cold and High-Voltage Pulsed Current

High-voltage pulsed current (HVPC), along with ice, has become a popular therapy mode for reducing effusion (Fig. 11–1). Several preliminary reports have sug-

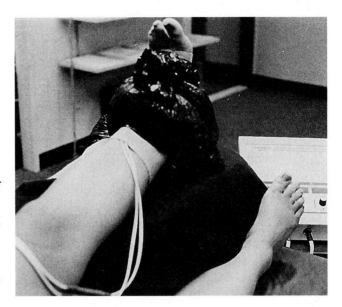

FIGURE 11-1. The use of cold, wet compression wrap, and elevation in combination with high voltage pulsed current for the acute management of an ankle sprain. Note that the stimulating electrodes are on the medial and lateral ankle under the cold pack.

gested that this combination appears to be effective in the management of musculoskeletal trauma, including sprains.[9,10,18] Lamboni and Harris[12] have reported good results in reducing edema using cold, compression, and HVPC at 30 pulses per second and negative polarity for 30-minute periods. Smith[21] reported similar results in one case postfracture. He used cold packs, elevation, and HVPC at 60 pulses per second (pps), negative polarity and reciprocal stimulation for 10 seconds per pad. A better controlled study,[22] however, comparing ice versus ice and HVPC (negative polarity) at 28 pps and 80 pps for the treatment of acute ankle sprains, found no significant difference in the treatment's effect on foot and ankle volume or range of motion in dorsiflexion. This study used sensory-level stimulation and did not take advantage of edema control via a muscle pumping mechanism.

Perceiving the need for controlled studies to verify the efficacy of use of this modality in edema management of trauma-induced inflammatory response, Mendel and Fish[23] conducted a series of experiments involving the use of HVPC analyzing the soft-tissue responses of frogs and rats. Most effective use of electric stimulation was application of cathodal HVPC delivered in immersion technique at 120 pps and voltages 90% of visible motor threshold. A 30-minute treatment significantly reduced edema for more than 4 hours. Polarity of stimulation was found to be critical since anodal stimulation did not produce a treatment effect. The authors could not address HVPC efficacy relative to use with other modalities or in application to chronic edema. Further clinical studies are evidently warranted.

CASE STUDY 1

A 19-year-old male soccer player sustained an inversion sprain to his right ankle. He was unable to fully bear weight on his right foot and required assistance to leave the field of play. He developed swelling about the anterolateral aspect of the foot and ankle, resulting in limitation of range of motion. Physical examination revealed no gross deformities, palpable tenderness distal to the lateral malleolus, and mild ligamentous laxity to anterior and varus stress. X-rays revealed no bony pathology and stress films revealed no remarkable talar tilt.

PROBLEMS

1. Swelling about the anterolateral aspect of the foot and ankle.
2. Limited ankle motion.
3. Pain with weight bearing.

ASSESSMENT TECHNIQUES

1. Volume measurement of right foot and ankle.
2. Pain quantity, quality, and location.
3. Range-of-motion measurements.
4. Functional activities assessment, including gait when appropriate.

GOALS

1. Decrease swelling and maintain the reduction.
2. Reduce pain.
3. Increase range of motion of the foot and ankle.
4. Increase functional activities.

SELECTION OF TREATMENT MODALITY

Thirty minutes of cold, intermittent compression (50 mm Hg) and elevation, followed by 30 minutes of cold, wet wrap compression with HVPS (120 pps and intensity 10% less than the level required to evoke visible muscle contractions). Elevation of the limb was continued at this time.

The patient was given crutches, a compression wrap, and a semirigid stirrup orthosis to eliminate varus stress. Weight bearing was as tolerated. As pain and edema abated, the patient was instructed in a cryokinetics regimen: cold whirlpool (9°C) for 15 minutes, followed by range-of-motion (ROM) exercises and gentle Achilles tendon stretching. HVPC and cold, wet wrap compression were applied to conclude the treatment sessions. On the 4th day postinjury, swelling and pain appeared stabilized and a program of alternating cold applications and light resistance exercises was implemented.

HOME PROGRAM

A home program of 20 minutes of ice, cold wrap compression, and elevation throughout the subsequent 24 to 48 hours was implemented. The athlete continued to wear the orthosis for focal compression and frontal plane support as he progressed to weight-bearing proprioceptive re-education activities. On the 9th day, he resumed activity with protection of an athletic tape support.

RATIONALE FOR CLINICAL DECISION MAKING

Pain and swelling appear to be the primary problems initially; these areas need to be addressed first. ROM is affected by pain and swelling. Cold/compression and HVPC address the pain and swelling. The decrease in strength was primarily caused by disuse, and regaining strength is not expected to be a problem, although progress may be limited by pain.

COLD FOR MUSCLE AND TENDON INJURY

Injuries that involve the tendon or its musculotendinous junction pose many challenges for the sports medicine practitioner. The joint must be kept mobile to avoid morbid complications during healing without producing further damage. Cold has been demonstrated to be effective in relieving pain and allowing both passive and active exercises affording early joint motion.[5,9,15,18] Grant[4] and Hayden[5] both reported that ice massage of 5 to 7 minutes' duration achieved sufficient anesthesia to permit ROM and mobilization exercises. Waylonis, who later repeated Grant's study under controlled conditions, measured some of the physiologic changes in ice massage—pain stimuli, blood flow, and skin temperature.[24] Waylonis reported that although numbness occurred at 5 minutes of application, those who received a 10-minute application had a greater reduction of temperatures to the deeper tissues. Prentice[25] evaluated the effectiveness of heat and cold using electromyography (EMG), along with some form of stretching for inducing skeletal-muscle soreness. The study involved a four-way comparison among heat and contract-relax stretching, cold and static stretching, heat and static stretching, and a control group. The findings indicated that those who received a combination of 20 minutes of ice pack followed by static stretching exhibited less EMG activity than did the three other groups. Therefore, the implications for using cold and stretching in such conditions as muscle spasm may have some validity, as shown by experimental research.

Lentell and associates[26] examined the influence of thermal agents with low-load prolonged stretch. They observed that persons treated with ice and low-load prolonged stretching demonstrated clinically substantial, long-lasting gains.

Yackzan and associates[27] investigated 15 minutes of ice massage for delayed-onset muscle soreness (DOMS) to determine the optimal time within a stated protocol. Three groups receiving cold were tested: (1) ice immediately after exercise; (2) ice 24 hours after exercise; and (3) ice 48 hours after exercise. Pain and ROM were assessed after the person performed eccentric-based exercises of the elbow flexor muscles. There were no consistent patterns of significant differences in various comparisons studied either between the treated versus the untreated arms or the treated arms that were iced at different times. This study failed to demonstrate that cold alone was effective in preventing the occurrence of, or in alleviating pain in, DOMS. Therefore, cold in combination with stretching exercises may be the preferred technique.

Isabell and coauthors[28] induced DOMS using eccentric training. Loss in ROM and strength output were observed. The elevated serum creatine kinase levels that were documented postexercise training indicated muscle-tissue damage. Use of ice massage, ice massage with exercise, and exercise alone were all ineffective in significantly reducing symptoms of DOMS. In fact, their results indicated an increase in soreness and serum creatine kinase levels, and production of lowest peak total ROM of all groups when ice and exercise were used compared to use of ice or exercise alone.

However, the authors could not say conclusively that the combination of ice and exercise was deleterious to the recovery from DOMS, but they did suggest that physiologic responses from muscle adaptation and repair may be adversely affected by cold application. Denegar and Perrin[29] attempted to examine the efficacy of using transcutaneous electrical nerve stimulation (TENS), cold, and a combination treatment including static stretching on pain, decreased ROM, and strength loss associated with DOMS. Their results suggested that these modalities were effective in the management of pain and muscle spasm associated with DOMS. However, despite the significant decrease in perceived pain after modality application, muscle weakness associated with DOMS remained. This finding further suggests that muscle weakness may not be caused primarily by pain inhibition but may be in response to tissue damage.

Cryostretch techniques may also involve the application of a topically applied cold spray (refer to Chapter 4 for a discussion of cold sprays). Theorized to be based upon the counterirritant principle, cutaneous afferent impules to the spinal cord alter the perception of sensory pain input via C-fiber transmission responding to an otherwise painful muscle stretch.[30] Reflex relaxation ensues. The clinician thereafter slowly imposes prolonged soft-tissue elongation but must remain cognizant to avoid a stretch reflex. This would prove counterproductive to muscle spasm inhibition.

Various forms of cold application can be used in pain reduction and subsequent inhibition of muscle spasm. However, the clinician must be aware of the perils in stretching "cold" connective tissues, muscle shortening, or soft-tissue contracture. The use of heat in the subacute phase may better enhance soft-tissue extensibility.

CRYOKINETICS

Cryokinetics, that is, cold and exercise, is an integral part of the initial phase of the athlete's rehabilitation. The key to success in this early stage of recovery is the use of cold for pain inhibition to allow greater effort with graded exercise. Cohn and associates[31] studied the effects of cold in the postoperative management of pain in patients undergoing anterior cruciate ligament reconstruction. Pads filled with 50°F fluid formed an ice blanket applied to either side of the operated knee postoperatively and remained in place for the initial 4-day course. Compared to patients in the control group, the treated group performed ROM exercises with greater ease and required less palliative therapy during their postoperative course. Miller and Webers[32] conducted a study to determine the effects of ice massage on an individual's pain tolerance to electrical stimulation. These authors' findings suggest that ice massage may increase an individual's tolerance to the noxious sensation that usually accompanies high levels of electric stimulation. Thereby, the patient can continue strength training without unnecessary pain.

Ice is used in cryokinetics to numb the affected area; 10 to 15 minutes of application is usually necessary to achieve the required analgesia (Fig. 11–2). The use of cryokinetics has a built-in safety valve, unlike the potential dangers involved when pain-alleviating pharmaceutical agents are injected to enable the patient to perform exercises. Although the clinical application of cold produces a degree of analgesia, judicious application is generally not enough to completely anesthetize the involved tissue. If an athlete is experiencing pain during analgesia of the injured part during exercises, this alerts the practitioner that the exercise is too vigorous. In order to avoid pain during exercise, the patient's activity level should be decreased.

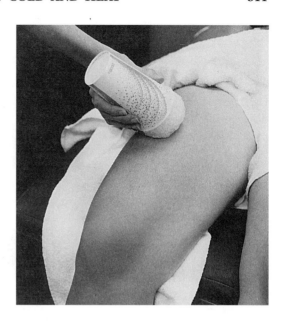

FIGURE 11-2. The use of ice massage on a thigh contusion to achieve analgesia prior to isometric exercise during the subacute stage.

Cold application can cause substantial pain before it moderates the injury-pain.[2] Carman and Knight[33] examined the potential habituation to cold-pain during repeated cyrokinetic treatment sessions and found that clinicians may be justified in their often-made claim that such discomfort will diminish with repeated applications. They found that habituation was temperature and body-part specific. The authors thereby concluded that the mechanism is predominately physiologic, but with a psychologic component. Ingersoll and Mangus[34] conducted a series of cold immersions over a 5-day period. The McGill pain questionnaire was used to measure pain during these treatments (see Chapter 2). Though the authors did not document habituation to perception of cold-induced pain, they did identify "hypalgesia" to describe their observed decrease—but not absence—of cold-induced pain. The effects of both hot and cold immersions on deep and superficial sensory perception were examined. The hypalgesic effect afforded the athlete the capacity to participate in a closed kinetic chain rehabilitation exercise regimen without altered proprioception and the resultant improper integration of neuromuscular input.

Cryokinetics is easily performed under proper instruction and supervision. Initially, cold is used to numb the injured part by applying ice massage, ice packs, or immersion baths (Fig. 11-3). If the therapist or trainer chooses to use an immersion bath, a technique sometimes employed for injuries of the distal joints, the duration of treatment should not exceed 15 minutes, and the clinician should ensure that the patient has intact peripheral circulation. Prolonged local exposure to cold has been reported to result in nerve palsies.[35] Sunderland's[36] study of peripheral nerve injury via cold applications indicates that motor function is affected first and to a greater degree than sensory functions. However, as warming occurs, sensory function is restored more rapidly than motor function. Clinicians must recognize the tremendous variation in the resistance of individual peripheral nerves to injury from cryotherapy. Total motor and sensory loss can occur at 0 to 5°C. The sensitivity of individuals to the duration and intensity of tissue cooling dictated by its method and location of application (degree of

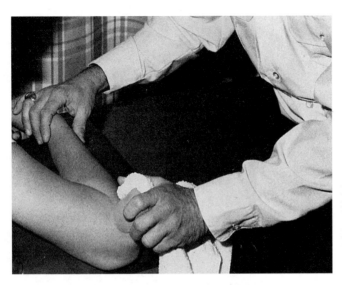

FIGURE 11–3. Cryokinetics in the management of tennis elbow. Ice massage is being applied to the area of lateral epicondyle to be followed by a slow, gentle stretch of the wrist extensor muscles.

relative insulation provided by the thickness of overlying subcutaneous fat) must be evaluated by the practitioner and modifications implemented accordingly.

Cold can be a valuable tool in the early management of rehabilitation of the injured athlete. Therefore, it is important that the trainer or therapist knows the specific effects of cold on the body, when to use this agent, where to apply it, and how it can assist in rehabilitation. Tables 11–1 to 11–3 provide the reader with the basic guidelines for the application of thermal agents in three common sports-related injuries. These should serve as guidelines only, and variations may be expected in application to specific cases.

CASE STUDY 2

A 19-year-old intercollegiate tennis player underwent plica resection of his left knee through an arthroscopic surgical procedure at semester's end. He had been rehabilitating his lower extremity through a home program without success for a subsequent 3-week period. At the second follow-up evaluation by his surgeon, he had continued pain with exercises and mild effusion. This precipitated a referral to physical therapy. The patient complained of medial peripatellar pain and pain with performance of quadriceps exercises both in terminal extension and at various points throughout knee flexion to extension arc of motion.

PROBLEMS

1. Medical peripatellar pain and pain with performance of quadriceps exercises.
2. Pain on knee flexion.
3. Mild effusion.
4. Limited functional activities.

TABLE 11-1 Therapeutic Guidelines for the Application of Cold and Heat in the Management of Ankle Sprains

Conditions	Management Phase	Basic Management	Combination Treatment	Objectives of Treatment
Inversion ankle sprain (grade 2–3)	Phase 1: Immediate, 0–72 hr	Cold Ice pack, 15–30 min Whirlpool, 12–20 min (13°C–21°C)	Compression Constant Intermittent HVPC stimulation	Reduce swelling and pain
	Phase 2: Subacute, 72–96 hr	Cold Cryokinetics, 7–10 min ice Whirlpool (13°C–21°C) Heat (edema controlled)	Passive/active exercising	Improve mobility; increase blood flow Same as above
		Whirlpool, 15–20 min (35.5°C–38°C) Ultrasound (dosage-dependent) continuous Phonophoresis	Mobilization	Same as above Selective heating of joint structures Tissue repair; induce medication to injury site
	Phase 3	Heat Whirlpool, 12–20 min (37°C–39°C) Ultrasound (dosage-dependent)	Isokinetic cycle Preprogram jogging Friction massage to fibular collateral ligament	Strengthening; improve blood flow Reduction of adhesions or scarring

TABLE 11-2 Therapeutic Guidelines for the Application of Cold and Heat in the Management of Thigh Contusions

Conditions	Management Phase	Basic Management	Combination Treatment	Objectives of Treatment
Thigh contusion (grade 2-3)	Immediate, 0-48 hr	Cold Ice pack, 15-30 min Cool whirlpool, 10 min (13°C-21°C)	Elevation crutches Compression wrap Rest HVPC stimulation	Control hemorrhaging Reduce muscle spasms and pain
	Subacute, 48 hrs (variable)	Cryokinetics, 10-min ice massage to injury site Ice pack, 15-20 min	Isometric exercise; passive ROM to tolerance Electrical stimulation; exercise	Improved flow; mobility; strengthening Muscle re-education; reduce stasis
	Phase 3 Injury site stabilized	Heat Whirlpool (38°C-39°C) Ultrasound (dosage-dependent)	Isokinetic cycle; preprogram Passive stretching	Strengthening injury site; improve blood flow Heat deeper tissues; clot reabsorption

TABLE 11–3 Therapeutic Guidelines for the Application of Cold and Heat in the Management of Achilles Tendinitis

Conditions	Management Phase	Basic Management	Combination Treatment	Objectives of Treatment
Achilles tendinitis	Swelling and redness present	Cold Ice pack, 15–30 min Cool whirlpool, 10 min (13°C–21°C)	Crutches ¼-in heel lift HVPC, 15–30 min	Reduce swelling; pain reduction
	Gradual onset: crepitation; pain present	Cryokinetics, 5–10 min ice massage	Non-weight-bearing Heel cord stretching; temporary orthotic ¼-in heel lift	Increase blood flow Mobility Biomechanical control
	Phase 3 Pain intermittent Edema not present	Ultrasound (dosage-dependent) Heat Whirlpool, 10–15 min (37°C–39°C)	Phonophoresis, active exercising, and flexibility program; consider permanent orthotic control	Induce medication Increase blood flow Biomechanical control if necessary
	Chronic (>3 wk) intermittent pain with excessive activities	Ultrasound (continuous) before friction massage or ice massage, ice pack, or whirlpool	Friction massage to Achilles tendon	Heat tissues Reduce adhesions Enhance tolerance prior to; reduce irritation after massage

315

ASSESSMENT TECHNIQUES

1. Pain quantity, quality, and location.
2. ROM measurements.
3. Girth measurements of knee.
4. Functional daily activities assessment.

GOALS

1. Reduce pain.
2. Maintain ROM of the knee.
3. Decrease pain on flexion.
4. Increase functional activities.

SELECTION OF TREATMENT MODALITY

Modifications were implemented to reduce pain and to block the quadriceps inhibition reflex. These included application of ice prior to biofeedback-monitored hip adduction isometrics, quadriceps isometrics sets, and subsequent short arc and terminal extension exercises (Fig. 11–4). Painful terminal knee extension range may be alleviated with reapplication of ice for 10 minutes. Patellar taping techniques may enhance extensor mechanism alignment; positioning the tibia toward internal tibial rotation decreases the Q angle and may lower the stress on

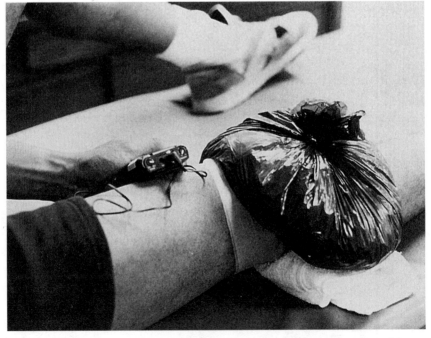

FIGURE 11–4. Ice used to reduce pain and block a quadriceps inhibition reflex while attempting to perform biofeedback monitored isometric contractions at terminal extension range of motion.

the medical compartment structures. Use of cryokinetics includes use of ice during electric stimulation–assisted maximal voluntary isometric contractions. This work is performed in 10-second intervals throughout the individual's pain-free range of flexion toward terminal extension (Fig. 11–5).

Closed kinetic chain exercises may also be instituted utilizing a pain-free range of quadriceps function. Exercises may include a leg press or partial squat work employing both lower extremities, thereby allowing contribution from the involved extremity as tolerated. Lateral step-ups also serve to retrain the quadriceps mechanism and to develop eccentric control. Such weight-bearing proprioceptive re-education exercises are gradually tailored to the movement patterns of the specific sport activity. The practitioner must exercise sound judgment in titrating the parameters of exercise progression with the patient's pain response to the treatment approach formulated.

HOME PROGRAM

A home program parallels that initiated in a clinical context and is instituted upon the re-evaluation of the athlete's tolerance for the initial program. Emphasis is placed upon the need for the athlete to take responsibility for his or her rehabilitation success, which is contingent on daily compliance to the tolerated program. The athlete is educated in detection, interpretation, and management of clinical signs of inflammation in order to safely proceed with the home program.

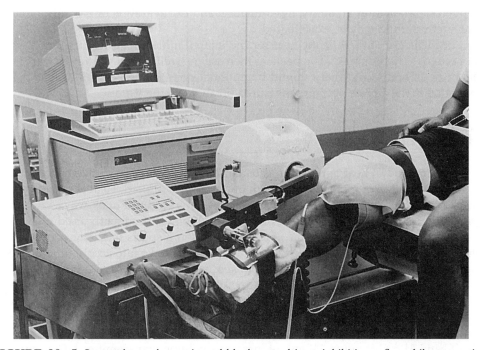

FIGURE 11–5. Ice used to reduce pain and block a quadriceps inhibition reflex while attempting maximal quadriceps recruitment isometrically, throughout the individual's range of pain-free extension.

The athlete may be instructed in patellar taping techniques and portable electric stimulator application for home use. Such devices are discontinued as extensor mechanism alignment and quadriceps recruitment improves.

RATIONALE FOR CLINICAL DECISION MAKING

The rehabilitative program continues until the intensity, frequency, and duration of athletic activity suffices to maintain the proper strength level required for the athlete to remain asymptomatic. The athlete must remain cognizant of the need to re-institute the program if the level of training fails to maintain proper extensor mechanism function as manifested by renewal of previous symptoms.

HEAT

The effects of heat on circulation, metabolism, and neural activity must be taken into account when beginning a new phase of rehabilitation. Heat improves capillary flow and increases the fluid quantity of tissues by speeding the blood flow and dilating the vessels in the heated areas. As a result, metabolism of heated parts is increased, hastening chemical changes and diminishing congestion brought about by the inflammatory process. The improved environment facilitates soft-tissue repair. Heat may reduce muscle spasm by directly increasing the threshold of sensory endings and indirectly by reflex inhibition: decreasing gamma motor neuron activity and inhibiting muscle-spindle excitability. Hence, it is a pain-relieving modality. However, if heat is applied too soon after an injury, inflammation and extravasation of blood from vessels and synovial fluid may be exacerbated.

Prudent use of therapeutic heat for the injured athlete requires fulfillment of certain criteria. There should have been no increase in swelling of the affected part within the prior 24 hours, and there should be minimal point tenderness, as well as marked reduction in the athlete's pain as measured on an analogue scale.

HYDROTHERAPY

The method of heat application is usually predicated on the convenience of application, availability of method, and depth of absorption desired. Heat is usually administered by either hydrocollator packs, hydrotherapy, or continuous-wave ultrasound. One author's experience is that hydrotherapy is the most frequently used modality in treating postacute sprains, strains, and contusions in a sports medicine setting. When choosing a therapeutic temperature, the therapist must take into account the disadvantages of, and the precautions necessary when using, whirlpools. Studies have shown that topically applied wet heat to raise superficial tissue temperatures is best produced when tissue temperatures between 37°C and 43°C are obtained.[37] Therefore, water should be within these temperature ranges, using variances that take into account the amount of edema and patient sensitivity. Whirlpool baths at temperatures between 40.5°C and 41.6°C result in 140 mL of increased volume in extremities.[38] Consequently, whirlpool baths at high temperatures are contraindicated in cases where edema is a potential problem.

The practice of full-body immersion for treatment extremities at high temperature should be avoided. Special care should be taken by the healthcare practitioner to avoid full-body immersion of an athlete who has just completed vigorous exercise. Two serious problems can result from this technique. First, because blood vessels throughout the body dilate, blood is drawn away from the parts not submerged. The change in blood pressure can result in the person fainting. Second, there is the danger of the athlete suffering from heat exposure. Because the body's surface is surrounded by water that is warmer than normal body temperature, heat may not be able to dissipate from the body through evaporation or radiation. A proper cool-down is first necessary for the athlete to dissipate the internal body heat that has resulted from exercise.

ULTRASOUND

The clinical application and guidelines for administration of hot packs and ultrasound have already been discussed in Chapters 5 and 7, respectively. The literature involving control studies using these modalities among the athletic population remains sparse. The significance of what is reported, however, can be applied to the population. Baker and Bell[39] found the application of hot packs can increase blood flow in the human calf up to 45 minutes following application. However, hot pack use prior to ultrasound administration did not enhance its effect on blood flow.

Ultrasound is commonly used by therapists and trainers as an adjunct in the management of soft-tissue injuries including capsular, ligamentous, or musculotendinous inflammation. Phonophoresis (Fig. 11–6) is becoming increasingly popular among

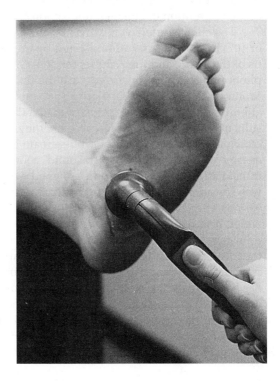

FIGURE 11–6. Ultrasound focused on the medial calcaneal tubercle and medial longitudinal arch in the management of plantar fasciitis.

practitioners. The notion is to enhance transdermal penetration of an anti-inflammatory medication while providing the therapeutic effects of ultrasound. The mechanism by which ultrasound facilitates transdermal drug transport has not been clearly defined; it may be advantageous over iontophoresis since the medications need not have a specific electrical charge.

Stimulation of tissue regeneration, increased blood flow, changes in cell metabolism, and promotion of pain relief are included as nonthermal effects of ultrasound produced by either continuous or pulsed mode.[40] The pulsed mode is beneficial in promoting healing with minimal thermal effects, and its effects on cell membrane permeability may enhance the depth of penetration of topical medication[41] in situations where it may be inadvisable to heat tissue.

Byl and colleagues[42] conducted a controlled pilot study involving determination of the effects of phonophoresis with corticosteroid administration. They reviewed a variety of medications that may be used particularly in this context: anesthetics such as lidocaine or menthol to create numbness to block pain perception; analgesics to relieve pain without impairment of other sensations; counterirritants such as methyl salicylate to relieve pain via stimulation rather than depression of sensory receptors; and anti-inflammatory medications such as dexamethasone or hydrocortisone acetate. Administered via ultrasound through the stratum corneum, the medication can bypass metabolism through the liver and enter the circulatory system directly. Acoustic streaming changes cell permeability, thereby enhancing the diffusion potential of tissues. This is also enhanced by heat-dilating blood vessels. Acoustic waves increase the kinetic energy of the medication molecules, allowing the drug to diffuse into the tissues. The effectiveness of drug administration via ultrasound could be inferred from the extravasation of plasma proteins, resulting in decreased fluid accumulation, tissue edema, local heat, and changes in polymorphonuclear cells and/or mononuclear phagocyte cells at the site of the lesion.[43] Interference with fibroblast division resulting in the retardation of collagen deposition was used to infer corticosteroid penetration.[44]

The clinical effectiveness has been reported by Kleinkort and Wood[45] in their use of 10% hydrocortisone administered by ultrasound in treating certain types of tendinitis of the elbow and the Achilles tendon. Griffin and colleagues[46] studied the efficacy of phonophoresis and concurred with the findings of Kleinkort and Wood. Cameron and Monroe[47] determined the relative transmission of ultrasound with various media and attempted to identify the group of media that transmit ultrasound well. Contrary to results obtained with other researchers, they found that the commonly used 10% hydrocortisone, administered either in its cream base or as a gel (the latter transmits acoustic energy well), transmitted ultrasound poorly. Drug-containing media were tested for transmission effectiveness and assigned a percentage relative to that of water, which was considered to rank 100% effective. In this regard, fluocinonide (0.05%) transmitted 97% as effectively as water; methyl salicylate (15%) conducted 97% as effectively as water; betamethasone (0.05%) conducted 88% as effectively as water; and lidocaine administered in a pad preparation was 68% as effective. The authors acknowledge that the ideal ultrasound power for the clinical application of ultrasound is unknown.

In application of ultrasound over an irregular surface, a water-filled latex glove has been suggested to enhance coupling; however, latex does not transmit acoustic energy and therefore will serve to insulate the area from ultrasound transmission.[48] An ultrasound gel pad (Fig. 11–7) can be used for effective ultrasound transmission over irregular surfaces and theoretically can serve as a conducting medium equivocal to gel–media-based phonophoresis treatments. The limited diameter of the pad (9 cm)

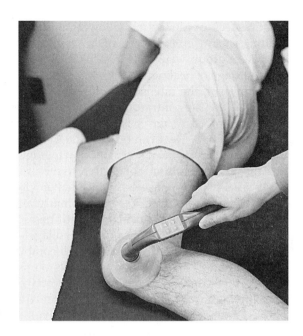

FIGURE 11-7. Depiction of the use of a gel pad for effective acoustic energy transmission with ultrasound applied over an irregular surface. (Aquaflex gel pad courtesy of Parker Laboratories, Inc., Orange, New Jersey.)

also serves to confine the treatment area, thereby disciplining the practitioner to focus effective energy delivery for maximal transdermal drug penetration.

Smith and coworkers[19] compared phonophoresis with other modes of treatment—ice, ultrasound, and iontophoresis—in treating shinsplint syndrome. Phonophoresis and the other modalities were effective for pain control, but none were significantly superior to each other.

When using this procedure in treating joint and tendon dysfunction, one must take the stage of inflammation into consideration. The clinician should consider the use of phonophoresis in treating subacute and chronic conditions rather than acute conditions if continuous-wave mode is used. Elevation of tissue temperature may exacerbate acute inflammation. Depth of penetration and anatomic positioning of the patient are also factors to keep in mind when using phonophoresis treatments. Intensities between 1.0 and 1.5 W/cm^2 for a 5-minute duration appear to have been commonly used. Conditions such as subdeltoid bursitis may be difficult to treat using phonophoresis, perhaps because of the excessive amount of tissue the drug must pass through to reach the inflamed area.

Plantar fasciitis, a common occurrence in runners, appears to respond to the therapeutic application of ultrasound. Clark and Stenner[50] studied the effects of ultrasound among patients who were diagnosed for plantar fasciitis. Of the 10 patients treated, eight reported improvement after nine applications of 15 to 20 minutes of 1.5-W/cm^2 continuous-wave ultrasound. Kleinkort and Wood,[45] however, related poor results after six phonophoresis treatments. They postulated that the thickened epidermis may have hampered delivery of the hydrocortisone to significant levels. The success of Clark and Stenner's[50] study may have been attributed to the thermal effects of ultrasound, that is, enhanced blood flow and tissue metabolism.

Ultrasound is often used to facilitate the healing of soft-tissue structures during the posttraumatic or postsurgical period. Frieden and associates[51] studied the therapeutic effects of ultrasound following partial rupture of Achilles' tendons in male rats. Through the use of electron microscopic analysis, ultrastructural changes within the treatment group were consonant with those changes that would occur in a more advanced stage of healing.

However, the intensity applied by the therapist must be a consideration. Histologic studies using ultrasound on traumatized tissues with hematomas indicated that intensities of 1.5 W/cm^2 were needed to effect the healing process via reabsorption of the hematoma.[52] Heat can be of value to the patient when it is used to warm connective tissue that has been scarred following injury or surgery. Strains involving the tearing of either muscle or connective tissue are a common occurrence in athletes. The body's cellular response is manifested in production of fibroblasts, which, in turn, leads to the production of collagen. Injury and subsequent immobilization can affect movement of tissues, causing joint stiffness. Studies have shown that, under heated conditions, the viscous properties of collagenous tissue can become altered, allowing residual elongation of this tissue when combined with a superimposed load. Noonan and associates[53] studied thermal effects on skeletal-muscle tensile behavior to determine if there is a significant correlation between temperature and length-tension relationship in muscle. Their findings confirm clinical perceptions that warmed muscle affords more deformation to attain a given load, and this decrease in stiffness is interpreted as a performance benefit that results in a lower risk of injury. Sapega and coworkers[54] suggested that prolonged, low-intensity stretching at elevated temperatures and maintaining that stretch while tissues cool can be effective in gaining ROM. The potential for lasting deformation of connective tissue is maximized, while the deterioration of tensile structural strength by heating prior to stretching is minimized. They suggested cold application to accelerate the tissue's returning to its preheat status. This notion needs testing, and, therefore, cannot be recommended at this point as a technique to use with "heat and stretch."

Lentell and associates[26] also examined the influence of thermal agents on the effectiveness of low-load, prolonged stretch involving the shoulder capsule and surrounding musculature. Their greatest consistent gains were produced when moist heat was used with initial deformation only. The application of heat and associated reflexive decrease in muscle tone results from the reduction of afferent spindle activity with an indirect reduction in alpha motor neuron activity. However, efforts to sustain these gains in ROM were actually inhibited with the use of ice. The authors postulate that ice acted as a facilitation technique, resulting in an increase in muscular activity acting to minimize the potential for retention of tissue elongation. This is in contrast to the results of the aforementioned researchers.[52-54] Lentell and coworkers[26] support the further study of strategies involving ice to reduce inflammation and to moderate pain in the management of musculoskeletal dysfunction involving shoulder pathology.

CASE STUDY 3

Six weeks after a 32-year-old woman began high-impact aerobics, she developed pain and tenderness along the plantar aspect of her feet bilaterally. This pain was intensified with repetitive stepping and jumping activities. She had taken nonsteroidal anti-inflammatory medication for 3 weeks without a marked change in her activity and without significant relief. X-rays were taken, and results revealed a mild periosteal reaction at the medial calcaneal tubercle bilaterally. The patient was referred for physical therapy. A gait evaluation revealed a prolonged pronation phase of her hindfoot from the heel strike through the propulsion phase, and limitation of midfoot supination and dorsiflexion. Non–weight-bearing dorsiflexion and extension of her toes increased her pain, which was localized to the medial longitudinal arch bilaterally.

PROBLEMS

1. Pain and tenderness along the plantar aspect of the feet bilaterally.
2. Intensified pain with repetitive stepping and jumping activities.
3. Limitation of midfoot supination and dorsiflexion.
4. Functional activities limited.

ASSESSMENT TECHNIQUES

1. Pain quantity, quality, and location.
2. ROM measurements.
3. Functional activities assessment, including gait.

GOALS

1. Reduce pain.
2. Increase ROM of the foot and ankle.
3. Increase strength of the foot and ankle musculature when appropriate.
4. Improve gait to normal.
5. Increase functional activities.

SELECTION OF TREATMENT MODALITY

Temporary orthotics were fabricated to moderate the tensile strain imposed on the fascia with repetitive forces incurred in a malaligned foot. The medial rear foot and forefoot were elevated to approximate a subtalar neutral position. Phonophoresis using dexamethasone in gel (1 MHz/0.8 W/cm^2/p 20% for 8 minutes) was focused on the medial structures involved. Manual deep massage of the fascia was followed with a regimen of flexibility exercises for the entire lower quarter. These exercises emphasized the gastrocnemius-soleus complex (with the foot in both supinated and pronated positions), the tarsal-tunnel tendon complex, and the foot's intrinsic musculature. This session was concluded with ice massage; then an ice immersion bath using high-voltage pulsed stimulation while the fascia was placed on gentle stretch. Following this technique, a brief period of manual massage may be reinstituted prior to weight-bearing activity.

HOME PROGRAM

The patient was instructed in self-stretches and massage techniques including rolling a lightly weight bearing foot onto a frozen golf ball. A posterior shell extending from the heads of the metatarsal bones to the proximal calf maintaining neutral dorsiflexion of the ankle may be fabricated from thermoplastic material. This orthosis is used as a night splint serving to place the plantar fascia on gentle stretch, rendering gradual deformation over time. During waking hours, if orthotics cannot be consistently worn in shoes, a "relative rest" dressing using athletic tape or moleskin is applied in approximation of the fascia length to support the longitudinal and transverse arches. As the patient began to be able to gradually dorsiflex the ankle and toes without pain, then strengthening and increased weight-bearing activities were gradually instituted. As with any home program, success is contingent upon the athlete's recognition of the signs and symptoms of renewed inflammation and employing the proper alteration of imposed stress to minimize tissue reactivity.

RATIONALE FOR CLINICAL DECISION MAKING

In the management of plantar fasciitis, a delicate balance is sought between the thermal agents employed in controlling the inflammatory response and the gradual reintroduction of the imposed forces needed to achieve adequate length-tension of the soft tissues to tolerate the athletic activity desired. Optimal biomechanical postures are attempted statically through the use of temporary orthoses or taping techniques and dynamically by strengthening the extrinsic and intrinsic musculature to dynamically support the plantar fascia. This is integral in definitive resolution to what is characteristically a prolonged period of pain and dysfunction.

CASE STUDY 4

A 23-year-old male distance runner developed left Achilles peritendinitis while participating in a 6-mile run. He was initially treated with ice and high-voltage pulsed current and given a 1/4-inch heel lift for a period of 72 hours. Swelling and pain subsided. He continued to have intermittent discomfort, however, 5 days' postinjury. Re-evaluation at that time revealed tightness in the gastrocnemius-soleus muscle complex with mild crepitation within the Achilles tendon.

PROBLEMS

1. Swelling in area of left Achilles tendon.
2. Pain at left Achilles tendon.
3. Mild crepitation within Achilles tendon.
4. Limited functional activities.

ASSESSMENT TECHNIQUES

1. Pain quantity, quality, and location.
2. ROM measurements.
3. Functional activities assessment, including gait.

GOALS

1. Decrease swelling and maintain the reduction.
2. Reduce pain.
3. Increase ROM of the foot and ankle.
4. Increase strength of the foot/ankle musculature, when appropriate.
5. Improve gait to normal.
6. Increase functional activities.

SELECTION OF TREATMENT MODALITY

Rehabilitation of the musculotendinous unit included ultrasound at $1 \text{ MHz}/1.5 \text{ W/cm}^2/\text{CW}$ for 6 minutes to the Achilles tendon, followed by 5 minutes of friction massage to alleviate scar tissue. Flexibility exercises of the complex consisted of weight-bearing stretches with the forefoot position in both abduction and adduction. Ice massage with the tendon in a lengthened position was employed after exercise sessions to minimize exacerbation of the inflammatory responses to higher levels of activity, as well as to encourage normalization of the proper length-tension posture of the soft tissue. The patient was able to resume activities 3 weeks after the onset of the initial injury.

HOME PROGRAM

A progressive strengthening program emphasizing eccentric loading of the tendon complex and instruction in the functional criteria of progression was outlined in detail. For each stage or progression, precautions for the recognition and management of renewed inflammation were included. Post-workout weight-bearing Achilles-tendon stretching for plastic deformation must become routine.

RATIONALE FOR CLINICAL DECISION MAKING

Optimal tolerance for the extreme forces generated and absorbed by the Achilles-tendon complex is best developed with a program that titrates initially the eccentrically, and subsequently the concentrically managed program that titrates managed forces with thermal agents. All muscle contractile work must be performed in a pain-free manner before the next phase is attempted. Gradual strengthening through triplanar motions on diverse terrains is imperative for normalization of musculotendinous tissue length. This will enhance full recovery and prevent further injury.

CASE STUDY 5

A 25-year-old female recreational middle-distance runner proved unable to sustain a more rigorous phase of premarathon training. Her limitations were imposed by right lateral femoral epicondylar pain. A marked increase in mileage involving hilly terrain and crested road running brought about a snapping sensation. Efforts to increase her stride length and efficiency seemed to contribute to her pain. Activity was limited by discomfort, even with daily activities of descending stairs. She developed localized swelling and point tenderness of the lateral femoral condyle, which was moderated by using new shoes and reducing her training regimen. Her symptoms persisted, however, for 10 days, at which time she sought medical intervention. She was placed on a course of anti-inflammatory medication and a rehabilitation course was recommended. Upon evaluation, pain and soft-tissue prominence was localized to 2 cm above the lateral joint line of the right knee. Pain was reproduced with active extension of her knee to 30 degrees both from a supine position and with an ipsilateral weight-bearing position. Structural abnormalities included a longer right limb, bilateral cavus feet that excessively pronated, and a tight iliotibial band evidenced by a positive Ober test. She had full ROM and her strength was good.

PROBLEMS

1. Swelling and point tenderness of the right lateral femoral condyle.
2. Limited weight bearing.
3. Pain of right knee on extension.
4. Limited functional activities.

ASSESSMENT TECHNIQUES

1. Pain quantity, quality, and location.
2. Strength measurements of knee, when appropriate.
3. ROM measurements.
4. Functional activities assessment, including gait.

GOALS

1. Decrease swelling and maintain the reduction.
2. Reduce pain.
3. Increase weight bearing.
4. Increase ROM of the knee.
5. Increase strength of the knee musculature, when appropriate.
6. Increase functional activities.

SELECTION OF TREATMENT MODALITY

Moist heat with high-voltage pulsed stimulation was applied for 20 minutes followed by phonophoresis (Fig. 11–8) at 1 MHz/1.5 W/cm^2/p 20% for 7 minutes using betamethasone and lidocaine. Flexibility exercises to improve the extensibility of the iliotibial band were instituted employing an Ober test position; a seated figure-four position of the hip and knee flexed; and standing wall leans in the frontal plane; all of which were held up to 1 minute for several repetitions. Cryotherapy involving ice massage for the width of this area on stretch completed these initial daily sessions. Structural corrections were implemented in-

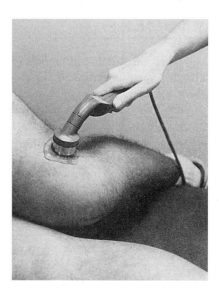

FIGURE 11-8. Depiction of the proper positioning for use of phonophoresis in the treatment of iliotibial band tendinitis.

cluding foot control via an orthotic device to alleviate excessive pronation bilaterally and to decrease the left limb length discrepancy. Her training involved a temporary shift to aquatics to retain cardiovascular gains to minimize weight-bearing overuse. Strengthening was gradually resumed as pain and inflammation abated, and weight-bearing training activities were initiated using a cross-country ski machine. This allowed a short knee flexion arc, thereby avoiding the 30- to 40-degree knee flexion friction point implicit in this syndrome's etiology. Ice massage or ice and cold wet wrap compression could precede and/or follow these sessions to minimize any antagonistic potential an increase in activity may elicit.

HOME PROGRAM

The athlete can renew jogging on a level surface with adequate shoe wear in the final phase. Proper warm-up and flexibility exercises must be continued. She was encouraged to maintain a disciplined stride length as she encounters hills in the last aspect of readaptation to her desired training regimen.

RATIONALE FOR CLINICAL DECISION MAKING

Because of the subcutaneous location of the inflamed tissue, superficial heat, ice massage, and phonophoresis are effective in managing the inflammatory phase of this syndrome. Definitive treatment is contingent upon normalization of the length-tension relationship of the iliotibial band complex. In addition, improving the posture of the lower kinetic chain to efficiently absorb the forces incurred in the repetitive pounding is inherent in training for middle distance running.

SUMMARY

Thermal agents can be effective when employed in a timely and prudent management of various stages of the cellular response to soft-tissue injury. When appropriately applied, further inflammatory changes are inhibited and pain is controlled, thereby minimizing the morbidity of neuromuscular dysfunction. The experienced healthcare practitioner will not only possess a working knowledge of the physiologic effects of thermal agents in application to the specific type and stage of injury, but develops the experience in evaluation of the motivational level and emotional status of the athlete, which has a bearing on the recovery process. Only through the integration of academic knowledge and clinical experience can the practitioner establish the expertise to guide subsequent judgment relative to treatment approach and progression to recovery.

Study Objectives

Having completed this chapter, the reader should now be able to:

1. Define cryokinetics and describe the technique.
2. Explain the neurophysiologic mechanisms by which cryotherapy techniques are effective in pain control.
3. List the common signs and symptoms of soft-tissue inflammation associated with tendinitis.
4. Describe the three stages of tendinitis and correlate what activity level is permitted with each.
5. List several forms of cryotherapy and compare their efficacy in edema control.
6. Explain the mechanisms by which edema control is thought to be achieved through cryotherapy techniques.
7. List several forms of heat application and explain its optimal employment in terms of the stages of inflammatory response.
8. Describe the deleterious effects of premature application of heat in the management of soft-tissue inflammation.
9. Explain the mechanisms by which phonophoresis may be effective in the management of soft-tissue inflammation.
10. Describe the means by which ultrasound or phonophoresis treatments can be applied over irregular surfaces.

REFERENCES

1. Kraus, H: Evaluation and treatment of muscle function in athletic injury. Am J Surg 98:353, 1959.
2. Knight, K: Cryotherapy Theory, Technique and Physiology, ed 1. Chattanooga Corporation, Chattanooga, TN, 1985.
3. Wise, D: Physiotherapeutic treatment of athletic injuries to muscle-tendon complex of the leg. Can Med Assoc J 8:117, 1977.
4. Grant, AE: Massage with ice (cryokinetics) in the treatment of painful conditions of the musculoskeletal system. Arch Phys Med Rehabil 45:233, 1964.
5. Hayden, CA: Cryokinetics in early treatment program. Am J Phys Ther 44:990, 1964.
6. Knight, K: Cryostretch for muscle spasm. Phy Sports Med 4:129, 1980
7. Bennett, D: Water at 67° to 69° to control hemorrhage and swelling encountered in athletic injuries. J NATA 1:12, 1961.

8. Lewis, T: Observation upon the reaction of the vessels of the human skin to cold. Heart 15:177, 1930.
9. Hocutt, JE, et al: Cryotherapy in ankle sprains. Am J Sports Med 10:316, 1982.
10. Cote, W, Prentice, W, and Hooker, D: Comparison of three treatment procedures for minimizing ankle sprain swelling. Phys Ther 68:1072, 1988.
11. Brown, S: Ankle edema and galvanic muscle stimulation. Phys Sports Med 9:137, 1981.
12. Lamboni, P and Harris, B: The use of ice, Airsplints, and high voltage galvanic stimulation in effusion reduction. Athletic Training 18:23, 1983.
13. Esterson, P, Knortz, K, and Wallace, L: Immediate care of ankle injuries. J Orthop Sports Phys Ther 1:46, 1979.
14. Starkey, J: Treatment of ankle sprain by simultaneous use of intermittent compression and ice pack. Am J Sports Med 4:142, 1976.
15. Quillen, WS and Rouillier, LH: Initial management of acute ankle sprains with rapid pulsed pneumatic compression and cold. Orthop Sports Phys Ther 4:39, 1982.
16. Klein, M, et al: Treatment of lower extremity lymphedema with the Wright linear pump: A statistical analysis of a clinical trial. Arch Phys Med Rehabil 69:202, 1988.
17. Merrick, M, et al: The effects of ice and compression wraps on intramuscular temperatures at various depth. J Athletic Training 28:236, 1993.
18. Sloan, J, Giddings, P, and Hain, R: Effects of cold and compression on edema. Phys Sports Med 8:116, 1988.
19. Wilkerson, G and Horn-Kingery, H: Treatment of the inversion ankle sprain: Comparison of different modes of compression and cryotherapy. J Orthop Sports Phys Ther 17:240, 1993.
20. Rucinski, TJ, et al: The effects of intermittent compression on edema in postacute ankle sprains. J Orthop Sports Phys Ther 14:65, 1991.
21. Smith, W: High galvanic therapy in the symptomatic management of acute tibial fractures. Athletic Training 16:59, 1981.
22. Michlovitz, S, Smith, W, and Watkins, M: Ice and high voltage pulsed stimulation, a treatment of acute lateral ankle sprain. J Orthrop Sports Phys Ther 9:301, 1988.
23. Mendel, G and Fish, D: New perspectives in edema control via electrical stimulation. J Athletic Training 28:63, 1993.
24. Waylonis, G: The physiological effects of ice massage. Arch Phys Med Rehabil 48:37, 1967.
25. Prentice, WE: An electromyographic analysis of the effectiveness of heat or cold and stretching for inducing relaxation of injured muscle. Orthop Sports Phys Ther 3:133, 1982.
26. Lentell, G, et al: The use of thermal agents to influence the effectiveness of a low-load prolonged stretch. J Orthop Sports Phys Ther 16:200, 1992.
27. Yackzan, L, Adams, C, Francis, K: The effects of ice massage on delayed muscle soreness. Am J Sports Med 12:159, 1984.
28. Isabell, W, et al: The effects of ice massage, ice massage with exercise, and exercise on the prevention and treatment of delayed onset muscle soreness. J Athletic Training 27:208, 1992.
29. Denegar, L and Perrin, D: Effect of transcutaneous electrical nerve stimulation, cold, and a combination treatment on pain, decreased range of motion, and strength loss associated with delayed onset muscle soreness. J Athletic Training 27:200, 1992.
30. Nielson, AJ: Spray and stretch for myofascial pain. Phys Ther 58, 1978.
31. Cohn, D, Draeger, R, and Jackson, D: The effects of cold therapy in the postoperative management of pain in patients undergoing anterior cruciate ligament reconstruction. Am J Sports Med 17:344, 1989.
32. Miller, C and Webers, R: The effects of ice massage on an individual's pain tolerance level to electrical stimulation. J Orthop Sports Phys Ther 12:105, 1990.
33. Carman, K and Knight, K: Habituation to cold-pain during repeated cryokinetic sessions. J Athletic Training 27:223, 1992.
34. Ingersoll, C and Mangus, B: Habituation to the perception of the qualities of cold-induced pain. J Athletic Training 27:218, 1992.
35. Drez, D, Faust, DC, and Evans, JP: Cryotherapy and nerve palsy. Am J Sports Med 2:256, 1981.
36. Sunderland, S: Nerve Injuries and Their Repair, ed 2. Churchill Livingstone, New York, 1991.
37. Abramson, D, et al: Comparison of wet and dry heat in raising temperature of tissues. Arch Phys Med Rehabil 12:654, 1967.
38. Magness, J, Garrett, T, and Erickson, D: Swelling of the upper extremity during whirlpool baths. Arch Phys Med Rehabil 5:297, 1970.
39. Baker, R and Bell, G: The effect of therapeutic modalities on blood flow in the human calf. J Orthop Sports Phys Ther 13:23, 1991.
40. Dyson, M: Therapeutic Application of Ultrasound. In Nyberg, WL, and Ziskin, MC (eds): Biological Effects of Ultrasound. (Clinics in Diagnostic Ultrasound). Churchill Livingstone, New York, 1985.
41. Henley, EJ: Iontophoresis, phonophoresis, transcutaneous drug delivery. In Critical Reviews in Physical Medicine and Rehabilitation, Vol II:3, CRC Press, Boca Raton, FL, 1991.
42. Byl, N, et al: Effects of phonophoresis with corticosteroids: a controlled pilot study. J Orthop Sports Phys Ther 18:590, 1993.
43. Tsurufuji, S and Sugio, K: Molecular mechanism in the manifestation of anti-inflammatory activity of glucocorticoids. Eur J Rheumatol Inflamm 1:226, 1978.

44. Harvey, W, Grahame, R, and Panayi, GS: Effects of steroid hormones on human fibroblasts in vitro. 1. Glucocorticoid action on cell growth and collagen synthesis. Ann Rheum Dis 33:437, 1974.
45. Kleinkort, J and Wood, F: Phonophoresis with one percent versus ten percent hydrocortisone. Phys Ther 55:1311, 1975.
46. Griffin, JE, et al: Patients treated with ultrasound driven hydrocortisone and with ultrasound alone. Phys Ther 47:594, 1967.
47. Cameron, M and Monroe, LG: Relative transmission of ultrasound by media customarily used for phonophoresis. Phys Ther 72:142, 1992.
48. Behrans, B: Personal Communication, June, 1994.
49. Smith, W, Winn, F, and Parrette, R: Comparative study using four modalities as shinsplint treatments. J Orthop Sports Phys Ther 8:77, 1986.
50. Clark, GR, and Stenner, L: Use of therapeutic ultrasound. Physiotherapy 62:185, 1976.
51. Frieden, S, et al: A pilot study: The therapeutic effects of ultrasound following partial rupture of Achilles tendons. J Orthop Sports Phys Ther 10:39, 1988.
52. Stratton, SA, Heckman, R, and Francis, RS: Therapeutic ultrasound: Its effects on the integrity of a non-penetrating wound. J Orthop Sports Phys Ther 5:278, 1984.
53. Noonan, TJ, et al: Thermal effects on skeletal muscle tensile behavior. Am J Sports Med 21:517, 1993.
54. Sapega, A, et al: Biophysical factors in range of motion exercise. Phys Sports Med 9:57, 1981.

CHAPTER **12**

Use of Heat and Cold in the Management of Rheumatic Diseases

Judy R. Sotosky, MED, PT, and
Susan L. Michlovitz, MS, PT

**CHAPTER
OUTLINE**

Arthritis may well be one of the most common diagnoses seen by physical thera-pists.[1] The term "arthritis" actually refers to over 100 different diseases, more appro-priately called rheumatic diseases. These disorders can involve not only the muscu-loskeletal system, but potentially every organ system in the body. Different forms of rheumatic disease affect individuals from birth to senescence. The incidence of rheumatic diseases, either as a primary or secondary diagnosis, will continue to rise as longevity improves and the baby boomer population ages.

The ever-changing nature of many types of rheumatic diseases, such as rheuma-toid arthritis, osteoarthritis, and fibromyalgia syndrome, pose many challenges to patients, their families, and their healthcare providers. Although currently there are no cures for most rheumatic diseases, great advances have been made in recent years in understanding the underlying disease processes and in designing successful interventions. Physical therapy is an integral part of a successful management program.[1]

A well-planned therapy program is an essential part of the comprehensive management of the patient with rheumatic disease. The primary objectives for therapy include relieving pain, reducing impairment, improving or maintaining function, and preparing the patient in methods of self-care.[2]

GUIDELINES FOR EVALUATION AND TREATMENT PLANNING

The evaluation serves as a foundation from which the treatment program can be designed and future outcomes measured. Evaluating a patient with active polyarthritis involving many joints and functional difficulties can seem overwhelming. An organized approach, such as the form in Figure 12–1, can assist in the evaluation process and allow for clear prioritization of joint problems. Pertinent areas of assessment include pain at rest and on activity, range of motion (ROM), muscle strength and function, joint stability or deformity, posture, gait, neurologic status, functional status, cardiovascular status, and patient goals.

The treatment plan should reflect the priorities determined by the evaluation and include short- and long-term goals. Techniques for pain relief, exercise for improving range of motion, muscle strength, and cardiovascular conditioning are cardinal components of the treatment program. Assistive devices to improve gait and function along with patient education in joint protection and energy conservation should also be incorporated. Of fundamental importance is the education of patients in self-care in order to empower them to be self-managers.[2] Most forms of rheumatic disease are chronic. Patients are likely to experience a recurrence of symptoms and must be prepared to modify their activity and respond appropriately to their current status. Self-care education for patients with arthritis produces real, albeit clinically modest, improvement in health outcomes.[3]

Thermal agents, including ultrasound, are valuable when used to provide temporary pain relief and reduction of muscle spasm, as an adjunct to exercise or positioning, in order to improve ROM, muscle strength, or function. In most cases, the use of a thermal agent is a means to allow the patient to exercise more comfortably, thus achieving improved exercise results and joint nutrition. Modality use alone has generally not been shown to provide sustained benefit in the rheumatic diseases.

The purposes of this chapter are to (1) discuss the role of thermal agents in the total treatment strategy; (2) review previous work that has used heat or cold agents as an adjunct in the management of rheumatic diseases; and (3) suggest guidelines for application of these agents and evaluation of treatment outcome.

GENERAL CONSIDERATIONS REGARDING THERMAL AGENTS

All of the thermal agents have been incorporated at some point in the various treatment regimens for polyarthritis. The decision of which agent to use in which situ-

BRIGHAM AND WOMEN'S HOSPITAL
A Teaching Affiliate of Harvard Medical School
REHABILITATION SERVICES
MUSCULOSKELETAL EVALUATION

INITIAL ☐   INTERIM ☐   DISCHARGE ☐

Referring Service: _____ Dx: _____ Date: _____

EVALUATION KEY:	U.E. ROM Measured in: SUPINE (+) ROM = HYPEREXTENSION (−) = "LACKS"	SITTING (STRENGTH GRADED 0 THROUGH 5)

COMMENTS	LEFT			RANGES	DEG.[1]	RIGHT			COMMENTS
TM JOINT: (Aperture)	STR[2]	P	ROM	A		A	ROM	P	STR.	TM JOINT:
NECK:				**NECK**						NECK:
				Hyperextension	45					
				Flexion	55					
				Lat. Flexion	45					
				Rotation	80					
SHOULDER:				**SHOULDER**						SHOULDER:
				Hyperextension	45					
GH Flex:				Flexion (comb)	180					GH Flex:
GH Abd:				Abduction (comb)	180					GH Abd:
IR/ER (Add):				Ext. Rot. (Abd)	90					IR/ER (Add):
				Int. Rot. (Abd)	90					
ELBOW:				**ELBOW/FOREARM**						ELBOW:
				Extension	0					
				Flexion	145					
FOREARM:				Supination	85					FOREARM:
				Pronation	70					
WRIST:				**WRIST**						WRIST:
				Extension	70					
HAND:				Flexion	75					HAND:
				Radial Dev.	20					
				Ulnar Dev.	35					
HIP:				**HIP**						HIP:
				Extension (T.T.)	0					
				Flexion	120					
				Abduction	45					
				Adduction	10					
				Ext. Rot. (Ext.)	45					
				Int. Rot. (Ext.)	45					
SLR:				Ext. Rot. (Flex)	45					SLR:
				Int. Rot. (Flex)	45					
KNEE:				**KNEE**						KNEE:
				Extension	0					
				Flexion	135					
	Supine:	WB:		Varus/Valgus		Supine:	WB:			
				Lig. Laxity						
ANKLE/FOOT:				**ANKLE/FOOT**						ANKLE/FOOT:
				Plantarflexion	50					
				Dorsiflexion	20					
TOES:				Eversion (comb)	20					TOES:
				Inversion (comb)	35					

REFERENCES:
1. Academy of Orthopedic Surgery, AOA, 1972.   THERAPIST: _____
2. Muscle Testing by Daniel & Worthingham, 1972 by W.B. Saunders Co.

Rev. 12-83

FIGURE 12–1. Brigham and Women's Hospital, Rehabilitation Services, Musculoskeletal Evaluation form. (From Banwell, et al,[1] p 47, with permission.)

ation is not always immediately clear. Certain basic questions come to the forefront. Should a superficial or a deep-heating agent be applied? Is heat or cold the more effective in treating the patient? Will cold increase stiffness in persons with arthritis? Will deep heat accelerate the destruction of joint structures in patients with inflammatory arthritis? As will become evident in the forthcoming review and discussion, some of these questions have been partially or fully answered. Others still require further investigation.

The choice of when to apply a thermal agent and which to use is dependent on a number of factors, including some of the following:

1. *Acute versus chronic inflammation:* When a joint is actually inflamed (hot and swollen), heat application may exacerbate symptoms. During this time, cold application and/or electrical stimulation can be effective in reducing pain and inflammation. Cold can also be effective in order to provide pain relief prior to exercise, when the patient demonstrates evidence of chronic inflammatory changes, although some patients do report a short-term increase in stiffness following cold application.

2. *Inflammatory versus noninflammatory polyarthritis:* In rheumatoid arthritis, when one's goal may be to reduce joint inflammation and temperature, it may be best to choose a physical agent that will alter only skin and subcutaneous tissue temperature (such as hot packs or cold packs). These will provide pain relief and relaxation through reflex mechanisms and counterirritation. A deep-heating agent (such as continuous-wave ultrasound or diathermy) has the potential to increase joint temperature and inflammation. In the case of chronic osteoarthritis, when muscle-guarding spasm or joint contracture may be the primary problems present, heating can usually be more aggressive.

3. *Number of joints involved:* With multiple joint involvement, the use of some of the thermal agents may be impractical. For example, application of hot packs to more than four joints can be cumbersome. In this instance, hydrotherapy (especially heated therapeutic pools) can provide mild heating, assist in reducing the effects of gravity and stress on painful joints, and thus promote ease of motion. Recently, more facilities with heated pools have initiated programs for people with arthritis, providing an avenue for continuation of a pool-based treatment plan of care. One must be aware of the actual content of these programs before recommending them.

4. *Loss of range of motion. The origin of the limitation in motion must be delineated:* If joint capsular shortening or musculotendinous contracture is limiting mobility, deep heat in combination with a slow, gentle stretch can be more effective than heat or stretch used in isolation. If the patient can tolerate cold application, simultaneous use of cold and slow stretch may produce desired results. This technique should be used with caution, because cold analgesia prior to exercise may mask both pain and potential damage to soft tissue. Regardless of the type of rheumatic disease, the therapist *must* know what changes have occurred in the joint structures and joint space prior to applying any external forces, in order to avoid increasing inflammation or causing further joint damage.

5. *Precaution/contraindication:* Some medical conditions associated with certain rheumatic diseases and patient appliances preclude the choice of many of the thermal agents; thorough evaluation and good clinical judgment can screen for those cases when a thermal agent can be potentially harmful. These conditions have been discussed in earlier sections of this text, and some will be reiterated later in this chapter.

6. *Clinic versus home care:* All patients with rheumatic diseases should be placed on a home care program. Some thermal agents are more practical to use than others. A table-top paraffin unit can be purchased or rented (Fig. 12–2); this is more practical and safer to use than the suggested "home mixtures" that are prepared in a double boiler or crock pot. Hot packs can be heated as needed, often in a microwave oven. They may be difficult, however, for the patient to handle if arthritis affects their

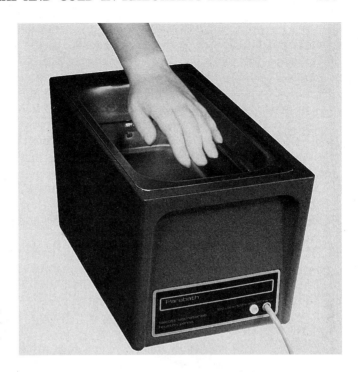

FIGURE 12-2. A home model paraffin unit. (Courtesy of Talcott Laboratories, Houston, PA.)

hands. Only electric heating pads with automatic shut-off features should be used in order to avoid the potential for falling asleep on the pad and producing a burn. Inexpensive cold packs are commercially available, or packs can be made from ice chips and a plastic bag. Diathermy and ultrasound should be applied only by or under the *direct* supervision of a qualified professional, which precludes their unsupervised application at home by the patient or a family member.

7. *Position for treatment:* Joints should be positioned so pain is not markedly increased. If one of the goals for treatment is to decrease pain, then the therapy administered should not increase pain. A sharp, aggravating pain must be differentiated from a more subdued aching of short duration (less than 2 hours), which can be expected when performing exercise or positioning to maintain or increase ROM.

8. *Preconceived notions:* Many patients with rheumatic diseases have experienced periods of pain and loss of function. They may have had previous treatments. They may also have been given advice by well-meaning neighbors and friends. It is not uncommon to hear a patient say, "Cold is bad for arthritis." Some people with arthritis respond favorably to cold, some to heat. Therefore, it is important to investigate patient beliefs and provide appropriate patient education regarding the disease process and principles of management.

Sources of Pain in Rheumatic Diseases

Understanding the specific pathophysiology, the actual status of the joint structures, and the potential sources of pain in a patient with rheumatic disease can help guide the therapist's choice of thermal agent and other interventions.

For the purposes of discussion, two different categories of polyarthritis are to be considered: disorders associated with systemic disease and inflammation (for example, rheumatoid arthritis), and disorders primarily associated with joint degeneration (for example, osteoarthritis with some local inflammation). An additional section briefly discussing the fibromyalgia syndrome, a syndrome characterized by complaints of diffuse musculoskeletal pain, is included at the end of this chapter.

In the clinical setting, the primary complaint of patients with rheumatic diseases is usually pain. However, not all pain emanates from the same source. It is essential to attempt to consider the factors that may contribute to it[4] in order to provide an optimal intervention.

A general list of potential sources of pain would include the following:

1. *Inflammation* causing chemical irritation of nerve endings, tissue destruction, and increased fluid pressure on joint structures.
2. *Articular cartilage loss* contributing to bone on bone pressure, and particulate matter in synovial fluid stimulating further inflammatory response.
3. *Muscle spasm* caused initially by pain and/or microtrauma perpetuated by decreased circulation and removal of irritants.
4. *Nerve/vascular compression* by swelling or chronic tissue thickening around the joint.
5. *Subchondral bony fracture* caused by osteopenia or collapse of bony cysts.
6. *Pathomechanical stresses on soft tissue and bone* resulting from increased fluid, joint malalignment, and deformity.
7. *Referred pain.*[2,5]

Other factors that can influence a patient's pain experience include changes in disease activity, changes in physical activity, altered joint status or posture, and psychologic or socioeconomic concerns.[2]

INFLAMMATORY AND NONINFLAMMATORY ARTHRITIS

Rheumatoid Arthritis

Rheumatoid arthritis (RA) is a systemic disorder of unknown etiology characterized by articular inflammation.[6] There is often a natural course of exacerbations and remissions causing varying symptoms from episode to episode. The synovial lining cells hypertrophy, forming a vascularized granulation tissue (pannus). Digestants in the synovial fluid and pannus destroy periarticular tissue and articular surfaces. Pannus causes periarticular adhesions as well as a weakening of capsular and ligamentous structures. The end result can be hypermobility, hypomobility, or hypermobility and deformity (Fig. 12–3). As a result of inflammation, joint temperature is elevated.[7] Treatment including medication, splinting, and thermal agents is aimed at reducing pain and inflammation. Exercise is important for preserving range of motion, joint nutrition, muscle strength, function, and cardiovascular status.

Other dysfunctions associated with RA include, but are not limited to, vasculitis, osteoporosis, bursitis, tendinitis, skin breakdown, rheumatoid nodules, and arteritis.

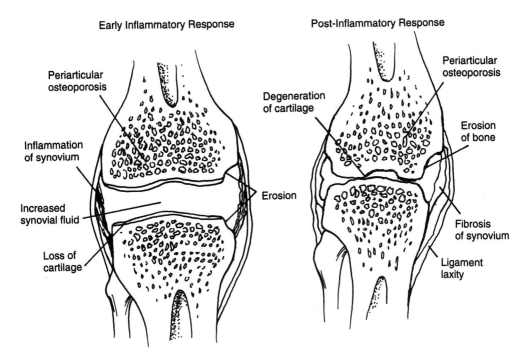

FIGURE 12-3. Inflammatory and postinflammatory response in the diarthrodial joint. (From AHPA Arthritis Teaching Slide Collection,[5] p 37, with permission of the American College of Rheumatology.)

Osteoarthritis

Osteoarthritis (OA) is a progressive disease primarily affecting the articular cartilage of diarthrodial joints, often accompanied by osteophytic spur formation at joint margins, asymmetrical joint space narrowing, and sclerotic bony changes (Fig. 12-4).[6] Localized soft-tissue inflammation may occur with disease exacerbation or trauma. OA can develop at any age secondary to trauma, joint abnormality, or metabolic disease. Other predisposing factors include advancing age, genetics, obesity, and excessive repetitive stress.[5] Pain is present on passive motion and during weight bearing. Morning stiffness generally lasts less than 30 minutes.

Table 12-1 depicts the clinical features and joints commonly involved in rheumatoid arthritis and osteoarthritis.

Superficial Heat and Cold

The activity of the disease process, particularly with inflammatory arthritis, must be taken into account. A patient with RA who has an acutely inflamed joint may find his or her symptoms further exacerbated by heat application. During this time, the application of ice packs may aid in reducing pain and inflammation. If the disease process is in the subacute or chronic stage, superficial heat or cold may be equally effective in reducing discomfort and in ultimately improving function.

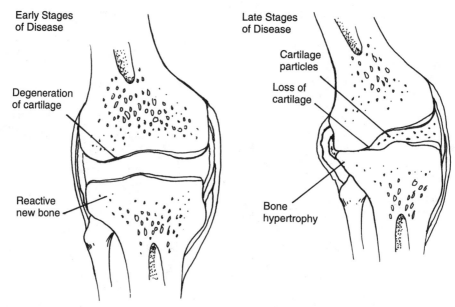

FIGURE 12–4. Early and late stage effects of osteoarthritis on the diarthrodial joint. (From AHPA Arthritis Teaching Slide Collection,[5] p 47, with permission of the American College of Rheumatology.)

Superficial thermal agents are probably the most commonly applied of the thermal agents for persons with RA or OA. The patient will usually report temporary relief of, or decrease in, pain following such application. Patients can be instructed in the use of hot packs, cold packs, and paraffin for home use, allowing carryover from the hospital or clinic setting.

Many studies have compared the effects of heat and cold on patients with RA and OA (Table 12–2). Curkovic and associates looked at the effects of superficial heat and cold on the pain threshold of the hands of 30 patients with RA.[8] A warm bath (38°C) was applied for 10 minutes to 15 patients. The other 15 patients received ice massage (1 to 3 minutes) to the fourth proximal interphalangeal joint of the right hand. Pain threshold was measured at baseline, posttreatment, and 10, 30, and 60 minutes following treatment. Both heat and cold application resulted in a pain threshold increase immediately following treatment, with no significant difference between the groups. However, the group receiving ice massage demonstrated an increased pain threshold at 10 and 30 minutes following treatment.

Yung, Unsworth, and Haslock[9] were unable to demonstrate any significant changes in metacarpophalangeal stiffness in 20 patients with RA, when measured by arthrogram. Ten received paraffin (dip and wrap, 50°C) and 10 an ice pack for 10 minutes. Arthrogram measurement before and immediately after treatment showed no significant changes. The findings of Dellhag, Wollersjo, and Bjelle[10] were similar.

In contrast, Harris and Millard[11] reported a slight increase in pain, tenderness, and swelling and an increase in grip strength, following daily paraffin applied to patients with RA. The treatment was given at a temperature of 44°C for a duration of 6 weeks. The results of treatment were not considered to be statistically significant.

The results of hot and cold packs on passive range of motion (PROM), swelling, and pain were assessed in a population of 36 OA patients, 14 days following total-knee

TABLE 12–1 Features of Rheumatoid Arthritis and Osteoarthritis

Findings	Osteoarthritis	Rheumatoid Arthritis
Joints commonly involved:		

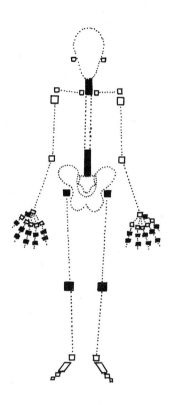 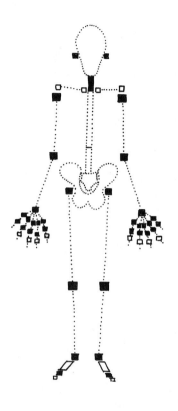

Joint swelling	Mild, hard tissue enlargement	Common, synovial, symmetric arthritis, >3 joints involved
Morning stiffness	Less than 30 minutes	Often greater than 1 hr
Joint changes	Osteophytes, asymmetric joint space narrowing	Pannus (synovial membrane proliferation), instability, erosion
Sedimentation rate	Normal or slightly elevated	Elevated
Additional findings	Heberden's and Bouchard's nodes	Rheumatoid nodules
		Baker's cysts
		Vasculitis
		Osteoporosis + Rheumatoid factor

Source: Adapted from Schumacher et al.[6]

arthroplasty.[12] The patients were divided into three groups: 10 receiving AAROM only, serving as the control group, 13 receiving hot packs for 20 minutes followed by AAROM, and 13 receiving cold packs for 20 minutes followed by AAROM. After 10 treatments over 1 week, the results showed no significant difference among groups for ROM. Application of cold did result in a significant reduction of swelling and significantly reduced patient report of pain with exercise.

TABLE 12–2 Clinical Studies Comparing Heat and Cold in Polyarthritis Management

Investigator	Subjects Treated	Heat/Cold Agent	Control Group	Conclusions
Curkovic, et al[8]	30 RA patients	Warm bath (38°C), 10 min, $n = 15$ Ice massage, 1–3 min, $n = 15$	None	Significant increase in pain threshold for both groups following treatment; significantly increased pain threshold maintained at 10 and 30 min post ice treatment
Utsinger, Bonner, Hogan[13]	RA knees	Hot packs, 2 times/day; cold packs, 2 times/day	Cross-over design (used same group of patients and compared results)	All showed clinical improvement in sleep duration, pain, timed functional tests. 50% preferred heat, 18% no preference
Hecht, et al[12]	36 OA patients, 14 days post-op total knee arthroplasty	Hot packs, 20 min, twice a day; cold packs, 20 min, twice a day; both followed by AAROM	10 patients who only performed AAROM	After 10 treatments, no significant difference in ROM; cold packs resulted in decreased swelling and pain with exercise
Yung, Unsworth, Haslock[9]	Patients with acute RA	SWD ($n = 9$), 20 min; paraffin (dip/wrap) 50°C for 20 min, $n = 10$; Pulsed US, 1 W/cm^2 in water bath, 35°C, $n = 8$; ice pack for 10 min, $n = 10$	Normal subjects in matching numbers	Significant decrease for RA patients following SWD and US only

Utsinger and associates[13] compared 1 week of ice packs (2 times a day) with 1 week of hot packs (3 times a day) applied to the same patients on alternating weeks. Fifty percent preferred hot packs to cold, and 18% had no preference of one over the other. All patients showed improvement in some of the measured variables (sleep duration, pain, timed function tests). In those patients who preferred cold, naloxone was administered prior to a subsequent cold application. In most of these patients, after the administration of naloxone, cold was no longer effective in reducing pain. The investigators suggest that cold may be effective in reducing pain by facilitating activation of endorphins.

One study of long-term effects of superficial heat application on the hands of patients with RA was undertaken by Mainardi and associates.[14] A 2-year study was conducted to investigate the long-term results of daily application of heat. Heat was applied to one hand through an electric mitten at 40°C for 30 minutes 2 times a day for 2 years. The other hand of each person served as the control. On x-ray examination, no further evidence of joint destruction could be attributed to the heat-treated hands. Therefore, more clinical investigations on the long-term effects of heat therapy to rheumatoid joints seem to be warranted.

Contrast baths have long been used in arthritis and sports rehabilitation. Documentation of short- and long-term effectiveness of this treatment is lacking. The presumed "vascular pumping" mechanism, enhanced by the analgesia of the warm or cool water and the ease of exercise in the water, continue to make this a less painful method for hand exercise, particularly in patients with inflammatory arthritis.

With its ability to reduce metabolism, increase the release of endorphins, and reduce blood flow and capillary pressure, cryotherapy is a logical choice for trying to decrease the inflammatory response and reduce joint swelling.[15] A few studies have looked at the response of patients with polyarthritis to cold therapy alone. Ice packs were applied for 20 minutes 3 times a day, for 1 month, to the knees of patients with RA.[16] An increase in ROM and sleep duration and a decrease in pain (as measured by visual analogue scale) and in oral analgesic intake were reported. There were no changes in synovial fluid composition. In this study, one knee was treated with ice, while the other knee had no cold application, thus serving as a comparison. Pegg, Littler, and Littler[17] used 5-minute ice-pack applications and exercise daily for 2 weeks in treating the knees and elbows of RA patients. Stiffness and pain were reduced in most patients, and ROM improved in 50% of the patients. When the same investigators changed the treatment to immersing patients' hands in cold water (dipping in and out for 10 minutes), the treatment was less effective.

Cold application can increase joint stiffness,[8,13] decrease joint stiffness,[18] or may have no effect on stiffness[9] in patients with inflammatory arthritis. Some patients with inflammatory arthritis will not tolerate cold application, particularly those with Raynaud's phenomenon, cold urticaria, vascular insufficiency, or cryoglobulinemia.[15]

Heat and cold both seem to be valuable adjuncts in the rehabilitation management of persons with polyarthritis. Ease of home application and patient preference should also be considered before choosing an agent.

EFFECT OF SUPERFICIAL THERMAL AGENTS ON INTRA-ARTICULAR TEMPERATURE

Weinberger and associates[19] evaluated the effect of hot packs on the intra-articular temperature of the knee in five patients with knee effusions. In four patients with RA and one with OA, surface thermal electrodes were attached and intra-articular temperature probes inserted in bilateral knees. One knee was treated with hot packs (42°C) for 30 minutes. The other knee served as the control. Although hot packs are considered superficial thermal agents, penetrating only a few millimeters into the skin, these researchers found an increase of 1°C in intra-articular temperature in the treated knee. The intra-articular temperature increased parallel to the increase in skin temperature under the hot pack. The joint temperature of the treated knee required 55 minutes to return to baseline temperature. The control knees showed a mild increase in skin temperature, but no change in intra-articular temperature. The investigators concluded that when there is evidence of acute inflammatory disease, superficial heat should be used with caution because an elevation of 1°C intra-articular temperature may enhance the inflammatory process.

Deep-Heating Agents

A series of studies involving the use of deep-heating agents have evaluated the effects of ultrasound (US), galvanic stimulation, shortwave diathermy (SWD), MWD, and pulsed US on populations of RA and OA patients.[9,20-23] (Table 12–3). Bromley, Unsworth, and Haslock[21] found reduced metacarpophalangeal joint stiffness in 13 patients with active RA following one application of paraffin (dip and wrap method, temperature unspecified) followed by pulsed US (1 MHz, pulsed with on-off 1:4 ratio, in water bath 35°C). Using a computer arthrograph to assess joint stiffness, these investigators assessed the effects of one application of paraffin/pulsed US ($n = 13$), paraffin alone ($n = 10$), pulsed US alone ($n = 11$), and AROM ($n = 6$). In addition, 12 persons without RA had their metacarpophalangeal (MCP) joint stiffness measured for baseline comparison. The persons with active RA were found to have significantly greater joint stiffness than their normal counterparts prior to treatment.

The results of the single application of paraffin/pulsed US were felt to be the potentiating effect of preheating the tissue with the paraffin, leading to an increased absorption of the US in the warmer tissue.

The research was extended to treating these same patients with the same series of modalities 2 times a week for 6 weeks. No significant difference was found with any of the treatments or combination of treatments, suggesting that with regard to stiffness, the effects of the agents are short lived. There was a positive trend toward reduced stiffness after 6 weeks in those treated with pulsed US alone, but it was not statistically significant.[21]

Yung, Unsworth, and Haslock[9] measured MCP joint stiffness by computer arthrograph in RA patients with acutely inflamed joints, following application of SWD (27 MHz, 20 minutes, $n = 9$), paraffin (dip and wrap, 50°C, $n = 10$), pulsed US (1 W/cm^2, 3 minutes, $n = 8$), ice pack (10 minutes, $n = 10$), and exercise (100 active flexion, extension, $n = 9$). They found significant difference between pretreatment and posttreatment in the groups receiving SWD and pulsed US. Other physical therapy interventions did not produce significant changes in stiffness. A group of 10 normal control patients showed no significant change in stiffness with any of the interventions.

Svarcova, Trnavsky, and Zvarova[20] evaluated the effects of thermal agents alone or in combination with ibuprofen in 180 patients with stage II through IV OA of the hip or knee. There were three groups of 60 patients. One half of each group received deep heat plus ibuprofen; the other half received placebo and deep heat. Ten treatments

TABLE 12-3 Studies Evaluating Deep Thermal Agents in Rheumatoid Arthritis and Osteoarthritis

Investigator	Study Population	Thermal Agent	Controls	Conclusions
Bromley, Unsworth, Haslock[21]	13 RA patients with acute MCP involvement	Single application of paraffin followed by pulsed US (1 MHz)	Compared with groups receiving paraffin, pulsed US, or exercise alone	Decreased MCP stiffness; however, after treating patients twice a week for 6 weeks, no significant changes were found
Yung, Unsworth, Haslock[9]	8 patients with acute RA	Single application of pulsed US, 1 W/cm^2 for 3 min	10 persons without RA	Decreased MCP stiffness posttreatment
Svarcova, Trnavsky, Zvarova[20]	180 OA of hip or knee	10 treatments at 2-day intervals with 15 min US, $n = 60$; galvanic stimulation, 20 min, $n = 60$; SWD, 2 min, $n = 60$	One half of each group received ibuprofen with the modality; the other half received placebo with modality	Significantly decreased pain by VAS following 10 treatments with all modalities; US or SWD with ibuprofen had better results than these modalities alone
Depreux[24]	OA hip	1.5–2.0 W/cm^2, 10 min/field, 10–20 sessions	None	Decreased pain, improvement in gait

343

were given at 2-day intervals with measurements of pain (by visual analogue scale) and global evaluation by patient and physician taken following the fifth and tenth treatment. The deep-heating agents used were 15 minutes of US (5 minutes per three fields), 20 minutes of galvanic stimulation (0.1 mA/cm, maximum intensity 700 W), and 4 minutes of pulsed SWD (46 MHz). Pain intensity on the visual analogue scale (VAS) reduced significantly by the tenth treatment for all groups. There was no significant difference in improvement among the groups receiving deep heat and placebo.

The combined effect of US or SWD and the ibuprofen was greater, however, than the deep heat alone. This may have been the result of increased temperature at the capsule, allowing for an increased effect of the ibuprofen on the disease process. The galvanic stimulation produced similar results with or without the addition of ibuprofen. The majority of patients and physicians rated the responses as excellent or good, with the exception of four patients who received SWD who rated their response as worse.

DePreux[24] administered US to patients' hips and reported a decrease in pain and improvement in gait. Ultrasound was delivered at an intensity of 1.5 to 1.0 W/cm^2, 10 minutes per field, for a total of 10 to 20 sessions. Unfortunately, no control group was used against which to compare the efficacy of this treatment.

Intra-articular steroid injections, nonsteroidal anti-inflammatory drugs (NSAIDs), and thermal agents have all been used in the management of OA of the knee. Wright[25] compared the effects of a placebo pill (one tablet, 2 times a day); a placebo injection (intra-articular normal saline, a total of four injections over an 8-week period); and SWD, 3 times a week for 6 weeks. Both the group receiving SWD and the group receiving a placebo injection improved in walking time, had a decrease in pain, and required fewer oral analgesics. These two groups showed a greater improvement than did those who had taken the placebo pill.

The overall improvement in symptoms and function seen in these studies may have resulted from the effects of deep heating on reducing joint stiffness, pain, and spasm by direct action on tissue temperature and circulation at the joint level. However, one must also consider the potentiating effect that increasing capsular and muscle blood flow has on the distribution and effectiveness of medications at the joint. Further investigation of this phenomenon seems warranted.

EFFECT OF DEEP THERMAL AGENTS ON INTRA-ARTICULAR TEMPERATURE

During the last two decades, controversy has arisen regarding the long-term effects of heat application in persons with inflammatory arthritis.[8,19] Persons with active RA can have elevated joint temperatures up to 37°C.[7] Normal intra-articular temperature is 3°C to 5°C lower. It has been determined that joint temperatures of 30°C result in decreased destruction by enzymes; those at 35°C to 36°C show increased enzymatic activity.[8] Therefore, one could consider that further elevating joint temperature with a thermal agent during the period of acute or subacute inflammation may be additive and thus more detrimental to joint structures. Intra-articular temperature increases of 1°C were found following hot-pack application by Weinberger and associates,[18] discussed earlier in this chapter.

Weinberger and coworkers[23] hypothesized that raising the temperature of joints with inflammatory arthritis to levels of 42°C will actually inhibit the enzymatic effects of collagenase, thus actually reducing inflammation. They treated seven patients having RA with chronic, stable knee effusions with MWD (15 to 35 W) for 1 hour 2 times a week for 2 weeks. The patient's other knee served as the control. MWD was specifically chosen for its ability to selectively heat the capsule, a tissue with a high water content in comparison to the surrounding structures.

Intra-articular temperatures of 41.3°C ± 0.9°C were obtained at the end of the 1-hour treatment. Significant improvement in 50-foot walking time and pain were noted at the end of the series. No significant changes were found in synovial fluid leukocyte count and prostaglandin E2 level, knee circumference, or ROM. Pain, walking time, knee circumference, and ROM remained stable at 6 weeks' posttreatment. No adverse reactions were seen.

Most of the studies looking at the effects of thermal agents on intra-articular temperature used small populations. Therefore, it appears that the jury is still out on the actual intra-articular effects of deep-heating agents. Caution must be used in selecting modalities for use when inflammation is present.

Another difficulty in drawing conclusions from the research on thermal agents is the language used to describe the joint status. *Disease activity* refers to the level of inflammatory activity present. *Disease stage* is a severity measure relating to the extent of anatomic damage.[15] Unfortunately, these terms are not always applied consistently, making direct comparison of studies difficult.

From a review of all of these studies, one can conclude that both superficial and deep heat and cold seem to have places in the treatment regimen of patients with degenerative or inflammatory polyarthritis. They act to provide relief of pain and spasm, increase circulation, and prepare the patient for exercise. In general, cold is still recommended for acute inflammation. Heat or cold can be used in subacute or chronic inflammatory situations. All thermal agents should be used very cautiously, in modified fashion, or not at all, in patients with vasculitis, skin ulceration, vascular insufficiency, impaired sensation, or Raynaud's phenomenon.

Deep-heating agents are generally reserved for joints without acute, or with great caution in subacute, inflammation in which one wishes to selectively heat a deep structure such as the capsule, ligaments, or muscles, in combination with slow, gentle stretching. Suggestions for patient positioning for stretching must provide stability of the joint, comfort for the patient, and maximum control of the limb for the therapist throughout the maneuver. Kottke and associates suggest several positions for different joint stretching.[26] Caution must be used in considering a stretch to an unstable joint (such as medial and lateral) or in a patient with osteoporosis. Prior to attempting stretching or splinting a hypomobile joint, x-ray findings should be reviewed to help the therapist determine if it will be realistic to expect an increase in ROM.

CASE STUDY 1

DIAGNOSIS

Rheumatoid arthritis

HISTORY/INTERVENTIONS

Newly diagnosed, 34-year-old woman, single parent of 10-year-old son, works for an insurance company. Just started on nonsteroidal anti-inflammatory (NSAID) medication and intramuscular gold.

PROBLEMS

1. Pain, swelling, stiffness of hands, feet, elbows, shoulders; 2-hour morning stiffness.
2. Difficulty with activities of daily living (ADLs) and job because of pain and fatigue.
3. Pain rated as 7/10 for hands and wrists, 6/10 for shoulders, and 5/10 for feet.

ASSESSMENT

1. +2 swelling and tenderness of both hands' metacarpophalangeal joints, proximal interphalangeal joints and wrists.
2. Elbows tender without swelling.
3. Shoulders with anterolateral swelling, tenderness, and redness.
4. Metatarsal phalangeal +1 tenderness.
5. ROM reveals full ROM throughout; however, pain present with AROM, particularly at end range of both shoulders, wrist and finger motion.
6. Strength is 4/5 for shoulders, elbows, and wrists; assessment influenced by pain.
7. Grip strength, measured with rolled sphygmomanometer cuff, was 165 mm Hg on right, 160 mm Hg on left.
8. Gait exam revealed decreased push off both feet. Patient wearing 1-inch pumps. No abnormal wear pattern observed.

DECISION MAKING FOR CHOICE OF TREATMENTS

Acute inflammation is present. She has multiple joint involvement. She works full time and is the sole breadwinner. A comprehensive home program, evaluation of social support system, evaluation of job setting, and referral to occupational therapy may be needed. Her arthritis is newly diagnosed, therefore patient education is important. Medications are not yet taking maximum effect.

DESCRIPTION OF TREATMENT

1. Patient supine with pillow under knees: ice packs to dorsal hands/wrists and shoulders for 20 minutes.
2. Paraffin dip and wrap to both feet for 20 minutes.
3. AAROM to shoulders, elbows, wrists, and hands for 10 repetitions.

TREATMENT OUTCOME

Patient reports pain reduced to 5/10 for hands, wrists, shoulders, and 4/10 for feet following treatment.

HOME PROGRAM

1. Education regarding use of commercially available cold pack for acutely inflamed joints.

2. Instruction in AROM for all joints after patient showers in the morning and in the evening when she returns from work.
3. Use of Spenco insoles and/or wearing sneakers recommended.

The patient was informed of the need for a brief series of sessions to accomplish a comprehensive management program. This would include education in pain control and about the disease process, joint protection methods, energy conservation methods, and evaluation of her work and home responsibilities in order to make recommendations and to provide an overall exercise program.

CASE STUDY 2

DIAGNOSIS

Osteoarthritis of knee

HISTORY/INTERVENTIONS

This 54-year-old male, moderately obese, originally injured his knee in a car accident approximately 10 years ago. He has had increasing difficulty over past 2 years. He has received intra-articular injections in last 12 months. The effect of the second shot only lasted about 2 weeks. His medical history includes mild high blood pressure. He is married with two grown children and two grandchildren, and he is a primary school principal. He has no regular physical activity.

PROBLEMS

1. Pain, gradually increasing by end of day so that he has difficulty standing/walking at work.
2. Stiffness with sitting or driving too long.
3. Difficulty squatting to talk with young children.
4. Morning stiffness less than 30 minutes.

ASSESSMENT

1. Knee pain at present at 5/10, describes knee pain at end of the day as 9/10.
2. Posture: Mild lumbar lordosis.
3. No significant leg length discrepancy, muscle atrophy, or medial/lateral knee deformity on weight bearing. The right knee +1 medial-lateral instability non–weight-bearing.
4. Mild hypertrophy of synovial tissue at right knee joint line with evidence of bony enlargement at the medial aspect of the knee. Left knee unremarkable.
5. Manual muscle test (MMT) reveals right quadriceps 4/5, hamstrings 3+/5, gluteals 4/5, hip abductors 4/5, and hip flexors 5/5.
6. ROM of R knee: Flexion = 115, extension = 0.

7. LLE = WNL for MMT and ROM.
8. Neurologic status intact.
9. Gait is antalgic on the right. Transfers to standard chairs with use of chair arms independently.

DECISION MAKING FOR CHOICE OF TREATMENT

This patient has subacute osteoarthritis of a weight-bearing joint and is moderately obese. He has muscle weakness, mild medial-lateral (M-L) instability. He has not been on any program before. There is flexibility in his job schedule.

DESCRIPTION OF TREATMENT

1. Hot pack or ice pack for 20 minutes to knees followed by instruction in quadriceps setting, gluteal setting, hamstring setting, straight-leg raises, and short-arc quadriceps exercises.
2. Instruction in use of cane; patient independent on level surface greater than 100 feet and on stairs with cane.
3. Discussed need to change position throughout the day, lose weight, use of a shock-absorbing insole to reduce forces on the knee joint, and strengthen the muscles around the knee to increase the support of the joint. Patient reports pain 4/10 following exercise and modality.

HOME PROGRAM

Isometric exercise, AROM, and gradual progression to resistive exercise in limited ROM. Use of cane and modalities to control pain and maintain function as muscles are strengthened and the patient loses weight. Investigate the possibility of pool exercise program in community or exercise bicycle at home. Limit activities that add stress on knees: kneeling, squatting, stairs, standing in one position for long periods. Plan to see once a week for 4 weeks.

FIBROMYALGIA SYNDROME

The fibromyalgia syndrome (FMS) is a common, chronic pain condition, characterized by widespread musculoskeletal pain, low threshold to pressure at tender points (Fig. 12–5), nonrestorative sleep, and morning stiffness.[27] FMS can be seen as the sole diagnosis, or the patient may have concomitant entities such as RA, OA, Lyme disease, or sleep apnea.[6] The patient-reported pain of FMS has been found to be similar or greater than that of patients with inflammatory arthritis and to involve a greater percentage of the body.[28]

Areas most commonly involved include the axial skeleton, shoulder, and pelvic girdles.[29] Symptoms are aggravated by cold or humid weather, tension, and inactivity.[28] Laboratory and x-ray results are generally negative. Although not deforming or life-threatening, FMS represents a significant source of disability. One study of 176 patients with FMS demonstrated that 30 percent had changed their jobs and 17 percent had stopped working because of their FMS.[30]

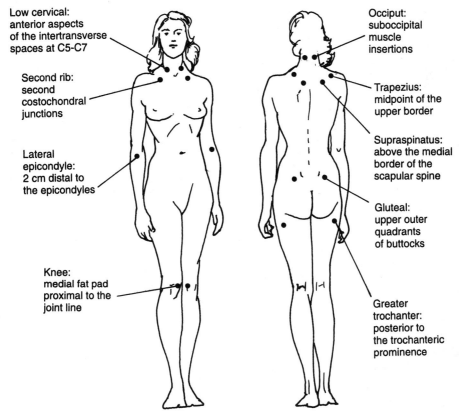

Low cervical:
anterior aspects
of the intertransverse
spaces at C5-C7

Second rib:
second
costochondral
junctions

Lateral
epicondyle:
2 cm distal to
the epicondyles

Knee:
medial fat pad
proximal to the
joint line

Occiput:
suboccipital
muscle
insertions

Trapezius:
midpoint of the
upper border

Supraspinatus:
above the medial
border of the
scapular spine

Gluteal:
upper outer
quadrants
of buttocks

Greater
trochanter:
posterior to
the trochanteric
prominence

FIGURE 12–5. Location of specific tender points in fibromyalgia. (From Schumacher, et al,[6] p 247, with permission.)

Use of Thermal Agents in Fibromyalgia Syndrome

To date no single thermal modality or combination of modalities has been shown to provide long-term improvement in FMS patients. As a source of temporary pain reduction, use of thermal modalities or massage, coupled with a gradual exercise program, appears to be the prevailing physical therapy treatment of choice.[28] It is important to note that emphasis needs to be placed on gradually increasing exercise from stretching problem areas to a gentle, low or nonimpact aerobic program.

In a 2-year study of 44 FMS patients by Granges, Zilko, and Littlejohn,[27] regular aerobic exercise was the only element correlated with lower FMS scores. Physical agent modalities alone all showed transitory effects. No combination of NSAIDs, analgesics, and/or antidepressants were superior in results or showed significant correlations with reduced FMS scores.

Although most patients with FMS experience a chronic disease, 24% of this population (all who met the standard criteria for FMS at baseline) actually demonstrated objective remission at the 2-year follow-up.

The range of modalities used with FMS is similar to that used in inflammatory arthritis: ice, heat, US, low-power laser, and electrical stimulation. It is likely that their role is primarily one of affording temporary relief of symptoms via the spinal gating mechanism and a sense of self-control for the patient. General consensus on the comprehensive management of FMS seems to include some combination of reassurance and explanation of the illness, symptomatic treatment with heat or massage (with instructions for independent home application), moderate physical exercise, evaluation of mechanical stressors, biofeedback/relaxation training, NSAIDs, antidepressants, nonaddicting analgesics, and psychosocial support.[28,31]

In a study of 35 patients with FMS, 22 of their primary physicians and 49 additional rheumatologists, Potts and Silverman[32] found a significant difference between the patients and all of the physicians on the importance of several aspects of care. These included stiffness, anxiety, instruction in the use of heat and massage, ways to improve mobility, and exercise instruction. The authors suggest that further attention to patient concerns in these areas may be warranted.

EVALUATING TREATMENT RESULTS OF THERMAL AGENTS

The results of treatment techniques for persons with rheumatic diseases are varied. A number of factors can influence the outcome of a particular treatment or combination of therapeutic modalities. The *disease activity*, often associated with spontaneous exacerbations and remissions of inflammation, has been mentioned earlier in this chapter. Because of the *variable course* of inflammatory arthritis, including its exacerbations and remissions, it may be difficult to claim the effectiveness of one particular treatment modality in a single patient. This is why control groups are so important in studies evaluating arthritis treatment.

The *stage of disease* is also important to consider. The extent of anatomic damage to the joints and surrounding tissues that cannot be reversed conservatively will influence treatment goals and expectations.

Concurrent use of medications with physical therapy management and/or changes in medication can change the patient's response to treatment. Patients respond individually to NSAIDs and, as was discussed earlier, their responses may be influenced by the potentiating effects of modalities. On the other hand, a patient may respond poorly to a new medication, which may be interpreted as a poor response to a program of heat and exercise. It is important to be aware of the medications and any changes occurring in the patient's medical treatment. Sometimes it is difficult to separate the individual components of a total management program in order to evaluate the efficacy of each.

Time of evaluation is also an important element and should be documented. Was the treatment applied and the patient evaluated at the same time each day? This is of particular importance with inflammatory arthritis, which may cause stiffness-related difficulties early in the day. A list of possible evaluation techniques can be found in Table 12–4.

Pain management in arthritis is a complex domain. It is often difficult to completely contain and thoroughly assess. Common methods of pain management used in arthritis therapy include heat, cold, electrotherapy, EMG biofeedback, relaxation and imagery, and medication. If the pain associated with the rheumatic diseases was easy to manage, there would not be so many different treatment modes used or tabloid claims of "miracle cures" printed.

Bradley[33] notes that the pain associated with arthritis has intensity and affective

TABLE 12–4 Outcome Assessment Techniques Used for Patients
with Rheumatic Diseases

Clinical	Research Facility/Laboratory
Amount and frequency of analgesic intake	Gait analysis (using force plates, EMG, high-speed photography, video)
Duration of morning stiffness	
Goniometric measurements	Joint fluid analysis
Gait analysis (stride length, step length, push off)	Sodium clearance
Isokinetic testing	Intra-articular temperature
Joint circumference	Sedimentation rate
Hand grip strength	Synovial prostaglandin and collagenase levels
Manual muscle test	
Sleep duration	
Timed functional tests (50-ft walk test)	
Patient reported functional abilities	
Visual analogue and other pain rating scales	
Arthritis health status questionnaires	
Affective pain measures	

and behavioral qualities. Using independent measures of pain intensity (such as a 10-cm visual analogue scale Fig. 12–6) and pain affect (such as the Descriptor Differential Scale, Fig. 12–7), along with provider-observed pain behavior, ROM, and function, can help distinguish between overall pain improvement and just an improved sense of well-being.[33]

SUMMARY

Most forms of thermal agents have been used, at one time or another, in the management of patients with rheumatic diseases. Although at the present none have been shown to have long-term effectiveness by themselves, their role as an adjunct to facilitate exercise, reduce pain and swelling, and improve function should not be ignored. The ability of the patient to control his or her symptoms, however temporarily, had great benefit in reducing a sense of helplessness common with chronic inflammatory disease. Reduction of pain can also provide comfort in performing routine, often painful exercises.

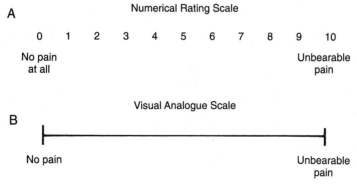

FIGURE 12–6. Several commonly used measures of pain intensity. (*A*) Numerical rating scale. (*B*) Visual analogue scale. These could be converted to measures of pain by altering the verbal descriptors for each of the scales. (From: Bradley, LA: Pain measurement in arthritis. Arthritis Care Res (6)4:178, 1993.

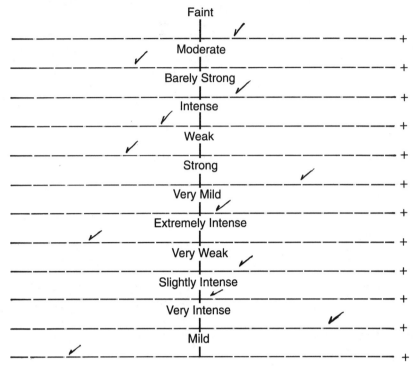

FIGURE 12–7. The pain intensity form of the Descriptor Differential Scale. (Adapted from Gracely, RH and Kwilosz, DM: The Descriptor Differential Scale: applying psychosocial principles to clinical pain assessment. Pain 35:279–288, 1988.

Patients must be well educated about their disease and methods of self-management such as exercise and the use of heat and cold. They will have been done a disservice if treatment is given without providing them with information and instruction in long-term management.

In addition, there are many educational and programmatic resources available through the Arthritis Foundation[34] that can provide community-based support to the patient and his or her family following discharge from physical therapy care. We recommend contacting your local chapter.

People with rheumatic diseases face daily challenges and a degree of unpredictability in their lives because of the nature of their illness. Their disease generally does not afford the physical therapist or other health professional the satisfaction that comes with providing a "cure" for their problems. The opportunity, however, is present for the physical therapist to work together with the patient as a partner, attempting to untangle and improve complex difficulties, to meet each challenge with positive support, and to encourage positive coping skills.

Study Objectives

Having completed this chapter, the reader should now be able to:

1. Name three sources of joint pain in inflammatory arthritis.

2. Describe which thermal agents should not be used in the presence of acute inflammation.

3. Identify the use of modalities as an adjunct to reduce pain, facilitating patient exercise.

4. State why education in self-management is a key component of treatment in the rheumatic diseases.

5. Describe the local effects of ice application on a patient with OA of the knee.

6. State that patients with inflammatory disease have intra-articular temperatures higher than normal individuals and why modalities that increase joint temperature may increase the inflammatory activity in the joint.

7. State why some modalities may have potentiating effects for medications and other thermal modalities used in treating arthritis.

8. State that no long-term benefit of modality use alone has been shown in FMS.

9. Name two possible influences on patient treatment outcome in rheumatic disease.

10. Name three techniques for pretreatment and posttreatment assessment in patients with polyarthritis.

REFERENCES

1. Banwell, BF and Gall, V (eds): Physical Therapy Management of Arthritis. Churchill Livingstone, New York, 1988.
2. Minor, MA and Sanford, MK: Physical interventions in the management of pain in arthritis: an overview for research and practice. Arthritis Care Res 6(4):197, 1993.
3. Mazzuca, SA: Economic evaluation of arthritis patient education. Bull Rheum Dis 43(5):6, 1994.
4. Mannheimer, JS: Nonmedicinal and noninvasive pain control techniques in the management of rheumatic disease and related musculoskeletal disorders. J Rheumatol (Suppl)14:26, 1987.
5. AHPA Arthritis Teaching Slide Collection, ed 2. Arthritis Foundation, Atlanta, GA, 1988.
6. Schumacher, HR, Klippel, JH, and Koopman, WJ (eds): Primer on the Rheumatic Diseases, ed 10. Arthritis Foundation, Atlanta, GA, 1993.
7. Hollander, JL and Horvath, SM: Intra-articular temperature as a measure of joint reaction. J Clin Invest 28:469, 1949.
8. Curkovic, B, et al: The influence of heat and cold on the pain threshold in rheumatoid arthritis. Z Rheumatol 54(5):289, 1993.
9. Yung, P, Unsworth, A, and Haslock, I: Measurement of stiffness in the metacarpophalangeal joint: The effect of physiotherapy. Clin Phys Physiol Meas 7(2):147, 1986.
10. Dellhag, B, Wollersjo, I, and Bjelle, A: Effect of active hand exercise and wax bath treatment in rheumatoid arthritis patients. Arthritis Care Res 5(2):87, 1992.
11. Harris, R and Millard, JB: Paraffin-wax baths in the treatment of rheumatoid arthritis. Ann Rheum Dis 14:278, 1955.
12. Hecht, PJ, et al: Effects of thermal therapy on rehabilitation after total knee arthroplasty. Clin Orthop Sep(178):198, 1983.
13. Utsinger, PD, Bonner, F, and Hogan N: Efficacy of cryotherapy and thermotherapy in the management of rheumatoid arthritis pain: Evidence for endorphin effect (abstr). Arthritis Rheum 25:S113, 1982.
14. Mainardi, CL, et al: Rheumatoid arthritis: Failure of daily heat therapy to affect its progression. Arch Phys Med Rehabil 60(9):390, 1979.
15. Hayes, KW: Heat and cold in the management of rheumatoid arthritis. Arthritis Care Res 6(3):156, 1993.
16. Kangilaski, J: Baggie therapy: Simple relief for arthritic knees. JAMA 247:317, 1981.
17. Pegg, SMH, Littler, TR, and Littler, EN: A trial of ice therapy and exercise in chronic arthritis. Physiotherapy 55:51, 1969.
18. Kirk, JA and Kersley, GD: Heat and cold in the physical treatment of rheumatoid arthritis of the knee: A controlled clinical trial. Ann Phys Med 9:270, 1968.
19. Weinberger, A, et al: Intra-articular temperature measurements after superficial heating. Scand J Rehabil Med 21(1):55, 1989.
20. Svarcova, J, Trnavsky, K, and Zvarova, J: The influence of ultra-sound, galvanic currents and shortwave diathermy on pain intensity in patients with osteoarthritis. Scand J Rheumatol (Suppl)67:83, 1987.
21. Bromley, J, Unsworth, A, and Haslock, I: Changes in stiffness following short- and long-term application of standard physiotherapeutic techniques. Br J Rheumatol 33(6):555, 1994.

22. Weinberger, A, et al: Deep heat in the treatment of inflammatory joint disease. Med Hypotheses 25(4):231, 1988.
23. Weinberger, A, et al: Treatment of articular effusions with local deep microwave hyperthermia. Clin Rheumatol 8(4):461, 1989.
24. DePreux, T: Ultrasonic wave therapy in osteoarthritis of the hip joint. Br J Phys Med 15:14, 1952.
25. Wright, V: Treatment of osteoarthritis of the knees. Ann Rheum Dis 23:389, 1964.
26. Kottke, FJ, Pauley, DL, and Ptak, RA: The rationale for prolonged stretching for correction of shortening connective tissues. Arch Phys Med Rehabil 47:345, 1966.
27. Granges, G, Zilko, P, and Littlejohn, GO: Fibromyalgia syndrome: Assessment of the severity of the condition 2 years after diagnosis. J Rheumatol 21(3):523, 1994.
28. Bucklew, SP: Fibromyalgia: A rehabilitation approach. Am J Phys Med Rehabil 68(1):37, 1989.
29. Wolfe F: Fibromyalgia: The clinical syndrome. In Bennett, RM and Goldenberg, DL (eds): The Fibromyalgia Syndrome. Rheum Dis Clin North Am 15(1):1, 1989.
30. Cathey, MA, et al: Functional ability and work status in patients with fibromyalgia. Arthritis Care Res 1:85, 1988.
31. McCain, GA: Nonmedicinal treatments in primary fibromyalgia. In Bennett, RM and Goldenberg, DL (eds): The Fibromyalgia Syndrome. Rheum Dis Clinics North Am 15(1):73, 1989.
32. Potts, MK and Silverman, SL: The importance of aspects of treatment for fibromyalgia. Arthritis Care Res 3(1):11, 1990.
33. Bradley, LA: Pain measurement in arthritis. Arthritis Care Res 6(4):178, 1993.
34. Arthritis Foundation (national office), 1314 Spring Street, NW, Atlanta, GA 30309. Phone 404-872-7100.

CHAPTER 13

Heat and Cold in Hand Rehabilitation

Jane Fedorczyk, MS, PT, CHT

Therapeutic heat and cold are commonly used as an adjunct treatment to exercise and splinting in hand rehabilitation. Thermal agents are also used to control edema, facilitate tissue healing, and reduce pain. In order for the application of heat and cold to be used effectively in hand rehabilitation, the clinician must be knowledgeable of the biophysical properties, and the precautions or contraindications, of each agent, especially those that apply to the injured hand. This chapter will emphasize the rationale and use of thermal agents in hand rehabilitation. Clinical applications specific to the injured hand will be described. The clinical decision making regarding the selection of the appropriate thermal agent will be addressed through case studies.

ANATOMIC AND PHYSIOLOGIC CONSIDERATIONS OF THE HAND

The hand is necessary for function in activities of daily living, vocational activities, avocational activities, and communication. Impairment of the hand can be devastating to the patient. Hand function is controlled by 27 bones, 33 muscles, three peripheral nerves, a complex vascular system, and many other supporting structures such as ligaments, joint capsules, tendon sheaths, and pulleys, all of which are located within the protective skin layer. There are many structures within a relatively small area which require freely uninterrupted gliding surfaces to maintain normal hand function. All of these structures are located within 1 to 2 cm of the skin surface. In comparison with other areas of the body, the superficial location of the structures of the hand allows for effective absorption of energy from superficial thermal agents.

Another important anatomic feature of the hand is the cutaneous tissue. The skin on the dorsum of the hand is fine, supple, and mobile. It can be completely separated from the deep fascia of the hand. This extensibility allows for the skin on the dorsum to adjust to extreme flexion and extension positions of the digits of the hand. The superficial venous system that runs together with the hand and digit lymphatics is also located within the skin on the dorsum of the hand. With the hand held in a gravity-dependent position, the veins become distended in the normal hand.[1] Damage to these superficial veins and lymphatic vessels can cause extensive edema on the dorsum of the hand. This is often seen with a crush injury. On the volar surface of the hand, the skin is rather immobile. It is firmly attached to the palmar aponeurosis, which prevents slippage during grasp. Although this is necessary for normal function, this anatomic arrangement can be problematic following injury and immobilization of the hand. Extensive scarring may occur within the palmar cutaneous tissue if full extension of the digits and palm cannot be achieved.

Second, the skin contains sensory receptors that respond to a variety of mechanical, thermal, and noxious stimuli. These mechanoreceptors and nociceptors are located in large numbers throughout the palmar surface of the hand, especially the fingertips. Because of the high innervation density of these sensory receptors, the cortical representation area of the cerebral cortex is much larger for the hand than for other body parts.[2] Sensibility contributes greatly to the function of the hand, especially when vision is occluded. In addition, when applying thermal agents to a patient, it is important to determine the status of the sensory receptors prior to treatment. The injured hand must have at least protective sensation to minimize the risk of injury from the application of heat or cold.

The hand is richly innervated and vascularized by a complex nerve and vascular system. The radial artery gives off a superficial branch that joins the ulnar artery to form the superficial palmar arch. The ulnar artery gives off a deep palmar branch that anastomoses with the radial artery to form the deep palmar arch. The superficial palmar arch has branches that form the common digital arteries, which then form radial and ulnar digital arteries. The palm is innervated by branches of the median and ulnar nerve, which form the common digital nerves before further division into the radial and ulnar digital nerves. Communication exists between the digital arteries and nerves through the nervi vasorum and vasa nervosum.[3] This connection controls the activity of the smooth muscle located within the arterial wall of the digital artery, allowing for vasoconstriction and vasodilation. When the innervation to the digits is interrupted, the communication within the digital neurovascular bundle is compromised. In this situation, the use of thermal agents is contraindicated. The digital artery may not be able to vasodilate or vasoconstrict in response to tissue temperature changes associated with the application of heat and cold.

Many of the structures within the hand are classified as dense connective-tissue structures that are composed of collagen. Chapter 5 discusses the effect of heat on the extensibility of connective tissue. Because most of these collagenous structures are located within 1 to 2 cm of the skin on the hand, generalized surface heating will often reduce joint stiffness and increase tissue extensibility. Cold, on the other hand, has been shown to increase joint stiffness (see Chapter 4). This may be an explanation for the low utilization of cold in hand rehabilitation.

GUIDELINES FOR EVALUATION OF THE HAND AND TREATMENT PLANNING

A thorough evaluation of the hand allows the clinician to determine the patient's functional deficits and generate hypotheses regarding the causes of the functional impairment. Once the problem statements are developed, then an appropriate treatment plan can be established.[4] In addition to establishment of a treatment plan, some components of the evaluation will assist the clinician in ruling out potential precautions or contraindications to the use of thermal agents. Some aspects of the objective examination will provide information regarding selection of a thermal agent and will serve as baseline measurements for evaluation of treatment effectiveness. Chapters 2 and 10 discuss methods of clinical evaluation used to determine the efficacy of applying thermal agents in the clinic. The emphasis of this section of the chapter is to highlight those aspects of a hand evaluation that will help the clinician select and apply therapeutic heat and cold effectively and competently. It is beyond the scope of this chapter to discuss the clinical assessment of the hand in detail. Concepts of the clinical evaluation of the hand have been described elsewhere.[5-7]

Subjective Examination, Observation, and Visual Inspection

The subjective examination is the initial step to begin clinical decision making regarding the use of heat and cold agents. Information gathered from the patient and medical chart can help with selection of the appropriate agent, but more importantly, it will assist the clinician with ruling out contraindications or identifying precautions for the use of thermal agents. The clinician should pay particular attention to complaints regarding decreased sensibility such as numbness and parasthesia. Relevant past medical history may provide information about potential vascular compromise such as Raynaud's phenomenon. The patient may have developed cold intolerance after a nerve or crush injury. A review of medications may alert the clinician to potential interactions or adverse effects with thermal agents.[8] Skin disorders such as dermatitis are a common problem in long-term use of antiepileptic drugs.[9] It has been recommended that any thermal agents that might exacerbate these skin disorders such as hot packs should be avoided. The patient may be aware of previous problems with the use of cold such as cold uticaria or cryoglobinemia. Chapters 4 and 5 discuss the precautions and contraindications to heat and cold that the reader should consider during the subjective examination.

The clinician should observe for any obvious signs of nerve or vascular compromise such as those listed in Table 13–1.[3,10–13] By identifying signs of vascular compromise and denervation, the clinician will rule out the use of inappropriate thermal agents or determine that if thermal agents are used, precautions are required.

The clinician should also observe the posture of the hand, the relationship of the hand to the body, and the patient's willingness to move the hand and upper extremity. The normal posture of the hand is relaxed flexion of the digits with greater flexion noted on the ulnar aspect of the hand. A disruption of the normal balance of the hand with deformities may indicate nerve injury.[10] If the patient holds the hand in a guarded position, he or she may be apprehensive about moving the hand secondary to pain. If the pain is severe, the clinician must determine if the patient would tolerate the application of heat or cold. The application of heat may reduce the patient's pain, but the patient may not be able to tolerate the weight of the hot pack. In this example, fluidotherapy or paraffin may be more appropriate than a hot pack. The analgesic effect of the thermal agent may then allow the therapist to do therapeutic exercises with the patient.

Range of Motion

Normal motion of the hand may be affected by pathologic changes to several structures of the hand, including the joint capsule, volar plate, intracapsular or extracapsular ligaments, intrinsic muscles, and tendons of the extrinsic muscles. Techniques for goniometry of the hand have been described.[5,14–16] An important aspect in the assessment of range of motion (ROM) of the hand is to determine which structure or structures are contributing to the loss of motion. By performing this differential diagnosis, appropriate decisions regarding treatment can be made.

The test for tightness of the intrinsic muscles of the hand was described by Bun-

TABLE 13–1 Signs and Symptoms of Nerve Injury or Vascular Compromise

Loss of Function	Observation
Motor	Presence of deformity: ape hand, claw, or wrist drop
	Abnormal hand posture; loss of flexion cascade
	Muscle atrophy of intrinsic or extrinsic hand musculature
	Presence of joint deformity
Sensory	Patient reports numbness or parasthesia
	Observe for burns or blisters usually on fingertips
Sympathetic	Skin color changes due to vasomotor instability
	Dry skin due to compromised sudomotor response
	Absent goose-bump response
	Atropy of fat pads in fingertips
	Skin is smooth and atrophic
	Curved fingernails, ridges in fingernails
	Increased or decreased hair growth
Vascular	Cyanotic or mottled skin color
	Skin is cool to palpation
	Patient reports throbbing pain
	Decreased capillary refill with blanching

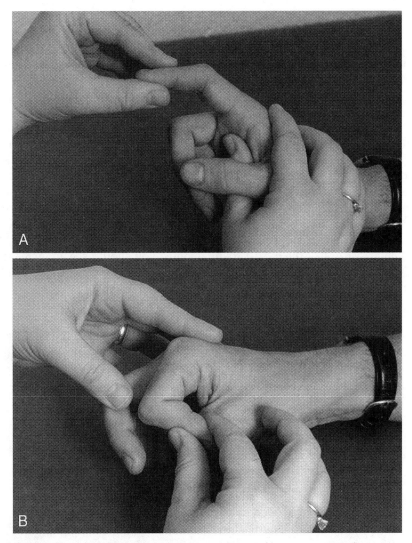

FIGURE 13–1. Intrinsic tightness is demonstrated if less passive PIP flexion is noted with MP passively extended (*A*) than with the MP passively flexed (*B*).

nell.[17] The test compares the amount of passive proximal interphalangeal (PIP) joint flexion obtained with the metacarpal phalangeal (MP) joint passively flexed simultaneously to the amount of passive PIP flexion available with the MP joint held in the extended position. If PIP flexion is greater with the MP flexed than with the MP extended, then this is indicative of intrinsic tightness (Fig. 13–1). Intrinsic tightness may be detected in one digit or all the digits.

The retinacular ligament attaches to the second annular (A2) pulley volar to the PIP flexion-extension axis and inserts into the terminal tendon of the extensor mechanism dorsal to the distal interphalangeal (DIP) joint flexion-extension axis. The retinacular ligament applies passive forces to the extensor mechanism to achieve simultaneous extension or flexion of the DIP and PIP joints. The ligament is taut with the PIP extended and the DIP joint flexed. Tightness of the oblique retinacular ligament is determined by the amount of passive DIP flexion available with the PIP joint extended (Fig. 13–2). If there is more passive DIP flexion available with the PIP joint flexed rather than with the PIP extended, then this would demonstrate tightness of the retinacular ligament.[18]

The tendons of the extrinsic flexor and extensor muscles of the forearm cross multiple joints to insert onto their distal attachments within the hand. Tightness of the extrinsic flexors or extensor tendons will result in a loss of passive composite motion. If the extrinsic flexors are tight, then there will be a loss of composite extension and the reverse occurs with tight extrinsic extensors. In general, as a stretch is applied across the digit in a composite manner, the wrist is passively moved in the same direction, and if tightness exists, decreased passive ROM of the distal joints should be observed. For example, if an extension stretch is maintained on the digits as the wrist is extended, then tightness of the extrinsic flexors would be detected if the fingers pulled into flexion as the wrist was passively extended (Fig. 13–3).[19] Also, when you eliminate stretch across one of the more proximal joints, you should see an increase in distal joint ROM. If no change occurs with the increased stretch on the extrinsic tendon, then the joint you are measuring has a contracture.

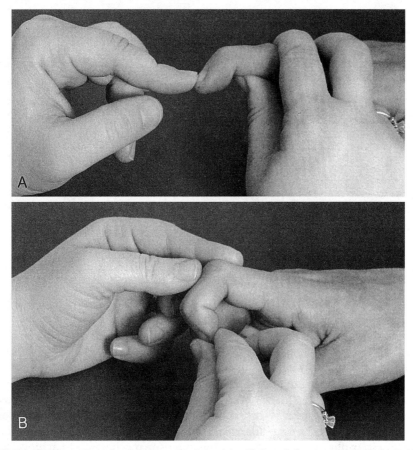

FIGURE 13–2. The retinacular ligament test is positive if there is less passive DIP flexion with the PIP passively extended (*A*) than with the PIP passively flexed (*B*).

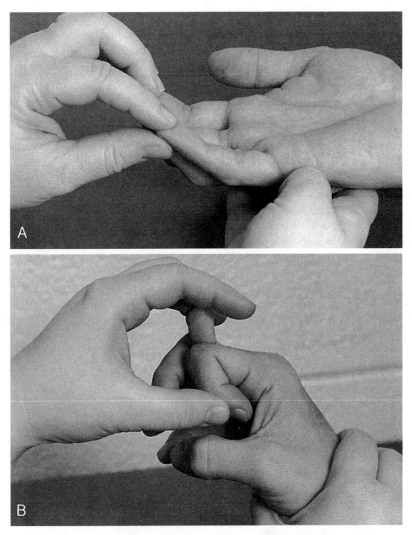

FIGURE 13–3. (*A*) Extrinsic flexor tendon tightness is assessed by performing passive composite extension of the digits. (*B*) Extrinsic extensor tendon tightness is assessed by performing passive composite flexion of the digits.

By determining the involved structures contributing to the loss of digital motion, the thermal agent can be selected and applied to the appropriate location of the hand. Typically, heat is used to increase joint ROM combined with passive stretch. If the loss of motion is caused by a joint restriction, the heat would be applied directly to the joint. If the loss of motion is caused by extrinsic tendon tightness, then this would require the application of heat to the area of tendon adherence with a passive composite flexion or extension stretch. For example, if a patient had extrinsic flexor tendon tightness causing a limitation in passive PIP joint extension, then ultrasound could be applied to the volar aspect of the forearm with a passive composite digital extension stretch with the wrist maintained in extension. If the ultrasound had been applied to the volar aspect of the involved PIP joint, this would have had no effect on the structures causing the restriction in ROM. Again, once the structure or structures causing the loss of motion are identified, the digit can be stretched in the most effective manner.

Edema

The assessment of edema is determined by comparing the involved hand to the noninvolved hand and by comparing the involved hand to itself over subsequent treatment days. Edema is usually assessed relative to time in response to activity or treatment. The tools commonly used are the volumeter (Fig. 13–4) for measuring water displacement and the tape measure for taking circumferential girth measurements.[20,21] The location and type of edema should be noted by the examiner. All subsequent measurements should be taken bilaterally to ensure that changes in values are brought about by treatment or activity and not just time of day or level of normal activity that would affect both hands. Girth measurements with a standard tape measure or tape designed to take circumferential measurements (Fig. 13–5) can be used on single digits, isolated joints, or areas proximal to the wrist. The volumeter is not sensitive to small areas of edema and is not capable of measuring edema proximal to the wrist.[20] The techniques and reliability of water displacement and girth measurements are discussed in Chapter 10 and other sources.[22,23]

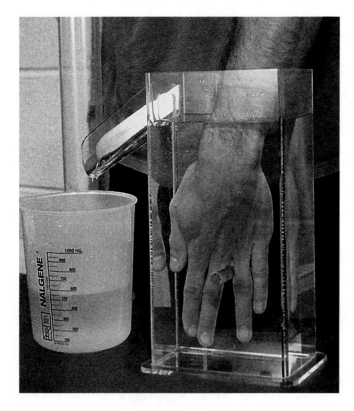

FIGURE 13–4. Hand volumeter to measure edema of the hand by water displacement.

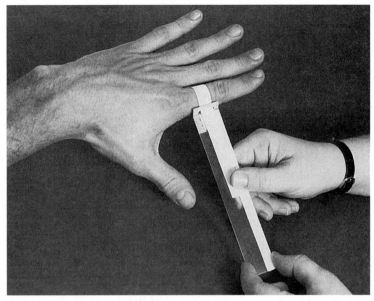

FIGURE 13–5. Circumferential tape measure for assessment of edema of the digits of the hand.

Circulation

Upon observation of the patient's hand, the examiner may note color changes that may be attributed to impaired circulation directly or to abnormal function of the sympathetic nervous system. Skin temperature may be assessed with palpation, especially over the dorsum of the hand or fingertips. Temperature biofeedback devices may also be used.[24] Allen's test has been described to assess the circulatory status of the ulnar and radial arteries.[25] A modification of the Allen's test has also been described to determine the function of the radial and ulnar digital arteries to each finger or thumb.[26]

Sensibility

There are numerous tests available to assess the integrity of the thermal, nociceptive, and mechanical sensory receptors. The threshold test for temperature recognition would be most applicable when using thermal agents. Failure to distinguish between hot and cold would require protection for the patient to prevent thermal injury. The use of thermal agents would be contraindicated. Two containers, usually test tubes, are used to perform the test. The temperature of the water in the cold test tube should be 40°F (4.44°C) and for the hot test tube 115°F to 120°F (46.11°C–48.8°C). The containers are alternated over the test area, and the patient is asked to determine if the temperature is hot or cold.[27] Temperature recognition kits are commercially available (Smith & Nephew Rolyan, Inc., Menomonee Falls, WI). Reliability and validity studies for this test are limited.[27] Threshold tests for light touch and protective sensation have been described.[28-34] Prior to the application of thermal agents, protective sensation should be established.

Pain

In general, clinicians need to assess pain for several reasons. If the nature of the pain is not straightforward, as it would be with a postoperative case, then we need to know the extent and location of the pain as a way to determine the underlying cause of the pain. In order for our treatments to be effective, we need to treat the source of the pain and manage the associated symptoms.[19] There are several methods of assessing pain in the patient with a hand injury. Chapters 2 and 10 review the clinical assessment of pain. Specific assessment tools have been developed for hand injuries. McCabe suggested a method to assess cold sensitivity in the hand.[35] Cold sensitivity occurs with traumatic injuries and increases the patient's perception of pain. Schultz has developed a pain assessment tool for the upper-extremity patient[36] (Upper Extremity Technology, Glenwood Springs, CO). The initial assessment of pain serves as a baseline for evaluating whether or not a particular thermal agent has been effective in alleviating pain.[37,38] The assessment of pain can assist clinical decision making to select the appropriate thermal agent.

CLINICAL APPLICATION

Superficial heat and cold can be used to manage a variety of clinical problems in the injured hand. Superficial agents penetrate to most structures of the hand. Continuous-wave ultrasound is used to provide focused heating to deeper structures. Diathermy is not a frequently used modality in hand rehabilitation, so it will not be considered in this discussion.

Pain Control

The rationale for the use of thermal agents in pain modulation has largely been based on clinical observation and experience, as well as information extrapolated from basic science. Thermal agents are known to promote pain relief, but their underlying mechanisms are not well understood.

The pain–muscle spasm–pain cycle can be the primary target to alleviate pain associated with hand trauma. When at least one component of this cycle is deactivated, pain can be reduced. It is well documented that muscle spasms and muscle guarding can be reduced with the use of either heat or cold, but the physiologic explanation remains puzzling. Therapeutic heat to a large surface area promotes generalized relaxation, which may decrease extrafusal muscle tension, which produces decreased muscle spindle activity. Increased cutaneous tissue temperature may cause decreased activity in the gamma-afferent fibers.[39] This may diminish the discharge rate of the muscle spindle by an indirect mechanism. The application of direct cold to muscle may decrease the firing rate of the muscle spindle by reducing the sensitivity of the spindle to stimuli.[40–42] Increased activity of the nociceptors can induce muscle spasm. An increase in activation threshold of nociceptors may reduce the transmission of painful stimuli. Both heat and cold have been suggested to increase the threshold stimulation of nociceptors.

The theory that heat or cold serve as a counterirritant is widely accepted.[43,44] It is proposed that the increased firing rate of thermoreceptors in the skin can block nociceptive input to the dorsal horn. The gate control theory is probably similar to the concept of counterirritation. The intensity of the thermal agent applied should not approach noxious levels.

The hemodynamic effects associated with the application of thermal agents are well documented in Chapters 4 and 5. Heat produces vasodilation and increased blood flow within the target tissue; cold reduces blood flow and causes vasoconstriction. Therapeutic heat may reduce pain by supplying essential nutrients for healing to the injured tissue and removing by-products such as chemical mediators. These substances are known to sensitize or activate nociceptors. Cold may alleviate pain by reducing excessive release of chemical mediators.[45,46]

The rationale for the use of superficial heating agents for pain control also applies to continuous-wave ultrasound. Ultrasound may be more effective in relieving joint and muscle pain than a surface heat agent. It has been demonstrated that an increase in muscle temperature to approximately 42°C can result in decreased activity of the muscle-spindle afferents and increased activity of the Golgi tendon organ afferents.[47] Muscle relaxation may be induced by decreased transmission of the alpha motoneuron in response to the changes in muscle spindle and Golgi tendon organ activity.[47] This explanation can lend support to the use of ultrasound.

Edema Control

Cryotherapy has been recommended for years for the management of acute inflammation and edema. Chapter 4 discusses the application of cold in rehabilitation, including the indications and contraindications for use. Cryotherapy is not commonly used in hand rehabilitation, since many patients with hand injuries are sensitive to cold. Other methods of edema control, including the application of heat with elevation and compression garments, are preferred.

The basic premise supporting the use of cold to control edema is that capillary permeability, blood flow, and tissue metabolism are reduced. Although the application of cold is discussed as part of the edema management during the acute phase of the hand injury, it is rarely used in isolation. Several authors have advocated the use of elevation, active exercise, compression wraps or garments, intermittent compression pumps, and string wrapping throughout the course of hand rehabilitation to control edema.[48–50]

Superficial heat, specifically paraffin, with the hand positioned in elevation has been suggested to control mild edema.[50] The heat is thought to assist venous return and lymph flow. Further explanation includes that heat provides an analgesic effect and increases collagen extensibility, thereby reducing joint stiffness. Active ROM exercises can be performed with greater ease once the pain and stiffness are reduced. This indirect response to reduce edema by providing a direct analgesic effect has also been associated with cryotherapy.[50] If pain is reduced via cold, it will be easier for the patient to perform active ROM exercises. The increased joint stiffness caused by cold is thought to be overcome after a few repetitions of an active exercise.

Tissue Extensibility

The effects of heat and cold on connective tissue are discussed in Chapters 5 and 4, respectively. In general, the elevation of tissue temperature will decrease the viscosity of the ground substance within collagen, the primary substance of connective tissue. This decreased viscosity combined with passive stretch can elongate connective tissue during the time the tissue temperature is elevated.[51] Once the tissue temperature has returned to normal, no further deformation is possible. This type of high-load brief stretch appears to have little long-term effect.[52] However, the technique of heat and stretch can be effective at preconditioning the tissue for ROM measurements and low-load prolonged-stress techniques such as splinting.[53]

CRYOTHERAPY

Cold can be applied in the form of ice packs, commercial cold gel packs, ice cups for ice massage, and cold whirlpools. Ice massage is commonly used in the treatment of localized problems such as tendinitis. Since the tendons of the hand are small, 35-mm film containers make adequate ice cups (Fig. 13–6) rather than larger paper or Styrofoam cups. The smaller surface area also helps to localize treatment. Cold packs and ice packs are usually applied to the hand with a moist towel interface. Hand patients generally tolerate commercial cold packs better than regular ice, since the cold pack does not seem to be as cold. If the towel is moistened with warm water, the patient may tolerate the more gradual temperature change better.

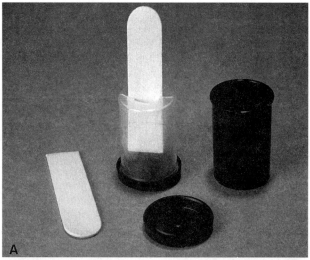

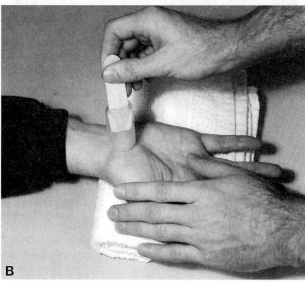

FIGURE 13–6. (A) 35-mm film containers can be used to make small ice cups for ice massage to the hand. (B) Ice massage to the flexor carpi radialis tendon.

SUPERFICIAL HEATING AGENTS

Hot Packs

Large square hot packs are difficult to wrap around the hand, but the "cervical" type works well. Another technique is to "sandwich" the hand between two small square hot packs. A passive stretch can be applied with any type of hot pack used. Coban (3M, St. Paul, MN) or an elastic bandage can be used to apply a comfortable, passive stretch into composite flexion of the hand. The hand may or may not be heated for approximately 10 minutes prior to the application of the Coban or elastic bandage. Depending on the size of the elastic bandage, it may be possible to eliminate one or two layers of toweling. Figure 13–7 illustrates the use of a dowel for the patient to grasp while the passive composite-flexion position is maintained with the elastic bandage.

A passive composite-extension stretch may be achieved with the use of the "sandwich" hot pack set-up (Fig. 13–8). The weight of the hot pack on the dorsum of the

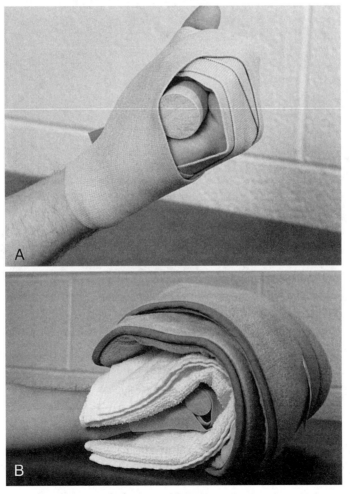

FIGURE 13–7. (*A*) Passive stretch technique for the hand to increase composite flexion. (*B*) Hand is placed in hot pack as a heat and stretch technique.

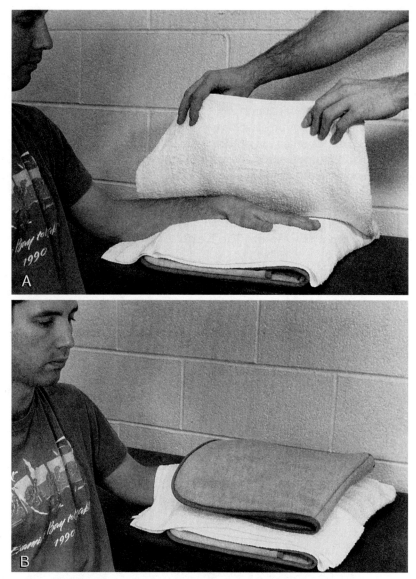

FIGURE 13–8. To increase composite extension of the digits (*A*), the hand may be sandwiched between two hot packs (*B*).

hand may be sufficient to promote an extension force on the digits. Extra towel layers may be required to protect the volar surface of the hand from thermal injury.

Paraffin

The dip-and-wrap method of paraffin application, as described in Chapter 5, is most commonly used in the treatment of hand patients. After the paraffin has been applied, the hand should be wrapped in plastic to avoid getting wax on the towel. A hot pack with towel layers may be wrapped around the paraffin-dipped hand for more vigorous heating. The hand may be placed in elevation above the level of the heart to minimize the risk of edema. Coban, adhesive paper tape, or Microfoam tape (3M, St. Paul, MN) can be utilized to increase composite flexion of a single digit or of all the digits. The tape or Coban is placed on the patient to apply a comfortable passive flexion stretch; then the hand is dipped in the paraffin in the usual manner (Fig. 13–9). An extension stretch could also be achieved with tongue blades taped to the dorsal aspect of the digits to maintain composite digital extension (Fig. 13–10). After removal of the paraffin, and tape, if any, the patient may squeeze the paraffin as a form of light resistive active exercise. In most clinics, for infection control purposes, the paraffin is not placed back into the paraffin tank.

Patients should not dip into the paraffin tank if they have a rash or open wound. Another way to apply the paraffin is to dip layers of rolled gauze such as Kerlix (Kendall Co., Manfield, MA) or Kling (Johnson & Johnson, New Brunswick, NJ) into the paraffin. The gauze is dipped in the same manner as the hand, and then wrapped around the hand or digit. The hand is then insulated with plastic wrap and towels (Fig. 13–11).

Fluidotherapy

This superficial heating agent can be used for the application of superficial heat and desensitization. The patient is able to perform active exercise while their hand is

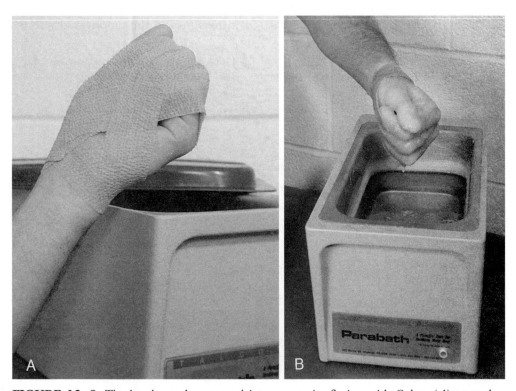

FIGURE 13–9. The hand may be wrapped into composite flexion with Coban (*A*) to apply a stretch prior to application of paraffin (*B*).

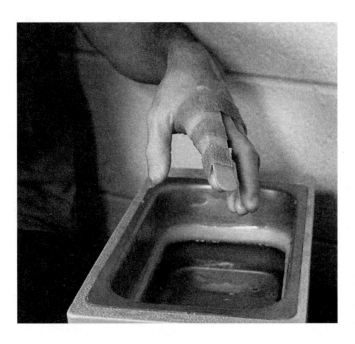

FIGURE 13–10. A digit may be taped to a tongue blade to provide a passive extension stretch with paraffin.

in the unit. If edema formation is of concern, then the temperature control should be placed on a low setting while still producing temperature elevation (100°F to 102°F). As with any heat agent, hand volume should be assessed pretreatment and posttreatment to determine if edema has increased in response to the biophysical effects of

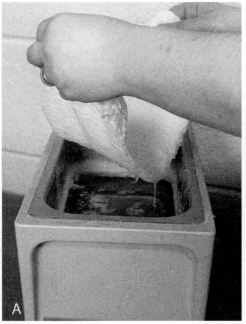
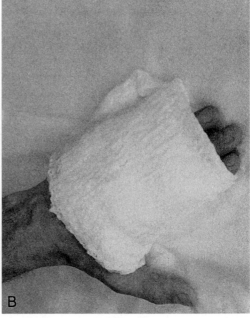

FIGURE 13–11. Gauze dipped in paraffin (*A*) and applied to the hand (*B*) for those patients that may have an open wound. It is contraindicated to dip in the paraffin unit with an open wound. The wound should be covered prior to wrapping of paraffin-soaked gauze.

heat. Patients with hypersensitivity of the fingertips from traumatic amputations, patients in the late stage of reflex sympathetic dystrophy, and patients with scar hypersensitivity may all benefit from the "bombardment" of the cellulose particles and heat combined.

Hydrotherapy

Warm and cold whirlpools were once utilized more frequently in the clinic as superficial heating or cooling agents. The benefit of such treatment is that the patient could perform active exercise during the whirlpool session. However, as clinics have developed more stringent guidelines for infection control, and efficient use of support staff is required, the use of the whirlpool in many hand clinics is now limited to the treatment of open wounds.

The whirlpool is an effective agent for cleansing and debriding superficial necrotic tissue in delayed primary or secondary wounds. The mechanical effect of the water assists to stimulate the formation of granulation tissue and to increase circulation within the wound, thereby facilitating tissue healing. In addition, the agitation of the water may provide an analgesic effect for the affected areas.[54]

A major concern regarding the use of the warm whirlpool is that the increased water temperature and dependent position of the hand will increase edema. Several studies suggest that if edema is a primary problem, discrimination should be used when selecting any heating agent, particularly a whirlpool.[55-57] If the patient's hand requires wound management, several steps can be taken to minimize an increase in hand edema. Hand pump exercises, such as opening and closing the fist with both hands completely overhead, every 2 to 3 minutes, have been suggested[58] and are illustrated in Figure 13–12. The appropriate positioning of the hand to minimize edema is demonstrated in Figure 6–3.

Additional information regarding whirlpools, whirlpool additives, and wound management is described[49] in Chapter 6.

Ultrasound

Ultrasound can be used selectively as a deep-heating agent in the hand. Because of its depth of penetration, the 3 MHz frequency is recommended for patients with hand problems. A smaller sound head (1 to 2 cm^2) maintains uniform contact with the skin surface (Fig. 13–13). The immersion technique is not necessary because of the availability of small transducers.

Ultrasound is routinely used in scar management to elongate adhesions that are inhibiting structures of the hand from freely gliding upon one another, particularly tendons. The use of ultrasound to reduce joint contracture and elongate scar tissue is described in Chapter 7. More investigation is needed to determine if continuous-wave ultrasound is effective in achieving a functional outcome in comparison to other techniques for elongating mature scar such as splinting.

Although further investigation is required, preliminary studies demonstrate that pulsed ultrasound can facilitate tissue healing and reduce inflammation (refer to Chapter 7). Another area of investigation has been the use of ultrasound over surgically repaired tendons.[59-63] Most of the studies have been conducted on a variety of animal models using pulsed ultrasound or continuous-wave ultrasound. The prelimi-

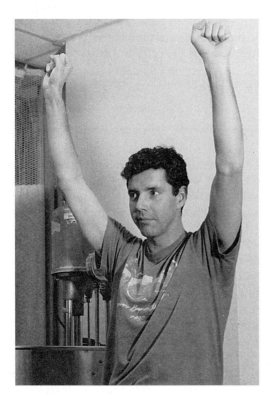

FIGURE 13–12. Hand pump exercises are done every 2 minutes to reduce the risk of edema formation in a warm whirlpool.

nary data are inconclusive. It is not practical to apply ultrasound in the first 10 days postoperatively because the sutures are still in place. Continuous-wave ultrasound is usually not applied to healing tendons until the late stages of fibroplasia (about 6 to 8 weeks postop). If ultrasound is being considered earlier after suture removal, the low-

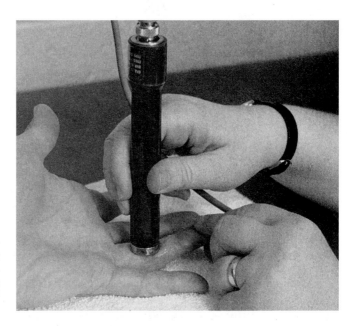

FIGURE 13–13. Small transducers have been designed for application of ultrasound to focused areas of the hand such as the volar aspect of the PIP joint.

intensity pulsed mode should be utilized to be consistent with wound and tendon healing studies.

COMMON CLINICAL PROBLEMS OF THE HAND

The Stiff Hand

A stiff hand is commonly seen after crush injuries to the dorsum of the hand and fractures of the hand or wrist. Aggressive early treatment is indicated to control pain, to control edema, and to promote ROM and tendon gliding. However, despite the best efforts of the patient and therapist, chronic joint stiffness of the hand may develop.

Treatment of the edematous hand should be aggressive, especially with crush injuries, since the superficial veins and lymphatics can be damaged. Immediately after injury, the application of cold may help minimize the formation of edema; however, to maintain the decrease in volume, the hand should be elevated above heart level at all times and compression wraps such as Coban should be applied. Active exercises should be added as indicated, depending on the involved structures. This will aid edema reduction through muscle pumping and promote increased ROM and tendon gliding.

As the stiffness becomes more chronic in nature, the differential diagnosis for ROM assessment is performed to determine which structures are contributing to the loss of motion. These tests are discussed earlier in this chapter. By identifying which structures are involved, appropriate therapeutic exercises and splinting regimens can be executed. Also, by determining the structures that are limiting joint motion, the selection of the appropriate thermal agent and its application can be made. For example, if a patient has a loss of PIP flexion to the right index and middle finger due to the adherence of his extrinsic extensor tendons to the fracture callus of his distal radius fracture, then continuous-wave ultrasound should be applied to the dorsum of the wrist, not the involved PIP joints. The application of heat and stretch to the stiff hand will help to reduce pain and enhance tissue conditioning prior to the application of hand splinting.

Superficial heating agents such as paraffin, hot packs, and Fluidotherapy can be used to reduce pain and increase collagen extensibility in the stiff hand. The application of heat prior to manual techniques such as passive stretch or joint mobilization frequently makes these techniques more tolerable to the patient and therefore easier for the clinician to perform.

CASE STUDY 1

HISTORY/INTERVENTION

The patient is a 40-year-old woman who is self-employed as a right-hand-dominant financial planner. She fractured her hand when she fell on vacation in Costa Rica. Her diagnosis included fractures of the shafts of the metacarpals of the right middle, ring, and small fingers. Because of allergies to most anesthetic drugs, the fractures were reduced by closed reduction without anesthesia. She was placed in a short arm cast that included the wrist in a neutral position and all four digits of the right hand. Digital flexion was blocked by the cast. By patient report, she had significant pain and edema for about 3 months' postinjury. She was followed by an orthopedic surgeon when she returned from her vacation, and one month after the injury she was sent to physical therapy. According to the patient, treatment consisted of paraffin, ultrasound, and an active therapeutic exercise program for 8 months. Since the patient had not regained functional use of the right hand, she was then referred to another physical therapist in a nearby hand clinic 9 months after the original injury.

PROBLEMS

1. Decreased active and passive ROM of the MPs, PIPs, and DIPs of the ulnar four digits of the right hand.
2. Decreased active and passive motion of the right wrist and thumb.
3. + Extrinsic extensor tendon tightness of the right ring and little fingers.
4. Contracture of the right thumb web space.
5. Residual edema of the right hand because of an inability to make a tight fist.
6. Pain noted after end-feel achieved at all joints. No pain at rest.
7. Decreased grip and pinch strength.
8. Decreased girth of the right forearm because of muscle atrophy.
9. Atrophy of the right hand intrinsic muscles.
10. Hypersensitivity of the right hand fingertips.
11. Pain noted after resistance to motion.

DECISION MAKING FOR CHOICE OF TREATMENT

1. Multiple joint involvement of the right hand involving joint and soft-tissue contractures.
2. Residual edema.
3. Hypersensitivity of fingertips.
4. Injury occurred 9 months ago. Previous PT for 8 months consisting primarily of thermal agents and active exercise.
5. Chronic stiff hand.

DESCRIPTION OF TREATMENT

The ulnar four digits of the right hand were stretched into composite flexion with Microfoam tape to patient tolerance and dipped in paraffin. A hot pack was wrapped around the hand. The patient was seated at a table with the right hand elevated above heart level. Paraffin treatment was 20 minutes. After removal of the tape, she was instructed to squeeze the paraffin glove into a ball until it had completely cooled. Joint mobilization and passive stretching were done to the right hand and wrist. Fabrication of a dynamic MP flexion splint was initiated. A web-spacer splint was fabricated for night use to stretch the web-space contracture. Additional splints to be fabricated included IP joint elastics to be worn with the dynamic MP flexion splint to maximize composite flexion. The patient was instructed in a home exercise program of passive ROM exercises, tendon gliding, and splinting.

Painful Hand (Reflex Sympathetic Dystrophy)

Reflex sympathetic dystrophy (RSD) is defined as a disorder of unknown etiology, typically affecting a single distal extremity with pain, edema, stiffness, vasomotor instability, and dystrophic changes to the skin. Pain is the overwhelming symptom in the early stages of RSD.[65-67] Functional impairment is significant because of sympathetic, sensory, and motor dysfunction as well as associated trophic changes to the involved extremity. The primary causes of RSD are trauma or surgical intervention.[65-67]

The clinical presentation is variable in history and physical findings. Both males and females are affected by the disorder, but it appears to be more prevalent in women.[65] Individuals known as "hypersympathetic reactors" appear to be prone to RSD.[65] There are usually confounding psychosocial problems; however, it is unclear whether these problems were present before or after the disorder.

RSD is a common painful condition of the hand. It can occur after trauma such as distal radius fractures or other fractures of the hand. It may also occur after surgery such as a carpal-tunnel release or palmar fasciectomy associated with Dupuytren's contracture. Three stages of RSD have been described.[65-68] These stages are helpful during communication with other clinicians and in prognosis. Table 13–2 describes the characteristics and duration of each stage.

The primary goal of treatment for RSD of the hand is to interrupt the pain cycle.[65-68] The therapist has the best chance of achieving this goal in the acute stage.[65,66] Other members of the medical team are also trying to achieve the same goal

TABLE 13–2 Stages of Reflex Sympathetic Dystrophy

Stage I (Up to 3 months)	Severe burning pain localized to site of trauma
	Allodynia, hyperesthesia, and/or parasthesia
	Localized, pitting edema
	Muscle spasm or muscle guarding
	Joint stiffness; difficulty initiating movement
	Vasomotor instability
	Increased sweat response (hyperhydrosis)
	Increased hair or nail growth
	Loss of function
Stage II (3–12 months)	Severe pain spreads to adjacent tissues
	Edema diffuses and becomes brawny
	Hair loss
	Cracked, grooved, or brittle nails
	Periarticular thickening
	Skin and muscle atrophy
	Spotty osteoporosis
	Vasomotor instability
	Initial radiographic findings of osteoporosis
	Loss of function
Stage III	Intractable pain may spread to entire limb(s)
	May see gradual resolution of pain once it peaks
	Joint and soft-tissue contractures
	Increased periarticular thickening
	Soft-tissue and muscle atrophy
	Significant bone deossification
	Loss of function

through medications and nerve blocks.[65] Secondary goals include edema reduction, increased joint mobility, and maximize functional activity.[65,67,69,70]

The use of thermal agents to treat the pain associated with RSD has been described.[65,67,69,70] Goodman[71] reported that 6 of 7 patients with RSD had control of pain and edema and return of function with the use of pulsed ultrasound over the location of stellate ganglion. Portwood and coworkers advocate the use of low-intensity ultrasound for the treatment of local tissues.[72] It should be noted that in each of the ultrasound studies, other treatment techniques such as stress loading,[73] superficial heating agents, and functional activities were utilized.

Walsh recommends that thermal agent selection vary depending on the vasomotor activity of the hand.[70] He has recommended the use of cold during phases of vasodilation to avoid the ill effects of heat. Heat promotes vasodilation, which in the case of RSD would only increase the amount of edema and subsequently pain through increased tissue distention. Heat is recommended during periods of vasoconstriction to stimulate blood flow and to alleviate pain.

As the disorder progresses and the pain begins to subside, heating agents are recommended to resolve residual edema, joint stiffness, and soft-tissue contracture. If hypersensitivity is evident, Fluidotherapy may be used. A passive stretch may accompany the application of heat, but care must be taken not to increase the pain. Compression garments and active exercise will help to reduce edema also. All therapeutic exercises should be simple. Exercise sessions should be short and should occur frequently throughout the day. Splinting and other techniques may be introduced as tolerated to restore motion, but care should be taken to keep treatment painless. Functional activities are emphasized.[65,67,69,70]

Although it is beyond the scope of this chapter, electrical stimulation to control pain has been suggested for the treatment of RSD.[65,67,69]

CASE STUDY 2

HISTORY/INTERVENTION

The patient is a 67-year-old man, right-hand-dominant attorney who underwent surgery for Dupuytren's contracture to straighten the contracted right ring and small fingers. Palmar and digital fasciectomies were performed 5 days ago on the right ring and small fingers with an open palm method.[74,75] The patient was referred 5 days after surgery by the attending physician to begin gentle active ROM, wound care, edema control, and splinting of the digits in extension. The splint would be removed periodically for bandage changes and active exercise.

PROBLEM LIST

1. Pain is primary patient complaint.
2. Patient holds hand in guarded position. (Hand held across chest; unwilling to move hand away from body.)
3. Decreased active and passive ROM of all the digits of the right hand.
4. Patient reports severe pain with palpation and joint motion.
5. Surgical incisions and small open wound in the palm that require healing.
6. As noted by visual inspection, edema is severe, but localized.

DECISION MAKING FOR CHOICE OF TREATMENT

1. Significant acute pain and edema.
2. Patient holds hand in guarded position and is apprehensive about movement of the hand.
3. Open wound on the palm of the hand.
4. Significant pain behavior observed. Unable to keep the patient calm, and the pain is worse than he expected.

DESCRIPTION OF TREATMENT

The patient was placed in a warm whirlpool at about 90°F (32.22°C). The hand was positioned in the tank in a gravity-minimized position. No water agitation for the first 10 minutes of a 20-minute treatment. After the whirlpool, a dry sterile dressing was placed to cover the wound on the palm. The patient was instructed in tendon-gliding exercises and to keep his hand elevated at all times. Compression wrapping for edema control was initiated by applying Coban lightly to the hand. To try to maintain the gains in digital extension, a static pan splint was fabricated to be worn at all times except for removal to perform active exercises and bandage changes. The extension position of the splint was tolerated by the patient. The patient was instructed to perform all exercises and splinting within his pain tolerance. If pain increased, the vigor of his exercises and splinting should be modified. As pain subsided, more vigorous exercise and splinting techniques were indicated to resolve joint stiffness. Heating agents were utilized in conjunction with passive stretching techniques to precondition tissues for ROM measurements and splint use.

SUMMARY

The use of heat and cold in hand rehabilitation can be effective in reducing the pain and edema of the hand. Heating agents used to precondition the tissues prior to exercise and splinting can reduce joint stiffness and tendon tightness. As outlined in this chapter, the appropriate selection of a thermal agent will depend on a review of the anatomic and physiologic concerns, and evaluation of the injured hand. Differential diagnosis in the ROM assessment will determine the structures contributing to the loss of motion and direct the appropriate selection and application heat. Thermal agents can be beneficial when applied in conjunction with therapeutic exercise and splinting.

Study Objectives

Having completed this chapter, the reader should now be able to:

1. Describe how specific anatomic features of the hand could affect thermal agent selection.
2. Discuss how components of the hand evaluation may influence the selection of thermal agents as part of the overall treatment plan.
3. Describe the effects of local cold application on edema following a crush injury to the hand.

4. Describe the effects of local heat on joint stiffness or soft-tissue contractures of the hand.
5. Discuss techniques to enhance the effect of heat and stretch in the injured hand.
6. Discuss edema concerns with the application of local heat and hydrotherapy.
7. Discuss the use of hydrotherapy in hand rehabilitation.
8. Describe the use of heat and cold as an adjunct to splinting and therapeutic exercise in the management of the stiff hand.
9. Discuss the clinical decision-making process of thermal agent selection with the painful hand.
10. Identify and discuss the precautions and contraindications to heat and cold in hand rehabilitation.

REFERENCES

1. Bowers, WH and Tribuzi, SM: Functional anatomy. In Stanley, BG and Tribuzi, SM (eds): Concepts in Hand Rehabilitation. FA Davis, Philadelphia, 1992, p. 29.
2. Kandel, ER: Central representation of touch. In Kandel, ER, Schwartz, JH, and Jessel, TM (eds): Principles of Neural Science, ed. 3. Elsevier, New York, 1991, p 372.
3. Sunderland, S: Nerves and Nerves Injuries, ed 2. Churchill Livingstone, New York, 1978.
4. Echternach, JL and Rothstein, JM: Hypothesis-oriented algorithms. Phys Ther 69:559, 1989.
5. Nicholson, B: Clinical evaluation. In Stanley, BG and Tribuzi, SM (eds): Concepts in Hand Rehabilitation. FA Davis, Philadelphia, 1992, p 59.
6. Clinical Assessment Recommendations, ed 2. Publication of the American Society of Hand Therapists, 1992.
7. Aulicino, PL: Clinical examination of the hand. In Hunter, JM, et al (eds): Rehabilitation of the Hand. CV Mosby, St. Louis, 1995, pp. 53–75.
8. Ciccone, CD: Pharmacology in Rehabilitation. FA Davis, Philadelphia, 1990, p 485.
9. Ciccone, CD: Pharmacology in Rehabilitation. FA Davis, Philadelphia, 1990, p 97.
10. Skirven, T: Nerve injuries. In Stanley, BG and Tribuzi, SM (eds): Concepts in Hand Rehabilitation. FA Davis, Philadelphia, 1992, p 332.
11. Callahan, A: Nerve injuries in the upper extremity. In Malick, MH and Kasch, MD (eds): Manual on Management of Specific Hand Problems. AREN Publications, Pittsburgh, 1984, p 19.
12. Callahan, A: Sensibility Assessment: Prerequisites and Techniques for Nerve Lesions in Continuity and Nerve Lacerations. In Hunter, JM, Macklin, E, and Callahan, A (eds): Rehabilitation of the Hand: Surgery and Therapy, ed 4, CV Mosby, St. Louis, 1995, p. 39.
13. Seddon, HJ (ed): Peripheral Nerve Injuries. Her Majesty's Printing Office, London, 1954.
14. Norkin, CC and White, DJ: Measurement of Joint Motion: A Guide to Goniometry, ed 2. FA Davis, Philadelphia, 1995, p 92.
15. Adams, LS, Greene, LW, and Topoozian, E: Range of motion. In Clinical Assessment Recommendations, ed 2. Publication of the American Society of Hand Therapists, 1992, p 55.
16. Cambridge, CA: Range of motion measurement of the hand. In Hunter, JM, Macklin, E, and Callahan, A (eds): Rehabilitation of the Hand: Surgery and Therapy, ed 4, CV Mosby, St. Louis, 1995, p. 93.
17. Bunnell, S: Ischaemic contracture, local, in the hand. J Bone Joint Surg 35A:88, 1953.
18. Nicholson, B: Clinical evaluation. In Stanley, BG and Tribuzi, SM (eds): Concepts in Hand Rehabilitation. FA Davis, Philadelphia, 1992, pp. 70–71.
19. Nicholson, B: Clinical evaluation. In Stanley, BG and Tribuzi, SM (eds): Concepts in Hand Rehabilitation. FA Davis, Philadelphia, 1992, p 71.
20. Nicholson, B: Clinical evaluation. In Stanley, BG and Tribuzi, SM (eds): Concepts in Hand Rehabilitation. FA Davis, Philadelphia, 1992, p 63.
21. Jaffe, R and Farney-Mokris, S: Edema. In Clinical Assessment Recommendations, ed 2, Publication of the American Society of Hand Therapists, 1992, pp. 13–19.
22. Waylett-Rendall, J and Seibly, D: A study of the accuracy of a commercially available volumeter. J Hand Ther 4:10, 1991.
23. Bear-Lehman, J and Abreu, BC: Evaluating the hand: Issues in reliability and validity. Phys Ther 69:1026, 1989.
24. Kader, PB: Therapist's management of the replanted hand. In Hunter, JM, et al (eds): Rehabilitation of the Hand. CV Mosby, St. Louis, 1990, p 823.
25. Allen, E: Thromboangitis obliterans: Methods of diagnosis of chronic occlusive arterial lesions distal to the wrist with illustrative cases. Am J Med Sci 178:237, 1929.

26. Ashbell, T, Kutz, J, and Kleinert, H: The digital Allen test. Plast Reconstr Surg 39:311, 1967.
27. Stone JH: Sensibility. In Clinical Assessment Recommendations, ed 2. Publication of the American Society of Hand Therapists, 1992, p 75.
28. Stone, JH: Sensibility. In Clinical Assessment Recommendations, ed 2. Publication of the American Society of Hand Therapists, 1992, p 76.
29. Tan, AM: Sensibility testing. In Stanley, BG and Tribuzi, SM (eds): Concepts in Hand Rehabilitation. FA Davis, Philadelphia, 1992, p 76.
30. Bell-Krotoski, JA: Sensibility Testing: Current Concepts. In Hunter, JM, Macklin, E, and Callahan, A (eds): Rehabilitation of the Hand: Surgery and Therapy, ed 4, CV Mosby, St. Louis, 1995, pp. 109–128.
31. Dellon, AL: Touch sensibility in the hand. J Hand Surg 9B:11, 1984.
32. Dellon, AL and Kallman, CH: Evaluation of functional sensation in the hand. J Hand Surg 8:865, 1983.
33. Dellon, AL, Curtis, RM, and Edgerton, MT: Evaluating recovery of sensation in the hand following nerve injury. Johns Hopkins Med J 130:235, 1972.
34. Dellon, AL: Evaluation of Sensibility and Re-education of Sensation in the Hand. Williams & Wilkins, Baltimore, 1981.
35. McCabe, SJ, Mizgala, C, and Glickman, L: The measurement of cold sensitivity in the hand. J Hand Surg 16:1037, 1991.
36. Schultz, KS: The Schultz structured interview for assessing upper extremity pain. Occup Ther Health Care 1:69, 1984.
37. Echternach, JL: Clinical evaluation of pain. In Herdman, SJ and Clendaniel, RA (eds): Phys Ther Prac 2:14, 1993.
38. Gersh, MR: Transcutaneous electrical nerve stimulation (TENS) for management of pain and sensory pathology. In Gersh, MR (ed): Electrotherapy in Rehabilitation. FA Davis, Philadelphia, 1992.
39. Fischer, E and Solomon, S: Physiological responses to heat and cold. In Licht, S (ed): Therapeutic Heat and Cold, ed 2. Waverly Press, Baltimore, 1965.
40. Knuttsson, E and Mattsson, E: Effects of local cooling on monosynaptic reflexes in man. Scand J Rehabil Med 1:126, 1969.
41. Eldred, E, Lindsley, DF, and Buchwald, JS: Effects of cooling on mammalian muscle spindles. Exp Neurol 2:144, 1960.
42. Newton, M and Lehmkuhl, D: Muscle spindle response to body heating and localized muscle cooling: Implications for relief of spasticity. J Am Phys Ther Assoc 45:91, 1965.
43. Parsons, CM and Goetzl, FR: Effect of induced pain on pain threshold. Proc Cos Exp Bio Med 60:327, 1945.
44. Gammon, GD and Starr, I: Studies on the relief of pain by counterirritation. J Clin Invest 20:13, 1941.
45. Jessell, TM and Kelly, DD: Pain and analgesia. In Kandel, ER, Schwartz, JH, and Jessell, TM (eds): Principles of Neural Science, ed 3. Elsevier, New York, 1991, p 385.
46. Cailliet, R: Pain: mechanisms and management. FA Davis, Philadelphia, 1993, p 67.
47. Mense, S: Effects of temperature on the discharges of muscle spindles and tendon organs. Pflugers Arch 374:159, 1978.
48. Sorenson, MK: The edematous hand. Phys Ther 69:1059, 1989.
49. Walsh, M and Muntzer, E: Wound management. In Stanley, BG and Tribuzi, SM (eds): Concepts in Hand Rehabilitation. FA Davis, Philadelphia, 1992, p 167.
50. Hunter, JM and Mackin, EJ: Edema: Techniques of Evaluation and Treatment. In Hunter, JM, Macklin, E, and Callahan, A (eds): Rehabilitation of the Hand: Surgery and Therapy, ed 4, CV Mosby, St. Louis, 1995, p. 83.
51. Lehman, J, et al: Effect of therapeutic temperatures on tendon extensibility. Arch Phys Med Rehabil 51:81, 1970.
52. Hamilton, G: Mobilization of the proximal interphalangeal joint: The influence of heat, cold, and exercise. Phys Ther 47:111, 1967.
53. Flowers, KR and Michlovitz, SL: Assessment and management of loss of motion in orthopedic dysfunction. Postgraduate Advances in Physical Therapy, published by the American Physical Therapy Association, 1988 copyright.
54. Walsh, M: Hydrotherapy. In Michlovitz, SL: Thermal Agents in Rehabilitation, ed 3. FA Davis, Philadelphia, 1990, p 113.
55. Walsh, MT: Relationship of hand edema to upper extremity position and water temperature during whirlpool treatments in normals. Unpublished thesis, Temple University, Philadelphia, 1983.
56. Magness, J, Garret, T, and Erickson, D: Swelling of the upper extremity during whirlpool baths. Arch Phys Med Rehabil 51:297, 1970.
57. Schultz, KS: The effect of active exercise on edema. J Hand Surg 8:625, 1983.
58. Byron, TM and Muntzer, EM: Therapist's management of the mutilated hand. In Mackin, EJ (ed): Hand Clinics 2(1). WB Saunders, Philadelphia, 1986.
59. Roberts, M, Rutherford, JH, and Harris, D: The effect of ultrasound on flexor tendon repairs in the rabbit. Hand 14:17, 1982.
60. Enwemeka, CS: The effects of therapeutic ultrasound on tendon healing. Am J Phys Med Rehabil 68:283, 1989.

61. Turner, SM, Powell, ES, and Ng, CSS: Effect of ultrasound on the healing of cockeral tendon: Is collagen cross-linkage a factor? J Hand Surg 14B:428, 1989.
62. Stevenson, JH, et al: Functional, mechanical, and biochemical assessment of ultrasound therapy on tendon healing in the chicken toe. Plast Reconstr Surg 77:965, 1986.
63. Huys, S, et al: Comparison of effects of early and late ultrasound treatment on tendon healing in the chicken limb (abstr). J Hand Ther 6:58, 1993.
64. Wehbe, MA and Hunter, JM: Flexor tendon gliding in the hand. Part II. Differential gliding. J Hand Surg 10A:575, 1985.
65. Lankford, LL: Reflex sympathetic dystrophy. In Hunter, JM, Macklin, E, and Callahan, A (eds): Rehabilitation of the Hand: Surgery and Therapy, ed 4, CV Mosby, St. Louis, 1995, pp. 779–815.
66. Schwartzman, R and McLellan, T: Reflex sympathetic dystrophy: A review. Arch Neurol 44:555, 1987.
67. Mullins, PT: Reflex sympathetic dystrophy. In Stanley, BG and Tribuzi, SM (eds): Concepts in Hand Rehabilitation. FA Davis, Philadelphia, 1992, p 446.
68. Betcher, AM and Casten, DF: Reflex sympathetic dystrophy: In Hunter JM, Macklin E, and Callahan A (eds): Rehabilitation of the Hand: Surgery and Therapy, ed 4, CV Mosby, St. Louis, 1995, pp. 817–833.
69. Waylett-Rendall, J: Therapist's management of reflex sympathetic dystrophy. In Hunter JM, et al: Rehabilitation of the Hand, ed 3. CV Mosby, St. Louis, 1990, p.787.
70. Walsh, M: Therapist's management of reflex sympathetic dystrophy. In Hunter, JM, Macklin, E, and Callahan, A (eds): Rehabilitation of the Hand: Surgery and Therapy, ed 4, CV Mosby, St. Louis, pp. 817–833.
71. Goodman, C: Treatment of hand shoulder syndrome: Combined ultrasonic application to stellate ganglion and physical medicine. NY State J Med, 1971, p 559.
72. Portwood, M, Lieberman, J, and Taylor, R: Ultrasound treatment of reflex sympathetic dystrophy. Arch Phys Med Rehabil 68:116, 1987.
73. Carlson, L and Watson, HK: Treatment of reflex sympathetic dystrophy using the stress-loading program. J Hand Ther 4:419, 1988.
74. McCash, CR: The open palm technique in Dupuytren's contracture. Br J Plast Surg 17:271, 1964.
75. Fietti, VG and Mackin, EJ: Open-palm technique in Dupuytren's disease. In Hunter, JM, Macklin, E, and Callahan, A (eds): Rehabilitation of the Hand: Surgery and Therapy, ed 4, CV Mosby, St. Louis, 1995, p. 995.

APPENDIX

Temperature Conversions for Fahrenheit and Celsius

To convert Centigrade to Fahrenheit: $\left(\frac{9}{5} \times {}^{\circ}C\right) + 32$

°C	°F		°C	°F
46	114.8		22	71.6
45	113.0		21	69.8
44	111.2		20	68.0
43	109.4		19	66.2
42	107.6		18	64.4
41	105.8		17	62.6
40	104.0		16	60.8
39	102.2		15	59.0
38	100.4		14	57.2
37	98.6		13	55.4
36	96.8		12	53.6
35	95.0		11	51.8
34	93.2		10	50.0
33	91.4		9	48.2
32	89.6		8	46.4
31	87.8		7	44.6
30	86.0		6	42.8
29	84.2		5	41.0
28	82.4		4	39.2

°C	°F		°C	°F
27	80.6		3	37.4
26	78.8		2	35.6
25	77.0		1	33.8
24	75.2		0	32.0
23	73.4			

To convert Fahrenheit to Centigrade: $\left(\dfrac{5}{9} \times °F\right) - 32$

°F	°C		°F	°C
120	48.9		76	24.4
119	48.3		75	23.9
118	47.8		74	23.3
117	47.2		73	22.7
116	46.7		72	22.2
115	46.1		71	21.7
114	45.6		70	21.1
113	45.0		69	20.6
112	44.4		68	20.0
111	43.9		67	19.4
110	43.3		66	18.9
109	42.8		65	18.3
108	42.2		64	17.8
107	41.7		63	17.2
106	41.1		62	16.7
105	40.5		61	16.1
104	40.0		60	15.5
103	39.4		59	15.0
102	38.8		58	14.4
101	38.3		57	13.9
100	37.8		56	13.3
99	37.2		55	12.8
98	36.7		54	12.2
97	36.1		53	11.7
96	35.5		52	11.1
95	35.0		51	10.6
94	34.4		50	10.0
93	33.9		49	9.4
92	33.3		48	8.9
91	32.8		47	8.3
90	32.2		46	7.8
89	31.7		45	7.2
88	31.1		44	6.6
87	30.6		43	6.1
86	30.0		42	5.6
85	29.4		41	5.0
84	28.9		40	4.4

°F	°C		°F	°C
83	28.3		39	3.9
82	27.8		38	3.3
81	27.2		37	2.8
80	26.7		36	2.2
79	26.1		35	1.7
78	25.6		34	1.1
77	25.0		33	0.6
			32	0

GLOSSARY

Absorption: The taking up by the body of radiant heat, causing a rise in tissue temperature.

Acute pain: A short, sharp, cutting pain. Usually associated with acute inflammation or inflammation of serous membranes; also posterior spinal-root pains.

Adhesion: 1. A holding together or uniting of two surfaces or parts, as in wound healing. 2. A fibrous band holding parts together that are normally separated.

Aeration: 1. Act of airing. 2. Saturation or charging of a fluid with gases.

Afterdischarge: The discharge of impulses from a reflex center after stimulation of the receptor has ceased. Results in prolongation of response.

Alternating current: Abbr: AC. An electric current that reverses direction at regular intervals.

Analgesia: Absence of normal sense of pain.

Anastomosis: 1. A natural communication between two vessels; may be direct or by means of connecting channels. 2. The surgical or pathologic connection of two tubular structures.

Anesthesia: Partial or complete loss of sensation, with or without loss of consciousness, as result of disease, injury, or administration of an anesthetic agent, usually by injection or inhalation.

Anoxia: Without oxygen. Term is often used incorrectly to indicate hypoxia.

Antidromic: Denoting nerve impulses traveling in the opposite direction from normal.

Arachidonic acid: A precursor of prostaglandin. It is metabolized in the body to produce a group of chemicals called eicosanoids. Included in these are prostaglandin, thromboxane, and leukotrienes. Synthesis of prostaglandin and thromboxane is directly inhibited by nonsteroidal anti-inflammatory agents such as salicylates, indomethacin, and ibuprofen.

Arteriovenous (AV) anastomosis: Anastomosis between an artery and a vein by which the capillary bed is bypassed.

Atrophy: 1. A wasting; a decrease in size of an organ or tissue. 2. To undergo or cause atrophy. Etiol: May result from death and resorption of cells, diminished cellular proliferation, pressure, ischemia, malnutrition, decreased activity, or hormonal changes.

Attenuation: 1. The change (decrease) in a beam of radiation as it passes through matter. 2. In acoustics, the reduction in sound intensity of the initial sound source as compared with the sound intensity at a point away from the source.

Axonotmesis: Nerve injury that damages the nerve tissue without actually severing the nerve.

Axon reflex: A reflex that does not involve a complete reflex arc, hence is not a true reflex. The afferent and efferent limbs of the reflex are branches of a single nerve fiber, the axon (axonlike dendrite) of a sensory neuron. An example is vasodilation resulting from stimulation of skin.

Bactericidal agent: Destructive to, or destroying, bacteria.

Bradykinin: A plasma kinin. See: kinin.

Buoyancy: The upward pressure exerted by the fluid in which an object is immersed.

Bursa: A padlike sac or cavity found in connecting tissue, usually in the vicinity of joints. It is lined with synovial membrane and contains a fluid, synovia, that acts to reduce friction between tendon and bone, tendon and ligament, or between other structures where friction is likely to occur.

Bursitis: Inflammation of a bursa, especially those located between bony prominences and muscle tendon, as the shoulder and knee.

Calibration: Determination of the accuracy of an instrument by comparing the information or measurement provided with that of a known standard or an instrument known to be accurate.

Capacitance: 1. State of being able to store electric charge. 2. Ratio of the charge transferred from one to the other of a pair of conductors to the potential difference between the conductors.

Capacitor: Electronic device for storing electric charges.

Cavitation: The vibrational effect on gas bubbles by an ultrasound beam.

Chemotaxis: Movement of cells in response to a chemical stimulus or message; for example, the movement of neutrophils to the site of injury or inflammation.

Chlorination: Treatment of water by addition of chlorine and its compounds for the killing of bacteria. For effective disinfection, a concentration of 0.5 to 1 part chlorine per million parts of water is necessary.

Chondroblast: A cell that forms cartilage.

Chronic pain: The persistance of pain beyond the usual or expected course of an acute disease, or after a reasonable amount of time for an injury to heal has elapsed.

Clonus: Spasmodic alternation of muscular contraction and relaxation.

Collagen: A fibrous, insoluble protein found in the connective tissue, including skin, bone, ligaments, and cartilage. Collagen represents about 30 percent of the total body protein.

Collimation: The process of making parallel.

Complement: A series of enzymatic proteins in normal serum that, in the presence of a specific sensitizer, destroy bacteria and other cells. Complement components and complement regulators include at least two dozen substances. Once activated, the components are involved in a great number of immune defense mechanisms, including anaphylaxis, leukocyte chemotaxis, and phagocytosis.

Compliance: Cooperative performance in relation to prescribed therapy or medicines.

Condensation: Making more dense or compact.

Conductance: The conducting ability of a body or a circuit for electricity. The best conductor is one that offers the least resistance, such as gold, silver, and copper. When expressed as a numerical value, conductance is the reciprocal of resistance. The unit is the mho.

Conduction: 1. The process whereby a state of excitation affects successive portions of a tissue or cell, so that the disturbance is transmitted to remote points. Conduction occurs not only in fibers of the nervous system but also in muscle fibers. 2. The transfer of electrons, ions, heat, or sound waves through a conductor or conducting medium.

Conductor: Medium transmitting a force, a signal, or electricity. (Examples: aluminum and copper.)

Connective tissue: Tissue that supports and connects other tissues and tissue parts. The cells of connective tissue are comparatively few in number, the bulk of the tissue consisting of intercellular substance or matrix, the nature of which gives each type of connective tissue its particular properties. Connective tissues are highly vascular, with the exception of cartilage. Connective tissue proper includes the following types: mucous, fibrous (areolar, white fibrous, yellow fibrous, or elastic), reticular, and adipose. Dense connective tissue includes cartilage and bone (osseous tissue).

Consensual: Reflex stimulation of one part or side as a result of excitation of another part or opposite side.

Consensual response: Any reflex occurring on opposite side of body from point of stimulation.

Contraction: A shortening or tightening, as that of a muscle, or a reduction in size; a shrinking.

Contracture: 1. A condition of fixed high resistance to the passive stretch of a muscle, as may result from fibrosis of tissues surrounding a joint. 2. Permanent contraction of a muscle caused by spasm or paralysis.

Contusion: An injury in which the skin is not broken; a bruise.

Convection: The transfer of heat by means of currents in liquids or gases.

Convergence: In reflex activity, the coming together of several axons or afferent fibers upon one or a few motor neurons; the condition whereby impulses from several sensory receptors converge upon the same motor center, resulting in a limited and specific response.

Cryoglobulinemia: Presence in the blood of an abnormal protein that forms gels at low temperatures. Found in association with pathologic conditions such as multiple myeloma, leukemia, and certain forms of pneumonia.

Cryotherapy: The therapeutic use of cold.

Debridement: The removal of foreign material and dead or damaged tissue, especially in a wound.

Debridement, enzymatic: Use of proteolytic enymes to remove dead tissue from a wound. The enzyme does not attack viable tissues.

Decubitus ulcer: Ischemic necrosis and ulceration of tissue, especially over a bony prominence, caused by pressure from prolonged confinement in bed or from a cast or splint.

Diathermy: The therapeutic use of a high-frequency current to generate heat within some part of the body. The frequency is greater than the maximal frequency for neuromuscular response and ranges from several hundred thousand to millions of cycles per second.

Dielectric: An insulating substance offering great resistance to passage of electricity by conduction.

Diffraction: The change that occurs in light when it passes through crystals, prisms, or parallel bars in a grating, in which the rays are deflected and, thus, appear to be turned aside. This produces dark or colored bands or lines or other phenomena. Term is also applied to similar phenomena in sound and electricity.

Dipole: 1. Two equal and opposite charges separated by a distance. 2. In chemistry, one portion of the molecule has a certain charge, and the other portion has an equal and opposite charge.

Direct current: Abbr: DC. An electric current flowing continuously in one direction.

Diuresis: Secretion and passage of large amounts of urine. This condition occurs in diabetes mellitus. It can be an early sign of chronic interstitial nephritis. May also be caused by hysteria, result of fear and anxiety, ingestion of large quantities of liquids, diabetes insipidus, or the action of drugs that have the ability to cause diuresis.

Dorsal rhizotomy (posterior rhizotomy): Section of the dorsal root of the spinal nerve for relief of pain.

Edema: A local or generalized condition in which the body tissues contain an excessive amount of tissue fluid.

Effusion: Escape of fluid into a part.

Elasticity: The quality of returning to original size and shape after compression or stretching.

Elastin: An extracellular connective-tissue protein that is the principal component of elastic fibers.

Electrode: A medium intervening between an electric conductor and the object to which the current is to be applied. In electrotherapy, an electrode is an instrument with a point or a surface from which to discharge current to the body of a patient.

Electromotive force: Abbr: EMF. Energy that causes flow of electricity in a conductor. The energy is measured in volts.

Emigration: Passage of white blood corpuscles through the walls of capillaries and veins during inflammation.

Endogenous opiate-like substance: Chemical substance, polypeptides, produced in the brain, that act as opiates and produce analgesia by binding to opiate-receptor sites involved in pain perception. The threshold for pain is therefore increased. (Examples: endorphins, enkephalins.)

Eschar: A slough, especially one following a cauterization or burn.

Evaporation: 1. Change from liquid form to vapor. 2. Loss in volume because of conversion of a liquid into a vapor.

Extravasation: The escape of fluids into the surrounding tissue.

Extravascular: Outside a vessel.

Exudate: Accumulation of a fluid in a cavity, or matter that penetrates through vessel walls into adjoining tissue, or the production of pus or serum. In comparison with a transudate, there are more cells, protein, and solid material in an exudate.

Fibroblast: Any cell or corpuscle from which connective tissue is developed.

Firbrosis: Abnormal formation of fibrous tissue.

Gate control theory: The hypothesis that painful stimuli may be prevented from reaching higher levels of the central nervous system by stimulation of larger sensory nerves.

Granulation tissue: 1. Formation of granules, or state or condition of being granular. 2. Fleshy projections formed on the surface of a gaping wound that is not healing by first intention or indirect union. Each granulation represents the outgrowth of new capillaries by budding from the existing capillaries and then joining up into capillary loops supported by cells that will later become fibrous scar tissue. Granulations bring rich blood supply to the healing surface.

Ground: In electronics, the negative or earth pole that has zero electrical potential.

Hemarthrosis: Bloody effusion into a cavity of a joint.

Hematoma: A swelling or mass of blood (usually clotted) confined to an organ, tissue, or space and caused by a break in a blood vessel.

Hemorrhage: Abnormal internal or external discharge of blood. May be venous, arterial, or capillary from blood vessels into tissues, into or from the body. Venous blood is dark red; flow is continuous. Arterial blood is bright red; flows in spurts. Capillary blood is of a reddish color; exudes from tissue.

Hertz: A unit of frequency equal to 1 cycle per second. Abbreviated Hz.

Histamine: A substance, produced from the amino acid histidine, that is normally present in the body. It exerts a pharmacologic action when released from injured cells. The red flush of a burn is due to the local production of histamine.

Homeostasis: State of equilibrium of the internal environment of the body that is maintained by dynamic processes of feedback and regulation.

Hyaluronic acid: An acid mucopolysaccharide found in the ground substance of connective tissue that acts as a binding and protective agent. Also found in synovial fluid and vitreous and aqueous humors.

Hydrotherapy: Scientific application of water in treatment of disease.

Hyperalgesia: Excessive sensitivity to pain. Opposite of hypalgesia.

Hyperemia: 1. Congestion. An unusual amount of blood in a part. 2. A form of macula; red areas on skin that disappear on pressure. 3. In physical therapy, increase in quantity of blood flowing through any part of the body, shown by redness of the skin caused by the application of heat.

Hyperreflexia: Increased action of the reflexes.

Hyperthermia: 1. Unusually high fever. 2. Treatment of disease by raising bodily temperature, accomplished by introduction of the malaria organism, injection of foreign proteins, or by physical means.

Hypertrophy: Increase in size of an organ or structure that does not involve tumor formation. Term is generally restricted to an increase in size or bulk not resulting from an increase in number of cells or tissue elements, as in the hypertrophy of muscle.

Hypotonic: 1. Pertains to defective muscular tone or tension. 2. A solution of lower osmotic pressure than another.

Immune response: The reaction of the body to substances that are foreign or are interpreted as being foreign.

Impedance: Resistance met by alternating currents in passing through a conductor; consists of resistance, reactance, inductance, or capacitance. The resistance caused by the inductive and condenser characteristics of a circuit is called reactance.

Inductance: That property of an electric circuit by virtue of which a varying current induces an electromotive force in that circuit or a neighboring circuit. The unit of inductance, or self-inductance, is the henry.

Inflammation: Tissue reaction to injury. The succession of changes that occur in living tissue when it is injured. The inflamed area undergoes continuous change as the body repair processes start to heat and replace injured tissue. Inflammation is a conservative process modified by whatever produces the reaction, but it should not be confused with infection; the two are relatively different conditions, although one may arise from the other.

Inflammation, acute: Inflammation in which the onset is rapid and the course relatively short.

Inflammation, chronic: Inflammation that progresses slowly, is of long duration, and usually results in the formation of scar.

Inflammation, subacute: A relatively mild inflammation that may become worse and then is severe or chronic.

Insulator: That which insulates. Specifically, a substance or body that interrupts the transmission of electricity to surrounding objects by conduction; anything that exerts great resistance to the passage of electric current by conduction. The electrical resistance of an insulator is expressed in ohms.

Intravascular: Within blood vessels.

Inverse-square law: Law stating that the intensity of radiation or light at any distance is inversely proportional to the square of the distance between the irradiated surface and a point surface. Thus a light with a certain intensity at a 4-foot distance will have only one fourth that intensity at 8 feet and would be 4 times as intense at a 2-foot distance.

Ischemia: Local and temporary deficiency of blood supply caused by obstruction of the circulation to a part.

Joule's law: The principle that the rate of production of heat by a constant direct current is directly proportional to the resistance of the circuit and the square of the current.

Kallikrein: An enzyme normally present in blood plasma, urine, and body tissue in an inactive state. When activated, kallikrein is one of the most potent vasodilators. It forms kinin, q.v.

Keloid: Scar formation in the skin following trauma or surgical incision. Tissue response is out of proportion to the amount of scar tissue required for normal repair and healing. The result is a raised, firm, thickened red scar that may grow for a prolonged period of time. The increase in scar size is caused by deposition of an abnormal amount of collagen into the tissue. Blacks are especially prone to developing keloids.

Kinin: A general term for a group of polypeptides that have considerable biologic activity. They are capable of influencing smooth-muscle contraction, inducing hypotension, increasing the blood flow and permeability of capillaries, and inducing pain.

Kininogen: Substance that produces a kinin when acted upon by certain enzymes.

Labile cells: Cells that continue to proliferate throughout life, replacing cells that are continually being destroyed.

Laser: Acronym for light amplification by stimulated emission of radiation. The instrument converts various frequencies of light into one small and extremely intense unified beam of one wavelength radiation.

Laser, high power: Emits intense heat and power at close range. A tool used in surgery and in diagnosis.

Laser, low power: The average power of a low-power laser is 50 mW or lower. Also known as "cold" laser.

Leukocyte: White blood corpuscle. There are two types: granulocytes (those possessing granules in their cytoplasm) and agranulocytes (those lacking granules). Granulocytes include juvenile neutrophils (3%–5%), segmented neutrophils (54%–62%), basophils (0%–0.75%), and eosinophils (1%–3%). Agranulocytes include lymphocytes, large and small (25%–33%), and monocytes (3%–7%).

Macrophage: Cells of the reticuloendothelial system having the ability to phagocytose particulate substances and to store vital dyes and other colloidal substances. They are found in loose connective tissues and various organs of the body. They include Kupffer cells of the liver, splenocytes of the spleen, dust cells of the lung, microglia of spinal cord and brain, and histiocytes of loose connective tissue.

Magnetic field: The space permeated by the magnetic lines of force surrounding a permanent magnet or coil of wire carrying electric current.

Margination: Adhesion of leukocytes of walls of blood vessels in first stages of inflammation.

Monochromatic: Having one color.

Monocyte: A large mononuclear leukocyte having more protoplasm than a lymphocyte.

Mottling: Condition that is marked by discolored areas.

Necrosis: Death of areas of tissue or bone surrounded by healthy parts.

Neovascularization: The endothelial response in small vessels of the connective tissue in wound healing that results in the formation of new capillary beds that invade the injured inflamed sites.

Nerve conduction velocity: The speed at which an impulse travels the length of a nerve.

Neurapraxia: Cessation in function of a peripheral nerve without degenerative changes occurring. Recovery is the usual outcome.

Neuraxis: The cerebrospinal axis.

Nociceptor: A nerve for receiving and transmitting painful stimuli.

Nonconductor: Any substance that does not transmit heat, sound, or electricity or that conducts it with difficulty. Strictly speaking, there is no perfect nonconductor. On the application of a sufficiently high voltage, current may be caused to flow through materials usually spoken of as nonconductors. Syn: Insulator.

Nonspecific immune response: Does not involve antibody stimulation, but includes the inflammatory reaction, phagocytosis of microorganisms, and complement activation.

Noxious: Harmful.

Oncotic pressure, colloidal: The total influence of the protein on the osmotic activity of plasma water.

Opiate receptor: Specific sites on cell surfaces that interact in a highly selective fashion with opiate drugs. These receptors mediate the major known pharmacologic actions of opiates and the physiologic functions of the endogenous opiate-like substance, endorphins, and enkephalins, q.v.

Oscilloscope: An instrument for making visible the presence, nature, and form of oscillations or irregularities of an electric current.

Osmotic pressure: 1. Pressure that develops when two solutions of different concentrations are separated by a semipermeable membrane. 2. Pressure that would develop if a solution were enclosed in a membrane impermeable to all solutes present and surrounded by pure solvent. Osmotic pressure varies with concentration of the solution and with temperature increase. Animal cells have an osmotic pressure approximately equal to that of the circulating fluid, the blood. Solutions exerting this osmotic pressure are said to be isotonic or isomotic; stronger solutions that cause cells to shrink are hypertonic; weaker solutions that cause cells to swell are hypotonic.

Osteoblast: Any cell of mesodermal origin that is concerned with the formation of bone.

Pain rating scale: Most commonly used for pain assessment.

Pattern theory: The pattern or coding of sensory information is the key element. It involves the temporal and spatial sequencing of action potentials in the periphery. This theory negates the idea of a specific pain receptor, but rather considers the intense stimulation of nonspecific receptors as the adequate stimulus for eliciting pain sensation.

Pearl-chain formation: A nonthermal effect of diathermy that is produced when microorganisms, unicellular organisms, fat globules in milk, or red blood cells in serum become oriented in chain formation parallel to the lines of force in the electromagnetic field.

Peripheral vascular disease: An imprecise term indicating disease of the arteries and veins of the extremities, especially those conditions that interfere with adequate flow of blood to or from the extremities, such as atherosclerosis with narrowing of the arterial lumen.

Permanent cells: Cells that cannot reproduce themselves after birth.

Phagocytosis: Ingestion and digestion of bacteria and particles by phagocytes.

Phonophoresis: Driving of medication into tissue by ultrasound.

Piezoelectric crystal: A transducer that converts electrical energy into sound energy, and vice versa. (Examples: Quartz, barium titanate, lead zirconate titanate.)

Piezoelectric effect: The vibration of a crystal as a result of receiving electrical current.
> **p.e., Direct:** The generation of an electric voltage across a crystal when the crystal is compressed. This effect is used for converting ultrasound into an electrical signal that replicates the sound pattern.
> **p.e., Reverse (indirect):** The contraction or expansion of a crystal in response to a voltage applied across its face. This effect is used to generate ultrasound at any desired frequency.

Photon: A light quantum or unit of energy of a light ray or other form of radiant energy. Generally considered to be a discrete particle with zero mass, no electric charge, and of indefinitely long life.

Presynaptic inhibition: This process does not involve any direct inhibitory effect upon the postsynaptic membrane, but instead causes a reduction in the release of transmitter substance at the presynaptic terminal of the excitatory synapse.

Prostaglandins: Abbr: PG. A large group of biologically active, carbon-20, unsaturated fatty acids that represent some of the metabolites of arachidonic acid. The PGs, all of which are short-lived in the circulation, have a wide assortment of biologic effects that are not mediated by plasma, but they act as local intercellular or intracellular modulators of the biochemical activity of the tissues in which they are formed. Thus, they are classed as autocoids rather than as hormones.

Pulse-average intensity: The maximal intensity of a pulsed sound beam during the "on" phase. Also known as the temporal peak intensity.

Pus: Liquid product of inflammation composed of albuminous substances, a thin fluid, and leukocytes; generally yellow in color. If red, it suggests rupture of small vessels. If blue or green, it indicates presence of *Pseudomonas aeruginosa*.

Radiation: 1. Process by which energy is propagated through space or matter. 2. Emission of rays in all directions from a common center.

Radiation, electromagnetic: Rays that travel at the speed of light. They exhibit both magnetic and electrical properties.

Radiation, infrared: Invisible heat rays beyond the red end of the spectrum. Near or short infrared extends from 7200 to 14,000 angstroms (AU); far or long infrared extends from 15,000 to 120,000 AU.

Radiation, ionizing: Radiation that either directly or indirectly induces ionization of radiation-absorbing material used for diagnostic or therapeutic purposes.

Radiculitis: Inflammation of spinal-nerve roots, accompanied by pain and hyperesthesia.

Rarefaction: Process of decreasing density and weight, as of air.

Reactive hyperemia: The increased presence of blood in an area after restoration of blood flow following a decreased supply.

Referred pain: Pain seeming to arise in an area other than its origin.

Reflection: The throwing back of a ray of radiant energy from a surface not penetrated.

Refraction: Deflection from a straight path, as of light rays as they pass through media of different densities; the change of direction of a ray when it passes from one medium to another of a different density.

Reliability: Suggests consistent dependability of judgment, character, performance, or result.

Resistance: Opposition to, or the ability to oppose, anything, such as the power of a fluid to retard that which is passing through it; of the air; or opposition of the body to passage of an electric current.

Reticulin: An albuminoid or scleroprotein substance in the connective-tissue framework of reticular tissue.

Serotonin: A chemical present in platelets. Serotonin is a potent vasoconstrictor. It is thought to be involved in neural mechanisms important in sleep and sensory perception.

Skin graft: Using the skin from another part of the body, or from a donor, to repair a defect or trauma of the skin.

Solenoid: A coil of insulated wire in which a magnetic force is created in the long axis of the coil when an electric current flows through the wire.

Somatotopic: Concerning the correspondence between a particular part of the body and a particular area of the brain.

Spasm: An involuntary sudden movement or convulsive muscular contraction. Spasms may be clonic (characterized by alternative contraction and relaxation) or tonic (sustained). They may involve either visceral (smooth) muscle or skeletal (striated) muscle. When contractions are strong and painful, they are called cramps. The effect depends upon the part affected.

Spasticity: Increased tone or contractions of muscles causing stiff and awkward movements; the results of upper motor neuron lesion.

Spatial average intensity: The average intensity of ultrasound as measured by dividing the total power output (in watts) of the ultrasound applicator by the effective radiating area (in cm^2) of the applicator face.

Spatial peak intensity: The greatest intensity of ultrasound anywhere within the beam.

Specific gravity: Weight of a substance compared with an equal volume of water. For solid and liquid materials, water is used as a standard and considered to have a specific gravity of one (1000). For gases, the weight per unit volume is compared with dry air at a specified temperature.

Specific heat: The number of calories required to raise the temperature of 1 g of a substance 1°C, or the number of BTUs per pound per degree Fahrenheit.

Specificity theory of pain: Proposed that a specific pain system existed. There is receptor specialization for each sensation (heat, cold, touch, pain).

Sprain: Trauma to a joint that causes pain and disability depending upon degree of injury to ligaments. In severe sprain, ligaments may be completely torn.

Stasis ulcer: See: Decubitus ulcer.

Stimulated emission: An issuance or discharge; the sending forth or discharge, such as of an atomic particle, exhalation, or of a light or heat wave.

Strain: Trauma to the mucle or the musculotendinous unit from violent contraction or excessive forcible stretch. May be associated with failure of synergistic action of muscles.

Subliminal: Below the threshold of sensation; too weak to arouse sensation or muscular contraction.

Substance P: An 11-amino acid peptide that is believed to be important as a neurotransmitter in the pain-fiber system. This substance may also be important in eliciting local tissue reactions resembling inflammation.

Substantia gelatinosa: Gray matter of the cord surrounding central canal and capping head of posterior horns of spinal cord.

Syncope: A transient loss of consciousness caused by inadequate blood flow to the brain. Fainting.

Temporal average intensity: The intensity of pulsed ultrasound obtained by averaging the intensity during both the "on" and "off" periods.

Temporal peak intensity: See: Pulse average intensity.

Tendinitis: Inflammation of a tendon.

Thermography: In medicine, the use of a device that detects and records the heat present in very small areas of the part being studied. When these multiple readings are accumulated, the relatively hot and cold spots on the body surface are revealed. The technique has been used to study blood flow to limbs and to detect cancer of the breast.

Thermostat: An automatic device for regulating the temperature.

Thrombophlebitis: Inflammation of a vein in conjunction with the formation of a thrombus. Usually occurs in an extremity, most frequently a leg.

Transducer: Device that converts one form of energy to another. Used in medical electronics to receive the energy produced by sound or pressure and relay it as an electrical impulse to another transducer, which can either convert the energy back into its original form or make a record of it on a recording device.

Transformer: A stationary induction apparatus to change electrical energy at one voltage and current to electrical energy at another voltage and current through the medium of magnetic energy, without mechanical motion.

Transformer, step-down: Transformer that changes electricity to a lower voltage.

Transformer, step-up: Transformer that changes electricity to a higher voltage.

Transudate: The fluid that passes through a membrane, especially that which passes through capillary walls. Compared to an exudate, q.v., a transudate has fewer cellular elements and is of a lower specific gravity.

Trigger point: Any place on the body that when stimulated causes a sudden pain in a specific area, especially a type of pain previously felt spontaneously at the same location.

Ultrasound: Inaudible sound in the frequency range of approximately 20,000 to 10 billion (10^9) cycles per second (hertz). Ultrasound has different velocities in tissues that differ in density and elasticity from others. Use of ultrasound for diagnostic and therapeutic purposes requires special equipment.

Urticaria: A vascular reaction of the skin characterized by the eruption of pale evanescent wheals, which are associated with severe itching.

Urticaria, cold: Cold-induced urticarial eruption, which may progress to angioedema.

Vasoconstriction: Decrease in the caliper of blood vessels.

Vasodilation: Increase in the caliper of blood vessels.

Viscosity: Resistance offered by a fluid to change of form or relative position of its particles due to attraction of molecules to each other.

Wavelength: The distance between the beginning and end of a single wave cycle, usually measures from the top of one wave to the top of the next one.

Index

Note: Page numbers followed by f indicate figures; those followed by t indicate tables.